Learning to Listen/
Listening to Learn

Teaching Listening Skills to Students with Visual Impairments

Lizbeth A. Barclay, Editor

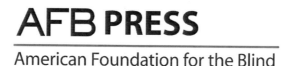

AFB **PRESS**

American Foundation for the Blind

Printed in the United States of America

Library of Congress Cataloging-in-Publication Data

Barclay, Lizbeth A., 1952–
   Learning to listen/listening to learn : teaching listening skills to students with visual impairments / Lizbeth A. Barclay.
      p. cm.
   Includes bibliographical references and index.
   ISBN 978-0-89128-491-8 (pbk. : alk. paper)—ISBN 978-0-89128-492-5 (asc ii cd)—ISBN 978-0-89128-493-2 (e-book)   1. People with visual disabilities—Education. 2. Listening—Study and teaching.   I. Title.
   HV1638.B37   2012
   371.91'1—dc23   2011040760

The American Foundation for the Blind—the organization to which Helen Keller devoted her life—is a national nonprofit devoted to expanding the possibilities for people with vision loss.

It is the policy of the American Foundation for the Blind to use in the first printing of its books acid-free paper that meets the ANSI Z39.48 Standard. The infinity symbol that appears above indicates that the paper in this printing meets that standard.

Contents

Foreword

As an individual with visual impairment, as well as a professional in the field of blindness, developing astute listening skills has always been an essential part of my life. One cannot assume that excellent listening skills are innate in students with visual impairments. Learning to listen and using listening skills effectively require systematic instruction, an array of experiences for practicing listening, and an ability to integrate cognitive, auditory, and visual cues to make sense of the world. Teachers of students with visual impairments and family members must encourage students to utilize these skills in school, as well as in home and community environments.

Learning to listen permeates every aspect of our lives. When one travels, listening to the auditory cues in the environment provides a memory map to assist with route planning and recognition of cues in the environment. In an academic environment one learns to take in valuable information by listening to key ideas and information presented by others. A good listener stores this information and retrieves it when needed. This is particularly true when one needs to gather academic information in a lecture setting. Listening to the speaker, determining the most salient information to record, and recording the information in braille or print ensures systematic organization of information.

For many years the topic of listening skills was not addressed by educators of students with visual impairments. Those of us who have been in the field for many years remember teaching listening skills with *Listen and Think Auditory Readiness*, the 1972 American Printing House for the Blind curriculum, but little else has been written about the topic. The information provided in *Learning to Listen/Listening to Learn* brings listening skills instruction to the fore. Barclay and her colleagues provide the reader with a strong case for teaching listening skills to students with visual impairments. They provide a strong literature base to justify the need for and importance of teaching listening skills. Most important, each chapter author provides practical strategies for implementing instruction for teaching listening skills to students with visual impairments, including those with additional disabilities.

This comprehensive text addresses listening skills as a critical area of instruction on numerous levels. The authors provide strategies for infants, toddlers, and preschool-age students, as well as for school-age students. Specific content is devoted to teaching listening skills to students who have learning disabilities and moderate to severe cognitive disabilities. The authors also offer guidelines for teaching listening skills to English language learners and to students who have hearing impairments.

It is unusual to find a text in which so much rich information is compiled into one volume. The organization and content of the text lends itself to the needs of the practitioner. Strategies are straightforward and easy to follow. They can easily be applied to the development of Individualized Education Program (IEP) goals. Barclay and her colleagues must be commended for a job well done and for providing the field with new and essential curricular material. This volume stands on its merits and adds significantly to the literature of the field.

Sharon Z. Sacks
Director of Curriculum, Assessment and Staff Development
California School for the Blind
Fremont, California

Preface

Sound has the potential to entice, inform, educate and entertain us. The whoosh of water from the faucet into the tub, the dripping of rain from a gutter, the rush of a creek under a bridge, and the crashing of waves at the beach represent just some of the sounds of water, for example. With repeated experiences with many aspects of water, in many contexts, including opportunities to hear, touch, label and compare it in various forms, children with visual impairments can begin to learn to understand the many sounds that water can make: they can develop listening skills and, in turn, comprehension of the world that surrounds them.

There is no doubt about the importance of listening for individuals who are visually impaired, yet it is a topic about which very little has been written. Every student with a visual impairment must rely heavily upon the distance sense of hearing, which, when paired with touch, provides the means for understanding the environment around them; it is evident that this bond of senses must be nurtured and developed. Learning to listen skillfully does not happen for our students without guidance and instruction. Skillful listening requires that parents and teachers devote attention to teaching listening skills.

It is clear to me, as a teacher of students with visual impairments for 20 years, first teaching in school districts and then as an assessor at the California School for the Blind, that much of what we must do as teachers has to do with supporting the development of listening skills. Understanding of language concepts, literacy, use of technology, grasp of orientation and mobility, and social skills all hinge upon the development of excellent listening skills. Yet finding guidelines, resources and curricula related to this area of the expanded core curriculum has been challenging. There are wonderful resources that address the literacy requirements of our students, but very little has been published within the last 25 years or more about listening. There is a need for a framework and teaching strategies that families and educators can utilize to more systematically and carefully teach listening skills.

Within the community of teachers of students with visual impairments, I knew that many of my colleagues were teaching listening skills to their students and that there was a wealth of information that needed to be organized, written about, and shared. *Learning to Listen/Listening to Learn* has been written to meet this need by educators in the field of visual impairment who place specific emphasis on the development of listening skills for students who are visually impaired. The contributors are seasoned teachers who have spent their careers meeting the educational needs of a diverse population of students with vision loss. *Learning to Listen/Listening to Learn* is a collaborative work that strives to cover the topic of listening skill development for students with visual impairments comprehensively through a variety of lenses, based upon development, grade level, and individual differences and learning requirements.

Learning to Listen/Listening to Learn emphasizes both the early development of listening skills at home and in school, as well as the shift that older students must make beginning in elementary school to utilizing listening skills to gain access to information in the classroom and the community. The book is presented in two parts. Part 1: The Development of Listening Skills, covers the importance of listening instruction, learning to listen for infants and toddlers, early skill development of preschool and kindergarten students, refining listening skills in elementary school, advanced skill development in middle school and high school, and listening skills for orientation and mobility. Recognizing that the majority of students with visual impairments have additional learning challenges that typically require a higher level of adaptation, Part 2: Unique Needs, deals with the more specific needs of students with additional disabilities, hearing disabilities, and learning disabilities as well as English language learners.

Throughout the book, the development of listening skills is described for all students with visual impairments. Each chapter includes many specific strategies that can be employed by parents and teachers to develop skills. An inventory of the listening skills that students with visual impairments ought to acquire over time, from infancy through high school, as well as a checklist of the same skills that parents and educators can use to document their students' acquisition of skills, can be found in the appendixes at the back of the book.

We hope that the interventions included in this text will provide both guidance and enrichment that will support teaching listening skills to our students. We strongly believe that the world provides an abundance of sound and auditory information that will engage, inform, and entertain students with visual impairments. It is up to us, as parents and teachers, to provide careful and thoughtful guidance and instruction in listening skills that will facilitate our students' understanding and provide full access to their curriculum and, in doing so, contribute to success in school, with social engagement and continual enjoyment, and later to satisfaction in work and daily life.

Acknowledgments

Learning to Listen/Listening to Learn has been the project of 11 authors for many years. Countless meals, conversations, and e-mails were shared by this group, but the community of collaborators extends far beyond the 11 writers. Support, guidance and tremendous patience have been provided throughout the years by our families, mentors, friends and colleagues. We are most appreciative for this support.

We would first like to dedicate this book to our dear teacher and mentor, Sally Mangold, who when the idea of a book on listening skills was first shared, enthusiastically exclaimed, "It is *time* for a book about such an important topic!" Sally's wisdom about the educational needs of children with visual impairments provided a constant beacon of inspiration as we moved through our process of exploration, collaboration, and writing.

The professionalism of AFB Press and the American Foundation for the Blind paved the way for the development and production of this book. We especially want to acknowledge Natalie Hilzen, Director and Editor in Chief, and Ellen Bilofsky, Managing Editor of AFB Press, for their editing expertise and tireless efforts on our behalf. Their knowledge of the field of education for students with visual impairments was evident throughout the entire process as was their attention to detail. We couldn't have done this without them!

Many of our colleagues supported this effort in a variety of ways. Specifically, we thank Frances Dibble, whose turn of phrase and expert eye was invaluable as she most willingly read and offered refinement to portions of *Learning to Listen/Listening to Learn.* Carol Martin shared her expertise as a counselor with Blind Babies Foundation, providing much of the spirit for Chapter 2, "Infants and Toddlers." Jerry Kuns, Technology Specialist at California School for the Blind, spent countless hours guiding us in our quest to address the important role that listening plays in learning to utilize technology, as well as sharing valuable perspectives about the importance of skillful listening from his personal viewpoint as an individual with visual impairment. We are truly grateful for these generous and skilled colleagues. In addition, we'd like to thank the following colleagues, mentors, parents and students for their support in countless ways: Nancy Akeson, Adrian Amandi, Lia Anderson, Kaitlyn Austin, Maurice Belote, Julie Bernas-Pierce, Alison Boswell, David Brown, Lisa Brown, Donna Carpenter, Jim Carreon, Steve Clark, Nancy Cornelius and the memory of her daughter Amy, Nita Crow, JoAnn DeJaco and the memory of her daughter Cassandra, Sue Douglas,

Delaine Eastin, Joy Effron, Kay Alicyn Ferrell, Dominic Gagliano, Mareva Gondfrey, Monica Hastings, Phil Hatlen, Helene Holman, Laurel Hudson, Ross Illingworth, Norm Kaplan, Amanda Lueck, Debbie Maine, Mike May, Donna McNear, Sue Melrose, Mary Pat O'Connell, Mary Ellen Pesavanto, Elizabeth Phillips, Anne Roeth, Sharon Sacks, Lore Schindler, Keegan Sheehan, and Linda Terry.

Finally, we wish to thank our students with visual impairment who have taught us about the importance of listening and our dear families who have been with us throughout this journey, providing complete support and always having time to listen.

About the Contributors

ABOUT THE EDITOR

Lizbeth A. Barclay, M.A., is Coordinator of the Assessment Program at the California School for the Blind in Fremont. A teacher of the visually impaired and an orientation and mobility specialist for 25 years, she has also taught classes in those areas at San Francisco State University and California State University, Los Angeles. Ms. Barclay was a contributor to *Collaborative Assessment: Working with Students Who Are Blind or Visually Impaired, Including Those with Additional Disabilities,* edited by Stephen A. Goodman and Stuart H. Wittenstein, and *Teaching Social Skills to Students with Visual Impairments,* edited by Sharon Z. Sacks and Karen E. Wolffe, and has also authored or co-authored many journal articles and conference presentations on the education of students with visual impairments.

ABOUT THE CONTRIBUTORS

Kathleen A. Byrnes, M.A., has been a teacher of the visually impaired and an orientation and mobility specialist for more than 37 years, most recently for the Marin County Office of Education in San Rafael, California, and the San Francisco Lighthouse for the Blind. She was editor of *A Future View: Quality Education for Those Who Are Blind and Visually Impaired,* prepared by the California Blindness Advisory Task Force for the California Department of Education in 2002, and was the 1995 California Teacher of the Year.

Laura Anne Denton, Ed.D., is an educational diagnostic specialist and consultant for Reading, Rhyme & Reason in Oakland, California, specializing in reading, language and learning disabilities, formal and informal assessment, and the effects of the learning environment. She has published in the *Journal of Visual Impairment & Blindness.*

Maya Delgado Greenberg, M.A., is an orientation and mobility specialist at the California School for the Blind in Fremont.

Stephanie Herlich, M.A., is a teacher of the visually impaired and an orientation and mobility specialist in Pleasanton, California; Low Vision Coordinator for the California School for the Blind in Fremont; and an educational consultant for Exceptional Teaching in Castro Valley. She is co-author of *Getting to Know You: A Social Skills*

Curriculum for Students Who Are Visually Impaired and Their Sighted Peers, to be published by the American Printing House for the Blind, and author of *Learning Braille Contractions,* as well as several journal articles.

Cheryl Kamei-Hannan, Ph.D., is Assistant Professor at California State University Charter College of Education, Division of Special Education and Counseling, Los Angeles. She is the author of numerous journal articles and conference presentations.

Madeline Milian, Ed.D., is Professor of Bilingual and ESL Education at the University of Northern Colorado, School of Teacher Education, in Greeley. She is the co-editor of *Diversity and Visual Impairment: The Influence of Race, Gender, Religion, and Ethnicity on the Individual* and has authored numerous journal articles, chapters, and conference presentations.

Theresa Postello, M.A., is a teacher of the visually impaired and an orientation and mobility specialist for the San Mateo County Office of Education, Redwood City, California. She received the 2010 Northern California Association for Education and Rehabilitation of the Blind and Visually Impaired Teacher of the Year Award.

Sandra Staples, M.A., is an orientation and mobility specialist and a specialist teacher for students with visual impairments in Lodi, California, and a lecturer at San Francisco State University. She received the 2006 Northern California Association for Education and Rehabilitation of the Blind and Visually Impaired Teacher of the Year Award.

Wendy Scheffers, M.A., is an orientation and mobility specialist and a teacher of the visually impaired for the Marin County Office of Education in San Rafael, California, as well as a lecturer at San Francisco State University. She is the author or co-author of several book chapters, journal articles, and conference presentations.

Marsha A. Silver, M.S., is a speech-language pathologist on the Outreach Assessment Team at the California School for the Blind, Fremont. She has contributed chapters to several books, including *Collaborative Assessment: Working with Students Who Are Blind or Visually Impaired, Including Those with Additional Disabilities.*

PART 1

THE DEVELOPMENT OF LISTENING SKILLS

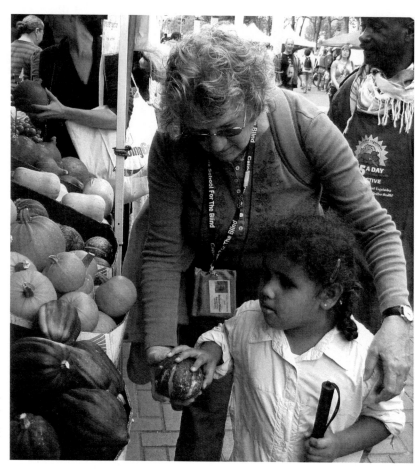

Theresa Maher

Chapter 1

The Importance of Listening Instruction

Lizbeth A. Barclay and Sandra Staples

Whereas hearing is the passive ability to receive sound, listening is a deliberate process by which sound is given meaning. Listening is a learned skill.

—G. Ferrington, "Soundscape Studies: Listening with Attentive Ears," 2003

CHAPTER PREVIEW

- ▶ Hearing and Listening
- ▶ Instruction in Listening
- ▶ Visual Impairment and Early Development
- ▶ Hearing and Auditory Perception
- ▶ The Importance of Experiential Learning
- ▶ Listening and Developmental Domains
- ▶ Students with Additional Disabilities

The ability to listen is essential to individuals who are visually impaired. In fact, the deliberate development of listening skills for all children with visual impairments needs to begin during infancy and continue throughout a child's development. This critical effort requires nurturing and attention from parents, educators, and related specialists in a collaborative approach that focuses on listening as it applies to the development of concepts and understanding, communication and social skills, preliteracy and academic skills, and independent travel.

The first listening experience begins the moment a child is born, as parents welcome their infant into the world in excited and loving tones, providing their baby's first combination of sound and touch. This communication begins the infant's integration of sensory information, which sets in motion the learning process. When a disturbance in the visual system blocks that important path of learning, the combination of sound and tactile and kinesthetic information needs to be interpreted without the benefit of vision. It is essential for children with visual impairments to learn how to take meaning from what they hear and feel; the deliberate development of listening skills will help them do this.

HEARING AND LISTENING

Hearing is the physiological process through which sound waves are collected through the ear and auditory information is transmitted to the brain. Listening, in contrast, is the act of assigning meaning to what is heard (Deshler, Ellis, & Lenz, 1996). Listening is a primary conduit by which individuals acquire information. Infants begin to attach meaning to what they hear by combining their senses of vision, touch, and hearing. Definitions of listening vary, but it has been called an "active cognitive process"

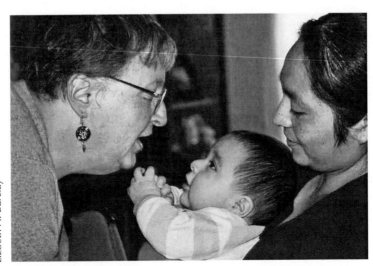

Lizbeth A. Barclay

Collaboration between parents and educators facilitates the deliberate development of early listening skills for children with visual impairments.

(Petress, 1999), and Hirsch described it as a neurological response and interpretation of sound that includes understanding and assigning meaning by reacting, selecting meaning, remembering, attending, analyzing, and incorporating previous experience (1986).

Researchers have discovered that during listening, the auditory cortex of the brain does not function in isolation; instead, it acts in tandem with other parts of the brain, integrating sensory input in order to interpret what is heard. Most people use visual cues to combine vision with sound to help them process what they are hearing (Ratey, 2001, p. 95). This reinforcing or clarifying effort happens when a child looks up to see an airplane fly over while hearing the whine of its engine, or when a student seated in the classroom glances around to see what classmates are doing to clarify the instructions that the teacher has given. For the learner with a visual impairment who does not receive visual input for clarification, this "active cognitive process," which involves attaching meaning to hearing, takes a unique path. It needs to be more deliberate and more experiential—that is, taught through experience, providing emphasis on the pairing of language and touch, action, and objects. Individuals' lack of opportunity for "incidental learning"—their ability to learn about the world by simply watching what goes on around them—necessitates a more conscious effort to help compensate for the visual information that is missing.

INSTRUCTION IN LISTENING

Although effective listening can and should be taught, systematic instruction in listening skills receives little attention in classrooms (Coakley & Wolvin, 1997). The teaching of listening skills for students who are visually impaired without additional disabilities is often perceived as consisting primarily of listening to recorded textbooks. For students who have additional disabilities, listening instruction can often rely on passive listening (Chen, 1999b), involving such activities as the shaking of a sound-making object near a student or the placing of headphones on a student and playing a recording of environmental sounds. At best, this experience for the student can be hearing sounds without the opportunity to understand what they are. At worst, a student may be overwhelmed with confusing auditory stimuli and lack the power to escape (Chen & Downing, 2006).

Vision and hearing are the two senses that allow individuals access to other people from a distance, to objects and actions around them, and to the environment. Students who have visual impairments, including those who have additional disabilities, need opportunities to become aware of, respond to, and understand information from their other distance-learning channel, hearing. Teaching effective listening within educational programs for students who have visual impairments with and without additional disabilities involves:

▸ emphasizing the functions of listening so that instruction in listening skill development has meaningful communication and functional relevance at its foundation

▸ considering a student's individual learning characteristics and sensory responsiveness

These principles are highlighted in various chapters throughout this book. In addition, Sidebar 1.1 lists some basic strategies for supporting the development of listening skills that are also addressed in Chapter 7 and elaborated upon in other chapters.

Active learning and active listening require that students be involved and have the opportunity to participate in what is happening (Jalongo, 1995). This requirement presents a unique set of challenges in designing instruction in listening skills for students who have visual impairments and additional disabilities. Sound can be an elusive stimuli—present and then fading, present and then absent—and may not be present long enough or with the saliency to spark awareness or inspire reaching forward and

---

((SIDEBAR 1.1
Strategies for Supporting the Development of Listening Skills

The following overall strategies are effective in helping children develop listening skills:

- Instruction in listening skills is embedded in the context of functional, everyday routines—for example, during a diaper change, while having a daily snack, or when performing an assigned job at school—so that these activities can have meaning for the child.
- Attention is paid to the child's learning characteristics and sensory responsiveness.
- A supportive listening environment is created, with attention to auditory distractions and the quality of sound.

The following targeted strategies, which will be explained and expanded upon throughout the book, can have a direct impact on a child's understanding:

- Pair touch and/or visual cues with sound.
- Allow time for the child to respond.
- Supply appropriate prompts to encourage a response.
- Be attuned to subtle behaviors that communicate a response.
- Reinforce the child's response.

actively exploring, particularly for students whose access to their environment and understanding of their environment are also compromised by other learning challenges. Ensuring that sound has sufficient saliency or relevance to the student with additional disabilities requires that it be judiciously paired with touch in the process of building awareness of sound and attaching meaning to sound.

According to Anthony and Lowry (2004), "Understanding auditory information from a distance . . . is tied to children's attainment of object permanence. Children must have developed an understanding that objects exist when they are out of immediate reach before out-of-reach sounds will be meaningful" (p. 136). In discussing the achievement of an understanding of object permanence, Bruce (2005) wrote, "This sense of permanency facilitates the children's gradual distancing of themselves from objects, which is important to holding an object in memory and to contemplation" (p. 467). She described "distancing" as a gradual process that includes separation of self from others, separation from objects, and separation of object and representation. Separation from others is dependent on first establishing attachment to others; separation from an object depends on understanding that object. To develop the memory of a person and attach meaning to his or her voice alone, or to develop the memory of an object and attach meaning to its sound alone, students who have additional disabilities need to know that people and objects continue to exist beyond their experience with them.

Children who are visually impaired, with or without additional disabilities, require tactile contact with someone who is interacting with them during meaningful activities or routines over time to develop attachment and to perceive that person as separate, someone who has "permanence." Similarly, they require tactile experience with an object, as well as meaningful exploration of the object together with someone else who is sharing the experience with them to build an understanding of the object and a sense of its permanence (Bruce, 2005). Just as sighted children share attention on an object with an adult by pointing and by both of them looking at, visually exploring and learning about the object's characteristics, children with visual impairments need to experience learning through joint attention—but, it will be through mutual touch, "the tactual equivalent of pointing" (Miles, 1999, p. 64). Together, and with the adult following the child's interest and movement, the adult and child tactually explore and learn about an object's features, which includes the sound it makes, as the child attaches meaning to the object, meaning to its sound—and develops interest in objects and a sense of object permanence. Acquiring these concepts is a process in which the student is actively learning; supporting the development of these concepts as they relate to sound teaches the student to learn to listen. The role of the understanding of object permanence and the capacity for joint attention is also discussed in Chapter 2.

VISUAL IMPAIRMENT AND EARLY DEVELOPMENT

The impact of visual impairment on development is highly individual and dependent upon a number of factors, including the extent of visual impairment, environmental opportunities for stimulation and support, and presence of additional disabilities (Liefert, 2003). With the complex and intense needs of many children who are visually impaired and have additional disabilities, there is tendency among adults to minimize the impact of a child's visual impairment (Hatlen, 1996; Miles & Riggio, 1999). However, for a child who has additional disabilities that influence memory, movement, or communication, a visual impairment can have a pronounced effect. To better illuminate the different learning needs and perspective of children who have a visual impairment and significant learning challenges as well as children who do not have these additional challenges, this section highlights not the visual system or the functional use of vision, but the role vision can play in learning and some of the ways in which that learning process differs when vision is compromised.

A visual impairment affects the following areas for a student:

▸ awareness of the world and objects in it
▸ opportunities to build understanding and knowledge by casual observation and imitation, also known as incidental learning
▸ curiosity about and movement toward something just out of reach
▸ opportunities to anticipate interaction or prepare for a change

Awareness and Understanding

Vision integrates information from the other sensory systems (Ward, 2000), synthesizing or pulling together elusive perceptions such as the squeak of a hinge, the scent of fresh air, a change in light or warmth, and the vibration of the floor with the visual image of a door opening and someone stepping over the threshold. Vision allows a child to both understand what is happening and simultaneously interpret the significance of the auditory, thermal, and tactile input. Without the integrating function vision offers, each piece of sensory information may be experienced as discrete and perceived sequentially. Sensory stimuli need to be woven together to create the "whole" of an event—a door opened and someone entered the room. This synthesis of the separate pieces of sensory input is a different cognitive task from interpreting the event visually. It requires processing time and memory of a previous experience, particularly so for children who have additional disabilities that complicate learning. Children with visual and multiple impairments may have fragmented impressions of their world, and their perspective may be limited to the discrete pieces of sensory information available to them. Developing concepts about their world and understanding events evolve from learning that is experiential, systematically structured, and carefully nurtured by educators, related specialists, and caregivers.

Children who are visually impaired but who have some usable vision have similar challenges to those experienced by children who completely lack vision in accessing and interpreting the world and events in it. While these children may respond visually, they are nonetheless using a compromised learning channel and perceive imperfect visual information. Their functional or usable vision may fluctuate, depending on such influences as their health, the impact of medications, and their neurological function. Students who have low vision often have the same requirement as those who are blind for extra time to process the perceptual information available to them and to draw upon previous experience and memory to unify discrete bits of sensory input (such as sound, scent, and touch, along with visual impression or color) into a whole construct.

Incidental Learning

Vision is a distance sense, allowing children access to objects not in direct contact with their bodies and to activities in which they are not directly involved. It is considered a primary sense for learning (Downing & Chen, 2003). Vision offers the opportunity for incidental learning—that is, learning accomplished or absorbed casually by watching someone else or by imitating what one has seen someone else do. Instruction is often presented in classrooms using what is called a "watch-and-then-do" approach (Nelson-Barber & Estrin, 1995); students learn by observing and then imitating a demonstration or another person's actions. Children who have visual impairments, with or without additional disabilities, need to learn from meaningful experiences using listening and touch, and through instructional strategies such as tactile modeling (Downing & Chen, 2003).

Curiosity and Movement

The visual world beckons and entices, prompting curiosity and offering children motivation for reaching out and using their hands to touch and manipulate objects, to reach forward for items just beyond their bodies, and to begin to move. Through engaging in these actions of reaching, touching, and moving, children build concepts about the environment and an awareness of the objects and people in it. Additionally, active movement provides kinesthetic feedback that is itself reinforcing (Jacobson & Bradley, 1997), intrinsically motivating children to continue to move and to explore. Visual cues for movement are either lacking or sometimes distorted for children with visual impairments. For those who have additional disabilities, the impact the visual impairment may have on active learning, on reaching and exploring, can be intensified by the ways in which the additional disabilities further complicate movement and curiosity.

Anticipation

Vision allows interaction with others from a distance as well as the opportunity to anticipate and get ready for change. As adults begin walking from across the room and in the absence of any other communication, children with unimpaired vision can anticipate their approach and prepare for interaction. Children who are visually impaired, with or without additional disabilities, miss these visual cues. They may be unprepared for being touched or picked up, for being given materials or for objects to be removed, or for a change in activity (Chen, 1999b). They may experience the world as unpredictable, even threatening, and events in it as happening randomly (Anthony &

((‹ SIDEBAR 1.2
How Do We Hear?

Hearing encompasses a series of events in which the ear converts sound waves into electrical signals and causes nerve impulses to be sent to the brain, where they are interpreted as sound. The ear has three main parts: the outer, middle, and inner ear (see Figure 1.1). Sound waves enter through the outer ear and reach the middle ear, where they cause the eardrum to vibrate. The vibrations are transmitted through three tiny bones in the middle ear called the ossicles. These three bones are named the malleus, incus, and stapes (and are also known as the hammer, anvil, and stirrup). The eardrum and ossicles carry the vibrations to the inner ear. The stirrup transmits the vibrations through the oval window and into the fluid that fills the inner ear. The vibrations move through fluid in the snail-shaped hearing part of the inner ear (cochlea) that contains the hair cells. The fluid in the cochlea moves the top of the hair cells, which initiates the changes that lead to the production of the nerve impulses. These nerve impulses are carried to the brain, where they are interpreted as sound. Different sounds stimulate different parts of the inner ear, allowing the brain to distinguish among various sounds, for example, different vowel and consonant sounds.

Source: Reprinted with permission from National Institute on Deafness and Other Communication Disorders (May 1999), "Otosclerosis," NIH Pub. No. 97-4234. Retrieved from www.nidcd.nih.gov/health/hearing /otosclerosis.html.

Lowry, 2004; Chen, 1999b), and they require meaningful communication using combinations of touch and sound to anticipate and prepare for change. It falls to educators, caregivers, and service providers to link touch and listening within learning experiences to foster meaningful communication and nurture understanding, to inspire movement and discovery, and to prepare children for change or for interaction.

HEARING AND AUDITORY PERCEPTION

To understand the development of listening skills, one needs to first consider the development of hearing, because this distance sense is essential in order for listening to occur. Hearing, a complicated process, is described in Sidebar 1.2.

When babies are born, their hearing, much like their vision and their motor systems, is not fully developed. Babies' brains develop the neural pathways that allow

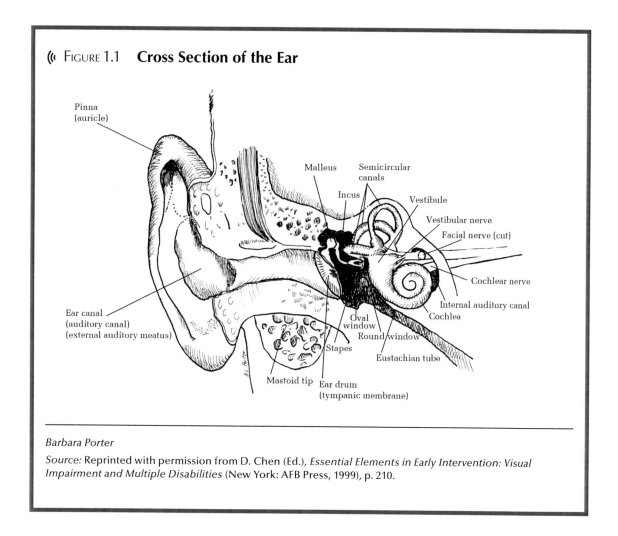

((FIGURE 1.1   **Cross Section of the Ear**

Barbara Porter

Source: Reprinted with permission from D. Chen (Ed.), *Essential Elements in Early Intervention: Visual Impairment and Multiple Disabilities* (New York: AFB Press, 1999), p. 210.

them to use the information coming in through their senses to comprehend themselves and the world around them (Moss, 1997). This is true especially in the first three years of life, but continues through childhood and adolescence (Brotherson, 2005; Ratey, 2001). Hearing and auditory perception develop and change in tandem with babies' other skills.

The term *auditory processing* refers to the way the brain recognizes and interprets the sounds that are heard. During auditory processing, the brain and the ear work together to interpret acoustical information, such as music, environmental sounds, and speech, including locating where sounds are coming from and discriminating between sounds even when there is background noise, such as a television at home or a noisy heating vent in a classroom (Morlet, 2010). Perception is our sensory experience of the world around us and involves both the recognition of environmental stimuli and actions in response to these stimuli. *Auditory perception* occurs when a child begins to associate meaning with various auditory stimuli and starts to seek out and classify sound. As a natural result of repeated instances of auditory perception, each new sound experience builds upon previous experiences, which allows for the development of categories of features of sound through which a child can compare and contrast new sound experiences (Ratey, 2001).

The components of auditory perception listed by Heasley (1974) are discussed in different chapters of this book as they apply to aspects of listening skills that emerge naturally at a particular developmental level or within a particular area of activity. For example, awareness of sound, auditory attending, and auditory attention span are featured in Chapters 2 ("Infants and Toddlers"), 3 ("Preschool and Kindergarten"), and 7 ("Students with Additional Disabilities") because these three components of auditory perception are the first to develop. While they are also discussed in Chapter 6 ("Listening Skills for Orientation and Mobility"), the auditory perceptual areas of sound localization and auditory projection ability are particularly emphasized there because of their importance to traveling skills. These components of auditory-perceptual development also establish a foundation for instruction in listening skills (Harley, Truan, & Sanford, 1997, p. 220), part of the expanded core curriculum for students who have visual impairments, including those with additional disabilities (Hatlen, 1996), in the area of sensory efficiency.

Components in the development of auditory perception that are addressed throughout the chapters of this book are defined in Sidebar 1.3. Stages in the early development of auditory skills are also discussed in Chapter 2.

Listening skills are described in many ways and in relationship to many developmental levels throughout this book. The Listening Skills Continuum—a listing of skills acquired throughout different developmental stages—has been compiled and provided in Appendix A at the end of the book for the reader's convenience. This continuum out-

---

((Sidebar 1.3

Components of Auditory Perception

Auditory awareness: Awareness of sound; demonstrated by the ability to change behavior based on the presence or absence of sound (Harley, Truan, & Sanford, 1997; Heasley, 1974)

Auditory attending: The ability to focus on a single source of auditory (hearing) information

Auditory attention span: The span of time that a person can attend selectively to language or nonlanguage sounds (Harley, Truan, & Sanford, 1997)

Sound localization: The ability to determine the direction from which a language or a nonlanguage sound originated (Harley, Truan, & Sanford, 1997)

Auditory discrimination: The ability to recognize and respond appropriately to similarities and differences in language or nonlanguage sounds (Harley, Truan, & Sanford, 1997)

Auditory memory: The ability to store and recall auditory material such as a sound or series of language or nonlanguage sounds (Harley, Truan, & Sanford, 1997; Northern & Downs, 1974)

Auditory memory span: The ability to remember the nature or characteristics of sound over increasing lengths of time (Harley, Truan, & Sanford, 1997)

Auditory sequencing ability: The ability to remember the order of items in a sequence of language or nonlanguage sounds (Harley, Truan, & Sanford, 1997)

Auditory projection ability: The ability to attend to and interpret language or nonlanguage sounds that come from a distance (Harley, Truan, & Sanford, 1997)

Auditory figure-ground discrimination (also called **auditory separation**): The ability to attend to a particular sound or series of sounds when other competing sounds are present (Harley, Truan, & Sanford, 1997)

Auditory blending: The ability to blend speech sounds or to synthesize isolated phonemic sounds, or the smallest units of sound, into a whole word (Harley, Truan, & Sanford, 1997; Northern & Downs, 1974)

Source: Adapted from B. E. Heasley, *Auditory Perceptual Disorders and Remediation* (Springfield, IL: Charles C Thomas, 1974).

---

lines the typical progression or sequence of skill development and is not intended as a guide to specific ages for skill acquisition. The Listening Skills Continuum is referred to throughout Chapters 2, 3, 4, and 5, which deal with the stages of childhood during which listening skills are developing. Within those chapters, skills relating to different chronological and developmental domains are listed, and they also can be found in the corresponding sections of the continuum to illustrate their location in the progression of skill development. Sidebar 1.4 provides a brief overview of the organization of the skills continuum.

The Listening Skills Continuum

The Listening Skills Continuum found in Appendix A at the end of this book was compiled to provide a list of the many listening skills that students with visual impairments need to acquire over time, depending on their individual differences in development, from infancy through preschool, elementary school, middle school, and high school. Although ages and grade levels are included in the continuum to provide a general guide for skill acquisition, it should be regarded as an outline of the progression of skill development for students with visual impairment, rather than a determinant of when during early development a child will acquire a skill. True developmental and age comparisons cannot be made because of the tremendous variation within the population of students who are visually impaired.

The items in the Listening Skills Continuum were selected from assessment tools that are used with children both with and without visual impairments to demonstrate a broad developmental range and variety of listening skills. The sources were chosen because of their relevance to listening skill development, a topic of importance for students with visual impairments about which little has been published. Consequently, some of the sources are older, such as the groundbreaking work of Selma Fraiberg (1977) from *Insights from the Blind: Comparative Studies of Blind and Sighted Infants*, yet they provide valuable information that still helps guide families and professionals with regard to the development of children with visual impairments. Skills selected include those pertaining to listening, such as "Quiets to sound; appears comforted by human voice" from the Oregon Project (Anderson, Boignon, Davis, & deWaard, 2007), and those that require listening for development, such as "Engages in discussion about a book/story that is heard" from the *Desired Results Developmental Profile (DRDP)* (2008).

INFANTS AND TODDLERS

The act of learning to listen, or develop auditory perception, enables infants and toddlers to interpret the world, act and move with intention, and communicate. Perception involves a lot more than just hearing sound. It requires a form of expectation, of knowing what is about to happen and preparing for it, and thus encompasses the initial formation of connections and comprehension. Beginning listening skills are organized within categories of auditory perception. The Listening Skills Continuum for infants and toddlers has been divided into the domains of auditory awareness, auditory attention, sound localization, auditory discrimination, auditory memory: concepts and vocabulary, additional receptive and expressive communication skills, and social listening.

PRESCHOOL AND KINDERGARTEN

Children in preschool and kindergarten need to develop listening skills that enable them to successfully understand and relate within the environments of home, school, and some aspects of the community, such as playgroups, day care, and when out and about with family members.

This section of the continuum has been divided into the domains of auditory attention: maintaining attention; auditory attention: figure-ground discrimination; auditory discrimination; auditory memory: concepts and directions; auditory memory: sequence, listening skills for reading readiness; and social listening.

ELEMENTARY STUDENTS

Listening requirements of children as they continue on to elementary school, from the first through the fifth grade, make the transition from the early childhood skills of learning to distinguish different sounds and identify their sources to the more refined abilities of attaching meaning to sounds and interpreting their more subtle and complex implications. Skills at these levels are focused primarily on listening in the classroom and have been divided into the domains of listening and literacy skills: phonemic and phonological skills, listening and literacy skills: listening comprehension of information that is orally presented or read, active listening, critical listening during oral instruction, listening and technology, and listening and social skills.

MIDDLE AND HIGH SCHOOL STUDENTS

For students in middle and high school, the continuum includes skills in the domains of listening in the classroom: active and critical listening, listening and organizing information, listening and technology, and listening during social interaction. Skills were chosen to illustrate the types of listening skills that can be found in state standards and in sources pertinent to students who are visually impaired.

   As already noted, the Listening Skills Continuum needs to be regarded as outlining a progression of skills rather than specifying rates of skill acquisition. While the continuum is not exhaustive, it is provided to guide families and professionals as they support the development of listening skills for children with visual impairments.

THE IMPORTANCE OF EXPERIENTIAL LEARNING

At the very beginning of a child's life, parents begin to combine touch and language and in this way provide the child's first meaningful experiences. The newborn learns through many repetitions of receiving and reacting to such stimuli. With each reaction to a stimulus, an infant's brain has the opportunity to store experience for future learning (Brazelton, 1983, p. 31). That experiential beginning is what launches a child's understanding of the world around him or her, and it is the linking of hearing and listening to tactile sensation that is the child's first opportunity for the development of listening skills.

   Experience plays a role in the development of listening skills in a variety of ways. Developmental research has revealed that contingency experiences, in which an infant's behavior elicits a response from the environment, encourage the infant's development and interactions with caregivers (Chen, 1999a). The uncomfortable or hungry infant begins fussing, which prompts the parent to pick up and cuddle the baby while softly cooing; the infant learns that behavior (fussing) will result in being picked up; therefore, being picked up was contingent upon certain behavior. The repeated experience teaches the infant that what is heard and felt can be elicited by behavior.

Experiential learning supports the development of concepts and language involving listening by linking what is heard to what is felt. The child is learning to listen to and understand language by connecting the words that are heard to touch, objects, and activities. Koenig (1996) wrote, "When a child has opportunities to actively experience things in the world, meaningful language will develop. It can occur when the child associates what she is experiencing with a word that already exists but which she has not experienced before" (p. 241). This makes it imperative to ensure that infants, toddlers, and young children have the opportunity to participate as fully as possible in daily routine activities and experiences that will allow them to connect what they hear to what is happening, helping them to develop an understanding of language concepts, an important aspect of listening skill development.

Repetition of experiences is especially important for students who are visually impaired. When one considers the many times sighted children casually observe objects and actions in their environment before they begin to use language functionally, this makes sense. Consider, for instance, the infant seated in the center of the kitchen as his mother or father prepares breakfast for the family. Each day the infant sees bread being popped into the toaster, eggs coming out of the refrigerator and going into the frying pan, and milk being poured into glasses, as language is paired with those activities. Now consider the experience of the infant who is visually impaired sitting in the center of the kitchen during the same set of breakfast preparation activities. Complete understanding of the vocabulary of the kitchen may take place only when the child has been able to actively participate many times in putting toast in the toaster, taking eggs out of the refrigerator and cracking them into the pan, and pouring milk into glasses. The importance of experiential learning to the development of listening skills is emphasized throughout this book.

LISTENING AND DEVELOPMENTAL DOMAINS

The development of excellent listening skills plays an important role in the continued development of a child's understanding of *concepts, communication skills, literacy skills, social skills,* and *skills of independent travel.* While listening does not take the place of vision, when listening is combined with touch and supported by intentional instruction, development and learning in these domains is possible and greatly enhanced. Throughout this book, listening skills are emphasized within those general developmental domains, which are described below.

Conceptual Understanding and Communication Skills

Listening skills are integral to the development of the understanding of concepts and the ability to communicate. They are developed primarily through the careful pairing of relevant experience with language. In *Blindness and Children*, Warren (1994) pointed out that "limitations in concept formation [in children who are visually impaired] may not be a necessary consequence of restricted visual experience, but instead may result from a limitation in the overall experience of the blind infant and young child" (p. 138). Learning word meaning, extending word meanings, and using words in sentences and questions for a variety of purposes and with greater and greater sophistication and understanding occur when listening is deliberately combined with experience. When hearing concepts such as *up, over, in,* and *on* emphasized within a meaningful context, such as during bathing or while making a snack, a child will more easily learn and retain those concepts because experience provides a meaningful context for understanding. When the activities are repeated over time and the concepts are reinforced each time, deliberate teaching is taking place. The development of listening skills within understanding of concepts, language, and communication is emphasized in Chapters 2 ("Infants and Toddlers"), 3 ("Preschool and Kindergarten"), and 7 ("Students with Additional Disabilities"). Chapter 10 ("Listening Guidelines for English Language Learners") focuses on the specific principles and issues with regard to listening for English language learners who are visually impaired.

Literacy Skills

Listening does not take the place of reading; rather, effective listening skills support the development of literacy skills. In fact, the development of listening skills is essential to the development of literacy skills. In *Foundations of Braille Literacy*, the authors stated, "Most authorities agree that children who enter school with well-developed listening and speaking language skills find it easier to learn to read and write" (Rex, Koenig, Wormsley, & Baker, 1994, p. 6). They continued by maintaining that reading, writing, listening, and speaking are components of an integrated language process and that they are not isolated components of language.

Well-developed listening skills provide the foundation for excellent reading and writing skills, and later, listening provides another important tool for students with visual impairments to acquire information while participating in the classroom during group activities, listening to audible curricular materials, and listening while accessing the ever-expanding array of technology tools, such as electronic braille note-taking devices and the computer. The development of listening skills in order to gain and support literacy skills is an important concept in this book, particularly in Chapters 3, 4, and 5, addressing school-age children. Again, it needs to be emphasized that listening is regarded as an important learning medium that supplements and supports literacy skills. It does not take their place.

Social Skills

Social skills are dependent largely upon well-developed listening skills. Preverbal communication (such as eye contact, pointing and reaching, laughing and crying, smiling and other facial expressions, babbling and using voice tones) combined with listening begins the first interactive dance of communication between infants and caregivers. Infants instinctively listen and respond to their parents' and caregivers' voices. This interaction between caregivers and their children is the first active turn taking that involves listening. Parents and caregivers are the primary source of this beginning social interaction, which will continue to grow at home and then at school.

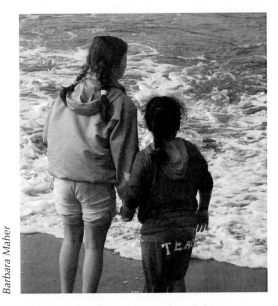

Barbara Maher

Listening is a key aspect of social interactions. Here the sound and feeling of the waves present a shared experience that provides a highly motivational topic for conversation.

Caregivers provide the environment for listening that will nurture children's ability to develop social language, which is dependent upon the understanding that grows with listening. Research has shown that intervention in this area is especially important. It was found that "the language of children who are visually impaired focuses more frequently on the children's activities, possessions and feelings and is less responsive to the interests of their partners than is the speech of sighted children. . . . These differences may affect both the quantity and quality of feedback from peers" (Sacks, Kekelis, & Gaylord-Ross, 1992, p. 27). Consequently, listening skill development as it applies to the development of social skills is extremely important, beginning at home and continuing in playgroups and preschool and then into elementary, middle, and high school. The development of listening skills as they apply to social skills is integrated throughout this book.

Movement and Independent Travel

Independent travel is highly dependent upon the sophisticated use of listening skills. In order to determine and maintain orientation in the environment, one needs to be knowledgeable about oneself in relationship to other objects, for example, cars, and about object-to-object relationships. Hearing facilitates this awareness by providing information that helps an individual identify known landmarks and information points (Wiener, Welsh, & Blasch, 2010). The ability to identify the features of the environment occurs through deliberate and systematic training in all environments. This training begins in the earliest stages of development, when a child starts to learn how to interpret what he or she hears.

Instruction in this area is routinely directed and carried out by an orientation and mobility specialist once a child has begun school, but it actually begins before that with caregivers. The auditory perceptual skills of sound identification and sound localization are the precursors to a child's ability to begin to interpret environmental sound, which begins to develop during infancy. The groundwork that parents and caregivers provide as they teach concepts such as *up, down, in, out, in front of*, and *in back of* within the context of daily routines such as bathing, dressing, and eating also prepares the foundation for this ability. Listening as it applies to movement is addressed throughout the book; Chapter 6 specifically focuses on the importance of listening skills in orientation and mobility.

STUDENTS WITH ADDITIONAL DISABILITIES

The population of students with visual impairments is extremely heterogeneous. Results from *Project PRISM: A Longitudinal Study of Developmental Patterns of Children Who Are Visually Impaired* (Ferrell, 1998) found that the development of a child who is visually impaired may progress at the same rate as that of sighted peers or may differ widely, depending on a variety of factors. These factors include:

- degree of visual loss
- age at visual diagnosis
- presence or absence of additional disabilities
- amount of early intervention
- network of support available to the child and family

The presence or absence of additional disabilities can be a particularly significant factor in a child's development. Estimates of the presence of additional disabilities in children with visual impairments vary between 60 percent (Ferrell, 1998) and 65 percent (Dote-Kwan, Chen, & Hughes, 2001; Hatton, 2001). This population of students is incredibly diverse, requiring a high level of specific teaching strategies to accommodate the individuality of each student and his or her constellation of learning challenges.

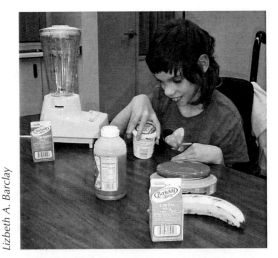

Lizbeth A. Barclay

Learning to listen through meaningful activities, such as making a smoothie, is a strategy that provides motivation and facilitates concept development for all students.

This book addresses the importance of the development of listening skills for all students with visual impairments, with an emphasis on this wide range of individual differences among children with visual impairments. Students with additional disabilities are the specific focus of Chapter 7. The listening requirements of students with hearing impairments are covered in Chapter 8, and listening and language and learning disabilities are discussed in Chapter 9.

CONCLUSION

The development of effective listening skills enhances the lives of all students with visual impairments. At the most basic level, these skills improve a student's awareness and understanding of the world, increasing security and encouraging curiosity. Refined listening skills are essential for understanding concepts and for accurate communication. In the social realm, they are a prerequisite for satisfying interactions. Strong listening skills provide the foundation for literacy skills.

Experience plays an important role in the development of listening skills in a variety of ways. The challenge falls to educators, caregivers, and related service providers to make the development of listening skills a priority by linking touch and sound within learning experiences to foster meaningful communication and nurture understanding and to inspire movement and discovery for all students with visual impairments.

REFERENCES

Anderson, S., Boignon, S., Davis, K., & deWaard, C. (2007). *Oregon project for visually impaired and blind preschool children* (6th ed.). Medford: Southern Oregon Education Service District.

Anthony, T., & Lowry, S. S. (2004). Sensory development. In T. Anthony, S. S. Lowry, C. Brown, & D. Hatton (Eds.), *Developmentally appropriate orientation and mobility* (pp. 125–240). Chapel Hill: Early Intervention Training Center for Infants and Toddlers with Visual Impairments, FPG Child Development Institute, University of North Carolina at Chapel Hill.

Brazelton, B. (1983). *Infants and mothers: Differences in development.* New York: Bantam Doubleday Dell.

Brotherson, S. (2005). Understanding brain development in young children. Retrieved from North Dakota State University (NDSU) website: www.ag.ndsu.edu/pubs/yf/famsci/fs609w.htm.

Bruce, S. (2005). The application of Werner and Kaplan's concept of "distancing" to children who are deaf-blind. *Journal of Visual Impairment & Blindness, 99*(8), 464–477.

Chen, D. (1999a). *Essential elements in early intervention: Visual impairment and multiple disabilities.* New York: AFB Press.

Chen, D. (1999b). Interactions between infants and caregivers: The context for early intervention. In D. Chen (Ed.), *Essential elements in early intervention: Visual impairment and multiple disabilities* (pp. 22–53). New York: AFB Press.

Chen, D., & Downing, J. (2006). Supporting interactions through touch. In D. Chen & J. Downing (Eds.), *Tactile strategies for children who have visual impairments and multiple disabilities: Promoting communication and learning skills* (pp. 30–44). New York: AFB Press.

Coakley, C., & Wolvin, A. (1997). Listening in the educational environment. In M. Purdy & D. Borisoff (Eds.), *Listening in everyday life: A personal and professional approach* (2nd ed.) (pp. 179–212). Lanham, MD: University Press of America.

Deshler, D., Ellis, E., & Lenz, B. (1996). *Teaching adolescents with learning disabilities* (2nd ed.). Denver, CO: Love Publishing Company.

Desired Results Developmental Profile Revised (DRDP). (2008). Sacramento: California Department of Education. Retrieved August 8, 2010, from www.wested.org/desiredresults/training/form_drdp.htm.

Dote-Kwan, J., Chen, D., & Hughes, M. (2001). A national survey of service providers who work with young children with visual impairments. *Journal of Visual Impairment & Blindness, 95*, 325–337.

Downing, J., & Chen, D. (2003). Using tactile strategies with students who are blind and have severe disabilities. *Teaching Exceptional Children, 36*(2), 56–61.

Ferrell, K. A., with Shaw, A. R., & Deitz, S. J. (1998). *Project PRISM: A longitudinal study of developmental patterns of children who are visually impaired. Final report.* Grant H023C10188, U.S. Department of Education, Field-initiated research, CFDA 84.023. Greeley: University of Northern Colorado. Available at www.unco.edu/ncssd/research/PRISM/ExecSumm.pdf.

Ferrington, G. (2003). Soundscape studies: Listening with attentive ears. *Telemedium: The Journal of Media Literacy, 49–50*(1), 42.

Fraiberg, S. (1977). *Insights from the blind: Comparative studies of blind and sighted infants.* New York: Basic Books.

Harley, R., Truan, M., & Sanford, L. (1997). *Communication skills for visually impaired learners.* Springfield, IL: Charles C Thomas.

Hatlen, P. (1996). The core curriculum for blind and visually impaired students, including those with additional disabilities. *RE:view, 28*(1), 25–32.

Hatton, D. D. (2001). Model registry of early childhood visual impairment: First-year results. *Journal of Visual Impairment & Blindness, 95*, 418–433.

Heasley, B. E. (1974). *Auditory perceptual disorders and remediation.* Springfield, IL: Charles C Thomas.

Hirsch, R. (1986). On defining listening: Synthesis and discussion. Paper presented at the Seventh Annual Meeting of the International Listening Association. Retrieved from ERIC database (ED 276 475).

Jacobson, W., & Bradley, R. (1997). Learning theory and teaching methodologies. In B. Blasch, W. Weiner, & R. Welsh (Eds.), *Foundations of orientation and mobility* (2nd ed.), Vol. 1, *History and theory* (pp. 211–237). New York: AFB Press.

Jalongo, M. R. (1995). Promoting active listening in the classroom. *Childhood Education, 72*(1), 13–18.

Koenig, A. (1996). Growing into literacy. In C. Holbrook & A. Koenig (Eds.), *Children with visual impairments.* Bethesda, MD: Woodbine House.

Liefert, F. (2003). Introduction to visual impairment. In S. Goodman & S. Wittenstein (Eds.), *Collaborative assessment working with students who are blind or visually impaired, including those with additional disabilities* (p. 4). New York: AFB Press.

Miles, B. (1999). Conversation: The essence of communication. In B. Miles & M. Riggio (Eds.), *Remarkable conversations: A guide to developing meaningful communication with children and young adults who are deafblind* (pp. 54–75). Watertown, MA: Perkins School for the Blind.

Miles, B., & Riggio, M. (1999). Understanding deafblindness. In B. Miles & M. Riggio (Eds.), *Remarkable conversations: A guide to developing meaningful communication with children and young adults who are deafblind* (pp. 20–37). Watertown, MA: Perkins School for the Blind.

Morlet, T. (Spring 2010). Auditory neuropathy spectrum disorder and (central) auditory processing disorder. *Deaf-Blind Perspectives, 17*(2), 1–4.

Moss, K. (Spring 1997). Are you listening? Auditory issues for children with visual impairment. *See/Hear Newsletter, 2*(2). Austin: Texas School for the Blind and Visually Impaired.

Nelson-Barber, S., & Estrin, E. T. (1995). Culturally responsive mathematics and science education for Native students (information analyses). San Francisco, CA: Far West Laboratory for Educational Research and Development. Retrieved from ERIC database (ED 388 483).

Northern, J., & Downs, M. (1974). *Hearing in children.* Baltimore, MD: Williams and Wilkins.

Petress, K. (1999). Listening: A vital skill. *Journal of Instructional Psychology, 26*(4), 261.

Ratey, J. (2001). *A user's guide to the brain.* New York: Vintage Books.

Rex, E., Koenig, A., Wormsley, D., & Baker, R. (1994). *Foundations of braille literacy.* New York: AFB Press.

Sacks, S. Z., Kekelis, L. S., & Gaylord-Ross, R. J. (1992). *The development of social skills by blind and visually impaired students, exploratory studies and strategies.* New York: AFB Press.

Ward, M. (2000). The visual system. In M. C. Holbrook & A. Koenig (Eds.), *Foundation of education* (2nd ed.), Vol. 1, *History and theory of teaching children and youths with visual impairments* (pp. 77–110). New York: AFB Press.

Warren, D. (1994). *Blindness and children: An individual differences approach* (pp. 17, 168). New York: Cambridge University Press.

Wiener, W. R., Welsh, R. L., & Blasch, B. B. (Eds.) (2010). *Foundations of orientation and mobility* (3rd ed.). New York: AFB Press.

Chapter 2

Infants and Toddlers: Learning to Listen

Lizbeth A. Barclay

Each newborn varies in an infinite number of ways from another—in appearance, in feeling, in reaction to stimuli, in movement patterns, in capacity to develop his or her own individual pattern.

—T. B. Brazelton, *Infants and Mothers: Differences in Development*, 1983

CHAPTER PREVIEW

- ▶ Infant and Caregiver Bonding: The Foundation for Social Listening
- ▶ Creating the Environment and Opportunities for Listening
- ▶ Cognitive Skills
- ▶ Language Development: Attaching Meaning to Listening
- ▶ Setting the Stage for Play
- ▶ Motor Development

Imagine an infant's first sensory experience: At birth he or she enters a new environment that seems to consist primarily of sounds and sensation. This new world feels foreign and less hospitable than the infant's previous home, the warm, comparatively quiet and comfortable womb. The infant arrives without knowledge and training, yet learning begins as he or she first experiences the combination of sound and touch. Each newborn is an individual, reacting to the environment with personal variation in reflexes and responses, evoked from the baby's senses of vision, hearing, touch, and smell. Individual differences in infant development were described by T. Berry Brazelton, internationally known expert on child development, in his classic, *Infants and Mothers*, in 1983. In the field of visual impairment, David Warren, author of *Blindness and Children: An Individual Differences Approach*, provided a summary and interpretation of the research literature on infants and children with visual impairments that described their individual differences based on variables such as environment and experiences (1994).

As indicated in Chapter 1, the impact of visual impairment on a child's development is highly individual and is dependent on factors such as the extent of his or her visual impairment, environmental opportunities, and presence of additional disabilities (Liefert, 2003, p. 4). The development of listening skills for infants who are visually impaired needs to be approached within this context of individual differences.

This chapter focuses on the youngest children who are visually impaired as they are learning to listen, exploring the development of that process, focusing on their listening needs, and offering strategies for teaching listening skills and creating environments and experiences that support learning to listen. Each section of this chapter focuses on the development of listening behaviors and skills within specific domains of early infant and toddler development: bonding and early social development, auditory awareness and attention, cognitive development, language development, activities, play, and motor development. In the beginning of each of these sections, relevant behaviors and skills are listed that parallel the skills outlined in the Listening Skills Continuum in Appendix A at the back of this book. This continuum is described in more detail in Chapter 1.

The development of infants and toddlers is an integrated and holistic process, with each developmental domain intertwined with and dependent on the others (Ferrell, 2011). Therefore, readers will observe that many of the skills relate to more than one domain. For instance, the skill "Responds to his or her name" can be found in both the "Social Listening" and "Language Development" sections of this chapter.

While the development of listening is the focus of this book, listening alone will not provide infants who are visually impaired with the sensory information that is necessary in order for them to make sense of their world. The combination of listening, touch, and movement is what provides a meaningful context on which to build. The beginning of that process is described in the next section.

INFANT AND CAREGIVER BONDING:
THE FOUNDATION FOR SOCIAL LISTENING

So often when a stranger comes in, a little blind baby will just quiet down and not do anything. The mom, of course, wants the baby to show off or be responsive, and the baby is quiet. But it's because the baby is listening and trying to figure out who the person is.

—Nancy Akeson, first counselor
of the Blind Babies Foundation, 2000

Emerging listening skills relating to bonding and early social development include the following:

▶ alerts to auditory stimulation
▶ responds pleasurably to the sound of the human voice
▶ smiles in response to a parent's voice
▶ demonstrates adverse reactions to the sound of a stranger's voice
▶ responds to his or her name

The early phase of infant development, in which the meaning of sound is mediated by the intimate bond provided by parents and caregivers, establishes the foundation for development in other domains of learning, including cognitive, communicative, and, in particular, social development. Infants with visual impairments depend on others to provide information about the physical world, the sounds that they hear, and the social world around them (Sacks, 2006). The early bond between infants and their caregivers is crucial in learning to listen because this connection supports a child's interest in and motivation to attend to environmental sounds. In turn, learning to listen to and interpret sound fosters social competence for these children as they broaden their circle of trusted family members and friends.

From the very beginning, each baby listens and responds to the sounds and voices that he or she hears based on personal style and temperament. A baby who has vision displays a variety of behaviors, including visual response, that naturally draw his or her parents into further interaction. Visually, the most important stimulus is the face of the caregiver, and vision enables the sighted infant to participate in an initial form of human partnership long before the infant is capable of intentional behavior (Fraiberg, 1977, p. 110). This ability makes establishing a bond with parents comparatively easy.

An infant who is visually impaired may demonstrate response to sounds and voices in a very different way, which parents need to learn to interpret and to which they learn how to respond. Through the work of Fraiberg (1977), we understand that babies who are blind develop a repertoire of communication through hand language or specific hand movements that expresses need and intention. Parents can begin to understand when their baby is paying attention from a variety of motor responses, such as when the baby stills (attention), wiggles (anticipation), quiets to a familiar voice, molds to his or her caregiver's body, or opens his or her mouth to sounds such as the microwave or the unbuttoning of a blouse before nursing.

While establishing the bond with their infant, parents can learn to interpret, respond to, and reinforce these early signs of attention, nurturing their child's listening behavior. Sometimes guidance from an early intervention specialist who has experience and knowledge in visual impairment and its effect on learning can be very helpful in learning to interpret indications of listening.

By recognizing these early and sometimes subtle signs of response, parents can begin to understand what they need to do to elicit responses that can be repeated. This pattern of response is the beginning of the dance of communication and is crucial to the establishment of the caregiver-infant bond that will create the foundation for development. Early intervention specialists can support families by helping them observe and document information about their infants through early in-home assessment.

A variety of factors may interfere with this seemingly natural process. It must again be stressed that as a population, infants with visual impairments are extremely diverse, and their development varies widely depending on the degree of vision loss, age at visual diagnosis, and presence or absence of additional disabilities. Many infants with visual impairments are born prematurely and may be medically fragile, enduring sometimes months in a hospital's neonatal unit before coming home. Consider the factors that can accompany having a newborn with special needs once he or she is at home. Many infants are often very irritable because of neurological immaturity (Brazelton, 1983). They often require many and frequent medical and specialist interventions, and their daily schedules may be constantly interrupted by appointments. These factors present a challenge to learning an infant's subtle signals of attention and beginning communication.

Within the many aspects of individual differences, some infants and toddlers who are visually impaired are extremely sensitive to sound, reacting fearfully in the presence of new and loud sounds, such as the vacuum cleaner or a loud voice, or overly busy and chaotic sound environments, such as a family birthday party or the grocery store. Adverse reaction to sound may be demonstrated by acute crying, or the infant or toddler may simply shut down and withdraw. Children with visual impairments also may sometimes create their own auditory environment by making sounds such as raspberries, unique squeals, or other vocalizations in order to gain control over or mask sounds that they find aversive. This sensitivity to sound may persist into preschool and sometimes even longer. When this is the case, collaboration between the family and an early intervention specialist is very important in helping strike a balance between continuing to introduce the child to novel sound and honoring the need to moderate the child's exposure to what he or she feels is jarring and disturbing. An infant's reaction to sound can be extremely individual, requiring parents to be sensitive observers. The ability to perceive sound is, of course, essential for establishing the bond between infant and caregiver, so screening of infants and toddlers is critical to ensure that their hearing is intact (see Sidebar 2.1).

((Sidebar 2.1
Hearing Screening for Infants and Toddlers

Hearing screening is critical for infants and toddlers in order to be certain that they are perceiving sound. Hearing loss is the most common birth defect in the United States (Audiology Foundation of America, 1999). Detecting any hearing loss as early as possible is also essential for the development of language and communication skills, since children begin learning speech and language in the first 6 months of life. Research suggests that children with hearing loss who get help early develop better language skills than those who do not. For children with visual impairments, early detection of any hearing loss is even more crucial because without vision, hearing is key to their motivation to move, explore, and learn.

Typically, infants' hearing is screened in the hospital, before they go home, through a program known as universal newborn hearing screening. Hearing screening can also be conducted through early intervention programs. The Individuals with Disabilities Education Act (IDEA) requires that infants and toddlers with disabilities be identified and provided with appropriate screening.

The two common screening methods used with infants are otoacoustic emissions and auditory brainstem response:

- The **otoacoustic emissions (OAE)** test shows whether parts of the ear respond properly to sound. During this test, a soft sponge plug is inserted into the baby's ear canal and emits a series of sounds to measure an "echo" response, which occurs in normal hearing ears. No echo could indicate hearing loss.

- The **auditory brain stem response (ABR)** test determines how the auditory brain stem (the part of the nerve that carries sound from the ear to the brain) and the brain respond to sound by measuring their electrical activity as a child listens. During this test, the baby wears small earphones in the ears and electrodes on the head. The baby might be given a mild sedative to keep him or her calm and quiet during the test. If the baby does not respond consistently to the sounds presented during either of these tests, the doctor will suggest a follow-up hearing screening and a referral to an audiologist for a more comprehensive hearing evaluation.

Source: Adapted from *It's Important to Have Your Baby's Hearing Screened* (NIH Publication No. 11-4968) (Bethesda, MD: National Institute of Deafness and Other Communication Disorders, May 2011). Retrieved May 25, 2011, from www.nidcd.nih.gov/health/hearing/screened.html.

CREATING THE ENVIRONMENT AND OPPORTUNITIES FOR LISTENING

Emerging listening skills relating to the development of auditory awareness and attention include the following:

- alerts to auditory stimulation
- quiets when presented with noise
- demonstrates listening attitude; reacts to sound source
- indicates attention to sounds by action of hands
- demonstrates selective response to sound
- responds to name

Seven-month-old Carlos is gently placed on the floor by his mother under a frame with sound-producing toys and objects that dangle from elastic within foot and hand distance from him. As he moves about, he inadvertently brushes against the hanging metal spoons that swing together with a bright clicking sound. Immediately, Carlos stills and remains quiet for a few seconds, processing what he has just heard, before moving again. This time Carlos stretches his foot to the side, which taps a tambourine that has been placed there. A slight frown of concentration appears on his face as he tries to discern the new sound. From the next room, Carlos hears the voice of his mother. Again, he quietly stills as he listens to her approach. As she nears, crooning, "Hello, little man . . . ," Carlos kicks his feet again, this time in excitement. He knows that he is about to be picked up.

The world provides a rich source of auditory information that we are constantly receiving and interpreting. In most home and community environments, opportunities abound for infants and toddlers to hear and listen. The act of learning to listen, or perception, enables us to interpret the world, act and move with intention, and communicate. Perception entails much more than just hearing sound. It requires a form of expectation, of knowing what is about to happen and preparing for it. Without this knowledge, or expectation, we would be quickly overwhelmed because every experience would be a new one (Ratey, 2001, p. 56).

The Infant's Response to Sounds

For infants who are visually impaired, the repetition of experiences and the modification of environment are especially important. To begin to make sense of the sounds around them, infants need to have many opportunities to hear and perceive sound in a calm and quiet environment. A conducive listening environment can be achieved at home by eliminating background noise, such as the television, radio, or appliances, as often as possible when engaging in communication or routines. This simplification of the sound environment helps a baby learn sounds without the challenge presented by competing noise and enables the caregiver greater opportunity to perceive the subtle ways that the child reacts to sound.

During infancy, input provided by parents and caregivers needs to be very simple and consistent, gently providing information about the noise that is heard and the sensations, objects, and experiences that are encountered. The complexity of communication needs to match the infant's developmental and cognitive levels. Parents can communicate about what the infant is doing as the baby is doing it, focusing on the most critical aspects of the activity (Chen, 1999). For example, a caregiver might tell a baby what is going on around him or what his hand brushed when he reached out, using simple language such as "Your hand hit the bells. Do it again," while making sure that the bell toy is in close proximity.

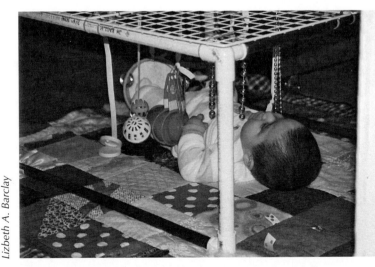

Lizbeth A. Barclay

Often, a baby who is blind will show he is listening by being still and quiet. This infant is concentrating as he listens to the tambourine he has accidentally kicked with his foot.

As babies begin to take the lead in attending and reacting to sound, we learn what is most important to them in terms of sound. This process can happen only if we give space for it to happen, and we can sometimes miss it because of the difference in the way that babies who are blind and visually impaired show response (Pogrund & Fazzi, 2002). Often, a baby who is blind will show a listening response by being still and quiet (Rowland, 1984). The response may be very subtle, such as accelerated breathing or a slight turn of the head. Therefore, it is important to build into routines and communication exchanges opportunities for pausing and listening. The pause, when listening occurs, will happen in contrast to an infant's movement and vocalization. Sidebar 2.2 provides guidelines for deliberately responding to an infant's response. As noted earlier, the importance of infant-caregiver bonding cannot be overemphasized, and maintaining an environment that is conducive to learning to listen is essential.

((SIDEBAR 2.2

Suggestions for Interventions to Assist Caregivers

The following suggestions will help professionals assist caregivers in identifying their infants' communicative behaviors and cues and provide natural ways of responding to infants' behaviors that the infants will perceive. Through careful observations, caregivers can become accurate and responsive interpreters of their infants' behaviors and can develop mutually enjoyable interactions.

1. IDENTIFY AND INTERPRET THE INFANT'S CUES

Observe the infant and identify the infant's range of behaviors and nonverbal cues. For example, what does the infant do when he or she is alert, tired, hungry, wants interaction, or needs to rest? Some infants use subtle cues (such as a change in muscle tone), while others use clear signals (like crying or quiet attentiveness). Some behaviors (for example, a facial grimace of an infant with spastic cerebral palsy that may indicate pleasure or displeasure) are difficult to interpret without careful observation and knowing the infant well.

2. IDENTIFY WHEN THE INFANT IS ACTIVE OR ALERT AND READY FOR INTERACTION

Observe the infant's behavioral states during the daily routine. Note when the infant is alert (the time of day and during which activities) to take advantage of those opportunities

(Continued)

for learning and interaction. For example, some infants are more interactive after lunch, whereas others prefer to nap.

3. RESPOND CONTINGENTLY TO THE INFANT'S BEHAVIORS

Identify an infant's interest on the basis of subtle nonverbal signals (such as a calm, quiet, or alert state; hand movements or body orientation toward the object or person; or quiet vocalizations). Respond to these signals in a way that supports the infant's interaction and promotes turn taking; for example, move the object to touch the infant's hand, touch or pick up the infant, and imitate the infant's vocalizations.

4. IDENTIFY THE INFANT'S PREFERENCES FOR STIMULATION

Identify whether the infant responds to visual, auditory, tactile, olfactory, or kinesthetic stimuli during natural situations. Does the infant prefer brightly colored, shiny, or high-contrast objects or toys with lights? Does the infant attend to familiar voices, songs or other music on audiotape, or toys that make sounds? Does the infant enjoy tickling games, massage, or touching and handling objects? Does the infant seem interested in the odors of foods, soaps, and lotions? Does the infant enjoy finger plays, movement, or rough-and-tumble games? Observe the infant's responses to a variety of sensory cues by, for instance, having the adult tap his or her fingers on the high-chair tray to encourage the infant to pick up small crackers; having the infant smell the shampoo before putting it on his or her hair; gently rocking the baby before putting him or her in a hammock; or having the adult clap his or her hands before holding them out for the infant to anticipate being picked up.

5. PROVIDE CONTINGENT SENSORY STIMULATION

Carefully observe the infant's behaviors and provide preferred sensory stimulation that is contingent on the infant's particular actions. For example, when the baby vocalizes, respond consistently by imitating the sound and touching the infant; after diapering the baby, wait for the baby to reach out before picking him or her up; wait for the infant to look at the red puppet before making it dance; and wait for the infant to move his or her body before pushing the swing. In addition, provide toys and adaptive switches that the infant can activate easily to produce vibration, lights, movement, or music.

6. CREATE INDIVIDUALIZED GAMES THAT BOTH THE CAREGIVER AND INFANT ENJOY

Identify opportunities within the daily routine that are natural times for playing individualized games, such as peek-a-boo using a washcloth during bathtime; riding the horsey while the infant is sitting on the caregiver's lap; or tickling the tummy when the baby is being diapered.

7. USE FAVORITE ACTIVITIES

Begin with activities that are familiar to and preferred by the infant to provide opportunities for contingent stimulation and for the infant to realize that he or she can influence the adult's response. During familiar activities (like massage, riding horsey, rough-and-tumble or movement games, or mealtimes), pause and wait for the infant to indicate, through a body movement or vocalization, that he or she wants the activity to continue. Once the infant is familiar with the massage routine, the caregiver may pause to see whether the infant anticipates the next step in the routine or in some way requests that the massage continue. Begin the horsey ride and then pause and wait for the infant to request "more horsey ride." Learning experiences that are contingent, or dependent, on an infant's behavior are activities that naturally follow the infant's signals and interest and involve his or her active participation. Mealtime can become a contingency experience for an infant who loves to eat. The infant will be motivated to request another spoonful of applesauce by opening his or her mouth, saying "more," or signing MORE. The infant can also indicate a choice between applesauce and apple juice by reaching for the spoon rather than the cup.

8. DECREASE HAND-OVER-HAND GUIDANCE, OR COACTIVE MANIPULATION

After physically manipulating the infant through an activity a few times, guide the infant through the initial movement and then wait for a behavior to indicate an expectation of what will occur next. For example, place the infant's hand on a switch, remove your hand, wait for an indication (such as a finger movement) that the infant wants to activate the switch, and then provide the assistance. This strategy will be effective only if the infant likes the activity, so it is essential to choose a preferred sensory event (auditory, tactile, or visual). Furthermore, the switch should be the easiest type for the infant to activate, given his or her motor ability. Similarly, with other familiar activities, stop after initially positioning the infant and wait for the infant to indicate what will happen next. For example, place the infant on a large ball; wait for the infant's behavior, such as patting the ball, before bouncing the infant on the ball. If the infant does not respond, assist the infant to pat the ball. As physical guidance is gradually decreased, the infant will discover that he or she can elicit a reaction from the environment or make something happen.

9. PROVIDE OPPORTUNITIES TO MAKE CHOICES

Offer choices during natural situations, such as between food or drink or between two toys. At first, an infant may choose to participate or not to participate in a specific activity at a particular time or to eat or not to eat the particular food that is offered. When possible, the caregiver's responsiveness to the infant's preferences will assist the infant in learning that he or she can affect the environment. Next, an infant may develop an understanding that he or she can make a choice between a preferred and a disliked object like food. Finally, an infant will be able to choose between two preferred objects or activities. Through these experiences, the infant will learn that his or her behaviors can elicit a response from the caregiver.

Source: Reprinted from D. Chen, *Essential Elements in Early Intervention: Visual Impairment and Multiple Disabilities* (New York: AFB Press, 1999), pp. 43–46.

Early Listening Skills

There are various ways to organize and represent the many skills associated with listening. As infants and toddlers with visual impairments grow and develop, learning to listen begins in domains that are closely linked to the areas of auditory perception, described in Chapter 1.

Anthony and Lowry (2004) describe five stages in the development of auditory skills, linking early listening skills to examples of typical behavioral responses, based on work by Johnson, Benson, and Seaton (1997). Typically, children begin by demonstrating their recognition of loud or intense sounds, often by crying, at stage 1, eventually progressing to the ability to listen to and respond by conversing during conversation in stage 5. Table 2.1 provides examples of behavioral responses within stages of auditory

---

TABLE 2.1
Stages of Auditory Skill Development

Stage	Main Theme	Behavior Example
Stage 1	Sound awareness Early attending Sound as meaningful event	• obvious response to intense sounds • obvious response to soft sounds • obvious response to caregiver's voice
Stage 2	Beginning localization Early sound recognition Beginning deliberate vocalization	• search for sound, looking/reaching • increased vocalizations • responds to different voice tones • beginning vocal play
Stage 3	Accurate localization and tracking Meaningful sound recognition Deliberate vocalization	• manipulates toy to make sound • attends to and follows voice • searches for changes in sound • "calls" for caregiver for basic needs • unfamiliar sounds are upsetting • anticipates events based on sounds • makes gestures to familiar words
Stage 4	Increased sound comprehension Increased speech comprehension Improved vocalization control	• understands familiar phrases • responds to name • participates in familiar vocal play • vocalizations sound like words • better use of inflectional patterns • plays with complex sound toys
Stage 5	Early auditory comprehension Meaningful use of oral language Increased ability to converse	• follows one-step directions without gestures • expressive vocabulary increases • attends to people despite background noise

Source: Reprinted with permission from T. Anthony & S. S. Lowry, "Sensory Development," in T. L. Anthony, S. S. Lowry, C. J. Brown, & D. D. Hatton (Eds.), *Developmentally Appropriate Orientation and Mobility* (Chapel Hill: Early Intervention Training Center for Infants and Toddlers with Visual Impairments, FPG Child Development Institute, University of North Carolina at Chapel Hill, 2004), p. 139.

skill development. While not grouped according to these stages, the specific skills in the Listening Skills Continuum for Infants and Toddlers represent additional examples (see Appendix A at the back of this book).

By recognizing a child's listening behavior, parents and caregivers encourage and nurture early listening skills. Sidebar 2.3 provides some suggestions offered by Ferrell (2011) for ways that parents and caregivers can encourage their child's listening behaviors.

((SIDEBAR 2.3

Activities and Guidelines for the Development of Early Listening Skills

The following suggestions are useful for parents, other caregivers, and professionals in helping encourage a child's early listening skills, following a progression that begins with awareness of sound and continues to include attention to and turning to sound, localizing sound, attaching meaning to sound, and learning to utilize sound in the environment:

AWARENESS OF SOUND

- Look for an awareness of voices, loud noises, and, gradually, responses to more ordinary household noises such as a clock's ticking, the coffeepot's dripping, and water running in the shower.
- Alert your child to these sounds, tell him what they are, and make him more comfortable and relaxed with them.
- Explain sounds that are heard in the distance to help make connections with prior experiences. For example, when hearing water running in the kitchen, explain, "The water is running in the kitchen sink. Your brother is running the water in the sink so he can do the dishes."

TURNING TO SOUND

- Help your baby turn her head in the right direction by placing your hand on her cheek and pushing gently but firmly.
- Provide opportunities for your baby to turn to sound throughout the day, but try to make sure that there's a reason for doing it. If you make turning to sound simply a routine that you repeat over and over, your baby will become tired, will lose interest very quickly, and will not repeat the action. Then it may appear that he has not yet learned to turn to sound, when what he has actually learned is that turning to sound has no purpose.
- Show your baby that turning to sound has meaning by taking her hand to touch the object that made a sound. Use toys that have other sensory qualities, such as a two-color squeeze toy that has interesting textures and makes sound with very little hand pressure.
- Turning to your voice can be particularly rewarding for your baby if you give him a kiss when he does it.

(Continued)

LOCALIZING SOUND

- Choose a variety of squeak toys, rattles, bells, and other noisemakers that produce interesting sounds and are close in size to what your baby can hold. Be careful, however, that the noise is not too scary, shrill, or loud. (Sometimes the sound will overload a baby's senses and she will tune it out altogether.)

- Make the sound first at ear level and on your baby's side. Wait for your baby to turn his head toward the sound. If he does not turn his head the first time you make the sound, make the sound again and gently turn his face toward that side; then bring his hand up to touch the toy and make the sound again.

- Once your baby can turn her head to sounds made at the side, move the sound down, below ear level. Your baby will turn her head first to the side, and then down. Again, coordinate the sound with a reaching movement by taking her hand to touch the object.

- Continue to move the location of the sound once your baby has mastered each location. When your baby can localize—that is, identify where a sound is coming from—and demonstrates this by turning his head to sounds below ear level, the next position to establish familiarity with is above ear level. At this point, you can also start moving the sound out in front of your baby.

- If your baby is multiply impaired and cannot turn her head to localize sound, look for eye movement to sound. Even if your baby is totally blind, she will turn her eyes to sound, at least in the beginning. If your baby is not reinforced for this behavior, however—if you don't give your baby any feedback that it was good to turn her eyes toward the sound—she will not continue to do it.

- Try different sounds at different distances to see which sounds your baby likes best and how far away the sound is when he no longer seems to respond. You may want to use your baby's favorite sounds on days you know he needs a lot of motivation because he doesn't feel good or he is having a difficult day.

- If your baby does not seem to respond the first time, make the sound last a little longer. Sometimes babies with multiple impairments need a longer period of time to figure out where a sound is coming from, or their response may be delayed because of other difficulties.

- Check to be sure your baby's response is the same to sounds made at both ears. If it is not, check with your doctor to see if there is an ear infection in the ear that seems to be less responsive to sound. Everyone has a side that he or she likes or uses more than the other, so you might find that your baby simply has a preference.

- As with all other activities, turning to sound is not an exercise done in isolation. Every sound is an opportunity to find out more about your baby's abilities, so look for her response when playing, eating, dressing, walking outside, and reaching.

GIVING MEANING TO SOUND

- Your baby will learn more about sounds if you are able to name a sound for him and point out its other sensory qualities. The sense of touch is important here, because as a sound is made, a vibration is given off. The information gained from the vibration is helpful to your baby in identifying the sound in other situations.

- Remember that the word used to describe a sound often has many different meanings. Take *bell*, for example; it could refer to the bell sound of a telephone ringing, the doorbell, the church bell, the alarm clock bell, the school bell, and the bicycle bell, among others. You need to be specific about the words you use so your baby does not get confused. How confusing it would be to your baby if she had just learned about the bell that rings when someone is at the door of your home, and then in the park you tell her about another bell—but you are not at home, she doesn't hear the door open, and she doesn't hear anyone talking to you. The second bell was a bicycle bell, which you might be able to see, but your baby might not. So be specific and informative—use the words *doorbell*, *bicycle bell*, and other specific terms.

USING SOUND IN THE ENVIRONMENT

When you are helping your baby learn about the meaning of sound, you are usually concentrating on one sound at a time. Several sounds may actually be made at any one time, but you have chosen the sound that you want to tell your baby about. Your baby will also need to learn how to pick out the important sounds—those that will give him the most information—and to ignore the sounds that do not give meaning. This skill will become critical when your baby is learning to move about in the environment—for example, if he tries to pay attention to all the sounds in the environment, he may not hear a car coming. To help your baby learn to pick out the important sounds in the environment, consider the following:

- Start by helping him distinguish one sound from another. For example, the television may be playing when you call his name. Does he hear you call him, and does he show you, either by turning or with some other signal? If not, it may be helpful to touch his shoulder to make him aware that you called him and that this was an important sound that he needs to pay attention to.

- When you start working on distinguishing sounds, make the new sound you are introducing very different from the sound that is already in the environment. Gradually work your way up to sounds that are not much different (such as the sound of water dripping in the sink versus the sound of rainwater dripping from the gutter).

- Play games such as "What made that sound?" and "Can you find _____?" to see if he can identify the source.

- Different sounds can be important one time and not important the next. For example, the sound of the refrigerator's humming is not important if you are in the kitchen eating a meal. But if the refrigerator is located next to a down staircase without a door or gate and the baby is crawling around on the kitchen floor, the sound of the refrigerator can be very important; it can signal to him that he is close to a dangerous area.

Source: Adapted from K. Ferrell, *Reach Out and Teach: Helping Your Child Who Is Visually Impaired Learn and Grow,* 2nd ed. (New York: AFB Press, 2011), pp. 141–181.

The skills related to auditory perception that are developed in a child's first months are essential for the development of cognitive, communicative, social, and movement skills. The next sections of this chapter explore that link.

COGNITIVE SKILLS

Emerging listening skills relating to cognitive development include the following:

- ▸ makes a slight move toward a familiar sound
- ▸ recognizes familiar sounds, parents' voices, own toys, and so forth
- ▸ anticipates familiar daily events based on auditory cues
- ▸ responds to spoken request
- ▸ demonstrates appropriate response for familiar words or phrases
- ▸ selects a familiar object when it is named
- ▸ shows anticipation of events when a verbal cue such as "Let's go outside" is provided
- ▸ responds to simple phrases with specific nonverbal responses
- ▸ follows simple verbal directions accompanied by gestures or physical cues

Early Cognitive Skills

The development of listening skills is inextricably tied to the development of cognitive skills. One needs to listen to the world to understand it, but one needs to understand the world to make sense of what one hears. Because the perceptual information that infants who are visually impaired receive may be limited—and may be even more limited for children with additional disabilities, especially hearing impairment—it is necessary to provide early intervention that supports the development of cognitive skills. This support pairs listening with experiential learning; many skills associated with experiential learning and daily living skills also support the development of cognitive skills. (Chapters 7 and 8, which focus on children with additional disabilities and with hearing impairments or deaf-blindness, also address this important issue.)

Early cognitive skills can be organized in a variety of ways; the work of Jean Piaget, for instance, described these skills within considerations of the sensorimotor stage occurring between birth and age 2. In this stage, babies learn about the properties of objects and about their relationship to people and other objects by "doing," which includes looking, hearing, touching, grasping, and sucking (Wood, Smith, & Grossniklaus, 2001). Specific to children with visual impairments, Lueck, Chen, Kekelis,

((SIDEBAR 2.4

Opportunities for Learning

Cognitive skills can be promoted by the following opportunities for learning:

- Supporting the development of a strong, effective bond between infant and caregivers
- Providing appropriate levels of environmental stimulation
- Encouraging active involvement of the infant that allows control of the environment and builds intrinsic motivation
- Guiding the infant to investigate object features and actions with object. One should start with the child's current level of cognitive function and move to a slightly higher level.
- Encouraging the infant to examine and search near space and far space in meaningful ways
- Promoting the conceptual understanding built upon experience that includes specific training for concepts not learned casually by infants with visual impairments
- Promoting a more complete understanding of the organization of the environment by provision of direct experiences that demonstrate where functional objects originate and where they are returned during the course of daily routines. Also, the identification of primary fixed objects along usual travel routes in familiar areas should be a featured activity.
- Supporting an infant's active interaction with people and objects through meaningful visual, tactual, social, and communicative exchanges

Source: Reprinted with permission from A. H. Lueck, D. Chen, L. Kekelis, & E. S. Hartmann, *Developmental Guidelines for Infants with Visual Impairment: A Guidebook for Early Intervention,* 2nd ed. (Louisville, KY: American Printing House for the Blind, 2008), p. 125.

and Hartmann (2008) stressed the aspects of cognitive development that include attention, memory, properties of objects, causal relations, conceptual understanding, spatial relationships, and problem solving. They emphasized the importance of promoting cognitive skills early in life. Sidebar 2.4 provides their suggestions for supporting cognitive development.

Concepts and Object Permanence

Concepts are the thoughts or ideas that a person has about people, places, objects, physical properties, events, actions, and reactions. (The development of concepts is discussed in more detail later in this chapter.) According to Warren (1994), if a child has a concept of an object, then he or she need not have that object physically present in order to think about it. But this level of concept formation can take place only if a child has developed an understanding of *object permanence*, the idea that objects and people continue to exist even when they can no longer be seen, heard, or touched.

Research regarding object permanence has been mixed. As Warren described the work of both Fraiberg (1977) and Bigelow (1986), he pointed again to the individual differences among infants with visual impairments, saying that among the infants tested in the studies, there was considerable variability in skill acquisition (Warren, 1994). According to the findings from Project PRISM (Ferrell, 1998), a later longitudinal study of the early development of children with visual impairments, however, infants who are blind search for an object that has been removed—a sign that they have acquired the concept of object permanence—at 13 months of age, as compared with sighted infants, who do so at 6 months of age. This gap in acquiring an understanding of this concept highlights the importance of actively promoting early listening skills.

Touch and listening combine to give meaning to concepts that are acquired through experiential learning, that is, learning that takes place during real and meaningful experience, such as during eating, bathing, and dressing routines, or while going to a park or shopping with family members as a toddler. Repetition and consistency of experience are essential components of learning for children who are visually impaired. During bathing, for instance, a natural routine activity, the learning process might feel and sound like this:

> ▸ *(while touching the soap)* "Here's the soap for washing. Mmm, smell it . . ."
> ▸ *(while picking up the towel)* "The towel is for drying. It's soft."
> ▸ *(while turning on and touching the water)* "Let's turn on the water. That's the water. Let's touch the water. It's warm . . ."

Pairing consistent and simple language while helping a baby touch each item provides many opportunities to develop the object concepts associated with that activity. As the baby becomes a toddler, leaving the towel, washcloth, and soap in a consistent place for retrieval before the bath will provide the consistency that is needed for the child to intentionally find and touch them in anticipation of the bath, demonstrating understanding of some of the properties and uses for those functional objects. Concepts are developed in tandem with listening skills through this regular pairing of information with sound and touch.

LANGUAGE DEVELOPMENT: ATTACHING MEANING TO LISTENING

Emerging listening skills relating to language development include the following:

- ▶ imitates own sound
- ▶ imitates speech patterns
- ▶ responds to name
- ▶ listens selectively to two familiar words
- ▶ has an appropriate response for familiar words or phrases
- ▶ has an appropriate response to directions such as "Give it to me"
- ▶ demonstrates concepts of up and down when directed
- ▶ selects familiar object in response to naming

Harry, who is 9 months of age, is just beginning to enjoy solid foods. He was born with a rare retinal condition and has no vision. His mother tries to feed him his pureed vegetables and fruit each evening just before the family dinnertime so that he can be with the family afterward while they have dinner.

As Harry sits in his high chair waiting for his food, he hears the sound of the jar being popped open by his mother. As she does so, she tells him, "Mmm, time for dinner, Harry. It's squash." Harry hears the spoon as it touches the jar and the bowl while his mother is spooning it out. She says, "Harry, I'm scooping out the squash." While placing it into the microwave oven, she tells him, "I'm making it warm for you, Harry," and he then hears the sound of the microwave. Next, as his mother puts on his bib, she adds, "It's almost ready. Here's your bib, Harry," and he grabs for it as it touches his neck.

Once the squash is warm and ready to eat, Harry's mother brings it to his tray, gives him time to smell it, and then comments, "Mmm, smell the squash, time to eat. Open your mouth," as she touches the spoon with squash to his mouth. Listening to the pairing of simple language with objects, routine sounds in his environment, and experience helps Harry to learn language because the real and routine contexts provide meaning to him.

Vocalizations and Imitation

Babies begin babbling, a form of pre-speech characterized by the production of well-formed syllables, at around 7 to 10 months of age. Before that, from the very beginning of life if motorically capable, babies produce vocal sounds, or vocalizations, that start simply with an open vocal tract and then progressively become more complicated as their motoric abilities progress (Locke, 1995, p. 176). It comes very naturally for parents to immediately imitate these sounds, encouraging and providing incentive for the infant to continue. According to data from Project PRISM, children who are visually impaired with no other disabilities "produce one or more consonant-vowel sounds" during the same time frame as children without visual impairment (Ferrell, 1998).

The incentive for infants to continue to produce sounds has been classified by researchers in terms of the purpose or function of communicative intent. As noted by Lueck et al. (2008), Bruner (1981) identified three categories of early communicative function: *behavior regulation*, *social interaction*, and *joint attention*. Lueck et al. (2008) listed these categories along with additional classifications of early communicative functions proposed by Coggins and Carpenter (1981); Dore (1974); and Roth and Spekman (1984), as follows:

> *Behavior regulation*: Getting someone to do or cease doing something, including:
> - protest, refusal, or rejection
> - request for object
> - request for action
>
> Example: A baby cries when hungry or wet to get someone to attend to her needs.

> *Social interaction*: Gaining the attention of another, including:
> - greeting
> - attention seeking
> - request for social routine
> - request for comfort
>
> Example: A toddler shrieks with delight when his father enters the room.

> *Joint attention*: Sharing attention to an object or event.
> - comment on object
> - comment on action
> - request for information
>
> Example: A toddler says "cat" when the family kitten runs by.

This classification is commonly used as a guide when observing and encouraging communication in infants and specifically in analyzing the role that listening plays in these functions (Lueck et al., 2008, p. 75). Table 2.2 lists these categories along with examples of each and suggestions for interventions that support and expand a child's communicative behaviors.

Being mindful of these very elemental purposes for communication can help families observe and nurture listening behavior in infants. Infants are given many reasons to use communication for *behavior regulation* by the very nature of their dependence on others for safety, warmth, nutrition, and comfort. As they learn from their attempts at communication for behavior regulation, they realize that they can gain the attention of others (*social interaction*), which is also comforting. As their relationship to parents and caregivers develops and they begin to share reactions to toys and common noises in the environment, such as running bathwater, infants begin to utilize communication during *joint attention* with their parents—a situation that occurs when infants share an experience of an object or event with others, which is discussed in more detail later in this section. As indicated, maintaining an environment that is conducive to listening is particularly important for infants and toddlers who are visually impaired, as it is for their caregivers, so that a listening response that may be characterized by silence, stillness, turning to sound, or subtle vocalization can be observed.

In her work about preverbal communication of blind infants and their mothers, Rowland (1984) reminded us that "in a vocal exchange, each partner fills the pauses between vocalization with listening, signified by silence. Even before vocalization patterns emerge, normal infants seem to be good listeners." She continued, "A silent or listening response to a vocalization may be as powerful as a vocal response" (Rowland, 1984, p. 301). Knowledge of the importance of silence is significant information for parents and caregivers of children who are visually impaired, because the temptation is to provide constant verbal interpretation and stimulation, when it is the fine balance of interaction that is important. This approach to nurturing listening behavior in children requires that parents, caregivers, and practitioners make a conscious effort to observe, wait, and listen during early communications. Note that this may not feel natural to many caregivers and may require modeling by an early interventionist as well as practice. Sidebar 2.5 provides Rowland's guidelines for nurturing the listening response in infants.

Imitation and Turn Taking

The early encouragement and imitation with which parents respond to their infants' beginning sounds most naturally lead to the development of turn taking, a very important element of conversation. We initiate turn taking when we imitate the sounds that

TABLE 2.2
Communicative Functions during Infancy

Function	Clarification	Beginning Intentional Communication	Intentional Communication	Suggestions for Intervention
Behavior Regulation				
Protest, refusal, rejection	Commands parent to stop disliked activity, rejects activity or object	Infant whines and pushes at parent's hand with washcloth when parent is trying to wipe the infant's face	Says "no" and turns head	Acknowledge the infant's signals and provide words for their meaning (e.g., "ooh, don't like getting your face wet").
Request objects	Asks for objects	Infant reaches for cracker on plate or tactually searches tray for plate	Says "cracker" as leans toward plate (or as searches for plate)	Provide opportunities for the infant to indicate requests for favorite objects (e.g., give a small helping of a favorite food and wait for the infant to request another piece). Expand on the infant's words (e.g., "want cracker," "I like crackers").
Social Interaction				
Request action	Commands parent to do something	Infant puts parent's hand on CD player	Says "on" while pulling parent's hand to CD player	Interrupt a favorite activity (e.g., listening to music, being pushed on a swing), wait and interpret the infant's nonverbal behaviors (e.g., fussing) and model or expand verbal request ("music on").
Greeting	Uses social conventions, i.e. "bye," "hi," "mama"	Infant waves as father says "bye-bye" and leaves room	Waves and says "bye-bye"	Develop greeting and leave-taking routines. Expand the infant's language by providing a model (e.g., "bye-bye, daddy," "see you later").

Attention seeking	Seeks attention to self or aspects of environment	Infant pulls on dad's pant leg	Tugs on dad and says "dada"	Expand the, infant's language by saying "Up, want up?" Provide opportunities for the infant to initiate getting attention by delaying an anticipated event (e.g., the baby is on the floor by dad's feet. They have a favorite "horsey" game in which the infant gets a ride on dad's legs. Dad waits the infant to vocalize and responds "oh, you want to play").
Request for social routine	Asks for caregiver to participate in familiar game	Infant pulls up shirt and pats tummy	Pull up shirt, pats tummy, and says "tummy"	Provide model to expand the infant's language by saying "tickle tummy." Develop familiar social routines with ways for the infant to initiate them (e.g., pulling up shirt to request a "tickle tummy" game, sitting on dad's legs to request "ride horsey" game) and respond to the infant's efforts to initiate them (e.g., "I'm going to tickle your tummy").
Request for comfort	Seeks comfort from caregiver	Infant reaches toward caregiver while fussing	Reaches toward mother and says "mama" while fussing	Respond to signals of distress by holding and comforting the infant. Use quiet, repetitive vocalization to calm the child. Expand on infant's communicative behaviors (e.g., "you want up").

(Continued)

TABLE 2.2
(Continued)

Function	Clarification	Beginning Intentional Communication	Intentional Communication	Suggestions for Intervention
Joint Attention				
Comment on object	Calls attention to aspects of an object	Infants points to ball in toy store, looks at mother	Infant says "ba" and points to balls	Encourage joint attention by pointing out familiar objects that are beyond the infant's reach. When feasible, take the infant over to touch selected objects (e.g., to the basket of balls in the toy store). Expand on the infant's comments (e.g., "yes, that's a bumpy ball"). Tactilely explore the object together. If the infant is blind, use hand-under-hand guidance to support mutual tactile attention.
		Infant taps pillow on top of sofa	Infant pats pillow and says "nigh-nigh"	Comment on the child's action and expand the child's vocalizations (e.g., "You found a pillow. It is time to go night-night.").
Comment on action	Calls attention to action of object, self, and others	Infant says "uh-oh" when pushes blocks off high chair tray	Infant says "down" as pushed blocks off high chair tray	Expand on the infant's word and gestures (e.g., "blocks fall down"). Describe the infant's actions on objects.
Request for information	Wants to know about an object or event	Infant looks at front door and then at mother; infant crawls around living room floor	Infant says "dada, bye-bye"; infant says "meow, meow"	Interpret and expand on the infant's vocalizations (e.g., "Daddy went bye-bye. He's at work." Or "Where's that kitty cat? Let's look in the kitchen.").

Source: Reprinted with permission from A. H. Lueck, D. Chen, L. S. Kekelis, & E. S. Hartmann, "Communicative Functions during Infancy," *Developmental Guidelines for Infants with Visual Impairments: A Guidebook for Early Intervention,* 2nd ed. (Louisville, KY: American Printing House for the Blind, 2008), pp. 76–80.

((‹ Sidebar 2.5
Guidelines for Nurturing the Listening Response in Infants

The following principles can be used to guide caregivers and professionals in nurturing the listening response in infants who are visually impaired:

- The vocalizations of infants should be reinforced as frequently and consistently as possible. For example, when the infant responds to a sound, movement, or touch by making a vocal sound, imitate that sound to encourage turn taking.

- Vocal reinforcement should be provided a short time *after* the infant stops vocalizing so the infant is not interrupted and the turn-taking pattern is reinforced.

- Vocal reinforcement by parents should include the imitation of the infant's sounds, both verbal (words) and preverbal (nonword vocalizations).

- The infant should be cued to the appropriate moments for vocalization by emphasizing the difference between period of parental vocalization and silence. Cues can be given in two steps: (1) Parents can place their mouth on the infant's cheek or place the infant's hand on their mouth when they are speaking so the infant can feel the speech act. (2) Parents can continue to hold their mouth against the child's cheek or hold the infant's hand on their mouth between vocalizations; then the infant can "feel" the silence—the cue that the parent is providing a safe space for a response.

- A constant barrage of verbal commentary by parents in not advisable. Although language stimulation is important, the quality of such stimulation would be improved by offering short bursts of commentary interspersed with short periods of silence. (This may not feel natural to many caregivers and may require modeling by an early interventionist and practice.)

- This approach to nurturing listening behavior in children requires that parents, caregivers, and practitioners make a conscious effort to observe, wait, and listen during early communications.

Source: C. Rowland, "Preverbal Communication of Blind Infants and Their Mothers," *Journal of Visual Impairment & Blindness, 78* (1984), p. 302.

children make, when we clap and teach them to clap in response, or when we bang a drum and then encourage them to take a turn in banging. Early communication games such as pat-a-cake and "Itsy Bitsy Spider" set the stage for a predictable sequence of events for anticipation and listening. By following the infant's lead, caregivers can engage in parallel play—playing next to their child, doing the same activity, such as pouring water from a cup into the bathtub—and turn taking on a level that is motivating to their infant.

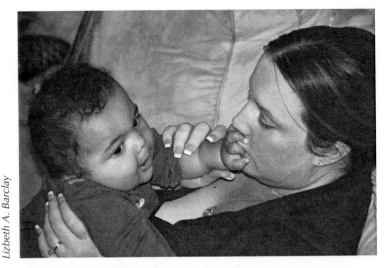

As his mother gently holds his hand to her mouth and repeats "ma, ma, ma," the baby begins to imitate her sounds.

Joint Attention

A very important stage and purpose of communication development for all infants is joint attention. Joint attention occurs when the infant's and caregiver's attention is on an object or event together and when the infant is able to share the experience of the object or event with others. For example, if the baby shakes a rattle or bangs a metal whisk on the floor, the parent can imitate the sound with another rattle or whisk and wait until the infant repeats the action. This stage of infant development is so important because it has been found that the combination of mothers' speech and joint attention facilitates the advancement in infants' early vocabulary. Reporting on a study about infants and joint attention, Bigelow, MacLean, and Proctor noted, "Sustained joint attention indicates infants' understanding of others as intentional beings, like themselves, whose attention to objects may be shared, followed or directed" (Bigelow et al., 2004, p. 518).

Typically, vision plays a large role in joint attention; however, in children who are visually impaired the shared attention can take place through touch and listening. The results from the previously mentioned study of infants and joint attention revealed the importance of maternal sensitivity to infants' play interests and to infants' scaffolding needs (that is, the degree to which parents need to provide support, such as by deliberately placing the infant's hand on an object), within joint attention (Bigelow, 2003). This study once again points to the importance of listening on the part of both parents and infant in this reciprocal process, as parents need to observe, wait for, and listen to their infant in order to understand his or her listening requirements.

Concepts

All the words we know, and the language that we speak and eventually read and write, have underlying concepts (Durkel, 2000). Language development is dependent on a child's concept development, and listening plays a key role in this process. As a baby's ability to produce a variety of sounds in response to people and objects develops, she or he begins to imitate and repeat the sounds and words that are paired with them. As the toddler imitates and repeats words that are paired with people, objects, places, and feelings, the deliberate and repetitive combination of hearing the word and at the same time touching the person or object, feeling the emotion or sensation, or being in the place helps cement the idea or concept of the person, object, location, or feeling into place. Many concepts that develop meaning within natural daily routines are easy to reinforce because they allow the child the full contextual experience that makes the concepts real.

The importance cannot be overstated of deliberately providing experiences (which children with vision observe every day) to babies and toddlers who are visually impaired in order to promote concept development. The routine activities of changing, feeding, and bathing are the structure in which a baby can learn to understand about the names, attributes, and functions of objects and predict the outcomes of activities. The pairing of sound and touch is provided within these routines in a way that is essentially repetitive. Consider the act of changing a baby. This activity occurs at least a dozen times a day for the first few weeks of an infant's life and continues, though with less frequency, through the toddler years. The simple activity of changing provides a reinforcing context for sound and touch to mesh in a consistent manner. The combination of auditory and tactile stimuli that reinforce each other, paired with the loving communication provided by parents, provides the baby with the reason to listen. For all these reasons, it is important to ensure that a routine is established in which activities can occur in a natural and relaxed manner.

Listening alone does not give meaning to activities such as washing the dishes, setting the table, or loading laundry into the dryer, but hearing and feeling the warm water as it pours from the faucet, feeling the soap bubbles as Mom washes them over the sticky plate, and listening to her words as she talks about washing dishes provide much more information than simply describing the experience. When seated in an infant seat at the table, the child only hears the sound of water pouring from the faucet

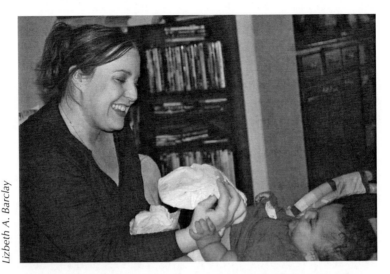

Lizbeth A. Barclay

This mother is holding the diaper close to the baby's hand so that he can touch it and begin to associate this object with the words and experiences of his diaper-changing routine.

and the clanking of dishes in the sink. The child who is in a front-facing baby carrier can participate in the activity along with Mom, by feeling the water, the soap bubbles, and the dishes as they are washed. The child is learning the activity that goes with the sounds and will recognize in the future what those sounds mean.

The opportunities to utilize sound for the development of concept understanding are literally endless, and it is up to parents and early interventionists to observe them and select them, a process that requires vigilant listening skills on their part. Using sound to reinforce concepts entails commenting on sounds paired with experiences occurring naturally within the environment, for example, listening together to the many sounds that water makes while it pours into the tub from the faucet during a bath, when the sprinkler is turned on from the spigot, when it is raining, or when the waves crash at the beach.

As a baby begins to demonstrate that he or she anticipates an activity by reacting to sound cues, it is easy to see how very important these associations of listening, activities, and objects can be. For example, a child may excitedly wave his hands and kick with his legs when he hears the sound of keys paired with the words "Time for our walk" before leaving the house to go for an afternoon walk with his mother. Providing sounds to promote anticipation is a powerful way to reinforce the beginning understanding of concepts. Eventually, this same technique can be extended by cuing toddlers about sounds that they hear in the community. For instance, before walking into the grocery store, asking "Do you think the store will be crowded?" will help guide a child's listening to the concepts of *busy, crowded,* and *noisy.* Sidebar 2.6 lists a number of other listening strategies that enhance the development of concepts and language.

((SIDEBAR 2.6

Enhancing Listening Comprehension during Everyday Experiences

The following strategies used in the course of a baby's everyday routines will enhance his or her understanding and development of concepts and language:

- Omit or reduce the sounds of background noise, such as from the television or radio, that will be distracting to the infant and mask listening and communication.

- Combine touch and talk to provide meaning to what the infant hears. For example, when she hears the words, "It's time to change you again. Here's your diaper," the diaper can be placed on her hand, providing a real object that she will learn to pair with words.

- When talking to the baby to introduce concepts, keep it simple, pairing words with the appropriate action or object. For example, when he is eating and the spoonful of bananas is going into his mouth comment, "Mmm, the bananas are going into your mouth."

- Talk to the infant about what she is doing and experiencing, what is happening in the environment, and what she is going to do (anticipation).

- Carry the baby in a front pack, sling, or backpack often as you participate in routine activities such as doing the laundry or preparing meals so that he can listen to natural routine sounds and touch the objects that are associated with them.

- Include the baby in family activities and routines, for example, keeping her in the kitchen during meal preparation and mealtime by placing an infant seat at the table. Talk to her and touch her during mealtime conversation.

- When the baby starts eating food, let him feel what he is eating and tell him about it. "Yum, you have cereal. It's warm and sticky, isn't it?"

- Teach environmental concepts by taking the baby outside to listen to many sounds, such as the sound of the wind in the trees, raindrops as they land on the umbrella, the cars that go by, a bouncing ball, and animal and bird noises, commenting on them as they occur.

- Gradually include the baby in as many trips in the community as possible, including the store, religious services, restaurants, the post office, and the laundromat. Tell the baby where you are going, talk about getting ready to go and why you are going, and describe, in simple language, any activity that takes place.

SETTING THE STAGE FOR PLAY

Emerging listening skills relating to play include the following:

▸ alerts to auditory stimulation

▸ bats at toys to hear something

▸ responds to music, making a physical response to rhythm

▸ makes a slight move toward a familiar sound

▸ orients to a sound source

▸ reaches toward a sound source in any direction

▸ reaches toward a sound source in the correct direction

▸ moves to obtain an object when given a sound cue

▸ cooperates in games

Sarah, who is now a chubby 1-year-old, was born two and a half months prematurely, weighing only two and a half pounds. Retinopathy of prematurity caused almost complete vision loss for Sarah.

Sarah enjoys playing with her favorite "toys," a metal cooking whisk, cake pan, mixing bowl, and set of metal measuring spoons. As she sits on the kitchen floor, whisk in hand and mouth, she periodically beats the whisk on the floor, enjoying the vibrating sound made by the wires. Eventually, she hits the metal mixing bowl that is beside her. Appreciating the effect of her action and using this new information, she again reaches out with the whisk, now using it as a tool to find the bowl again and enjoy the sound it makes as she strikes it. The bowl is then pushed out of reach, but she now locates the cake pan as she reaches with the whisk to find it. Delighted with her new discovery, she puts the whisk to her side and reaches for the cake pan, which she finds makes a different sound as she bangs it on the floor in front of her. Over time, becoming satiated with this sound, she once again reaches out and finds something wonderful: the set of measuring spoons, which are just perfect for shaking. She then finds that they are also cool and refreshing as she explores them with her mouth! (Adapted from Pesavento, 1986)

Play is the natural activity of children, providing a way for them to practice their cognitive, language, social, and motor skills. It is no wonder that parents and educators place so much importance and emphasis on play. In *Touchpoints: Birth to Three*, Brazelton stated, "Play remains a child's most powerful way of learning. She can test out many different situations and actions to find which one works for her. It is hard to overestimate the importance of play for a small child" (2006, p. 175).

The stages of play begin to develop during infancy with exploratory play, when infants manipulate toys to discover the way that they feel, taste, smell, and look. As babies mature and their motor and cognitive skills develop, they begin to play independently, using toys in a more functional way. *Parallel play*, when children play alongside each other, using similar toys but not sharing them, typically begins occurring at around 18 months of age, followed by *associative play*, in which children begin sharing their toys. In the preschool years, children engage in *cooperative play*, playing with others in an organized way with a common goal, usually role-playing and playing imaginative games (Johnson-Martin, Attermeier, & Hacker, 2004, p. 469).

Recent research about the development of play in children who are visually impaired is limited. What is clear about the individual differences of children with visual impairments is the tremendous variability in their development of play skills (Warren, 1994). The play skills of all infants are initially facilitated by mothers or other caregivers. During episodes of joint attention (discussed earlier in this chapter), a mother may typically gauge her infant's level of play during activities and provide new stimulation as she observes the infant's readiness to move on and respond to something new, and in this way she maintains the infant's engagement, leading to the learning of new play skills (Bigelow et al., 2004). For the baby who is visually impaired, this process requires that parents and caregivers observe and understand their child's behavior, as discussed earlier in this chapter. The development of an interest in play is enhanced by providing the optimal environment and tools for play.

Providing the Environment and Tools for Play

Because each infant with a visual impairment has a unique temperament and individual preferences, it is essential to discover what is interesting to the infant and allow him or her enough time to respond to it. In addition to keen observation and response, parents and caregivers can encourage and nurture listening skills during play by providing the opportunities and environment for play. Babies begin to feel capable through play when they learn that they can make something happen. Infants and toddlers who are visually impaired can learn to do this more easily in an environment that is familiar, quiet, and comfortable and with objects that appeal to their senses of touch and sound. Sidebar 2.7 provides some suggestions about creating an environment that is appropriate for play.

Attention and listening to sound-making toys play a big role in the development of interest in beginning play skills. Some traditional toys that are visually interesting may have little meaning or appeal for infants who are blind, while toys that make sound or are tactilely pleasing and that they can eventually learn to manipulate are preferable. Toys that are decorated with primary colors and that provide high contrast are attractive to babies who have some vision. (See Sidebar 2.7 for additional suggestions.)

Real objects are very special toys, especially when they can be used to produce sound and have interesting textures. They are important to infants and toddlers who

---

((SIDEBAR 2.7
Listening Strategies and Activities That Enhance the Development of Play Skills

These suggestions will help create a supportive and nurturing environment to encourage the development of play skills for a child who is visually impaired:

ENVIRONMENT AND TOYS

- Create play environments in many places throughout the house that have a variety of hanging, sound-producing toys and objects that the baby can reach and touch. Show the baby where they are and how to find them, talk about what they are, and demonstrate how they are used.

- Provide a variety of real objects for the baby to play with. Pots, pans, and wooden spoons, shoes, and boxes can provide interesting sounds, textures, and opportunities for exploration and concept development that are not provided by the pretty plastic toys that are commercially available in toy stores.

- When purchasing toys from mainstream toy stores, choose toys that produce sounds or talk, have bright colors and high contrast, emit light, and feature a variety of interesting surfaces and textures.

- Introduce new sound-producing toys carefully and slowly at first, especially if the sound produced is jarring to the baby. By going slowly and introducing for short increments, over time and with gentle encouragement, the baby will probably learn to enjoy the toy.

ENCOURAGING INTERACTION

When a child who is visually impaired begins to interact and play with other children, these suggestions will help make the interaction progress more smoothly:

- Control the play environment so that it is relatively quiet and contained.

- Help toddlers establish and maintain close proximity to their potential playmates when possible.

- Provide toys that are interesting to the child who is visually impaired.

- Provide verbal information and tactile guidance, when necessary, about toys that each child is playing with.

- Demonstrate what the other child is doing with a toy, or help the other child show what he or she is doing.

are visually impaired because they provide important information about everyday routine activities and concept and language development. They are real and solid objects, as opposed to representations of real objects, and thus can provide a child with concrete experiences. The wooden spoon, the metal mixing bowl, and the set of keys can be very appealing in their tactile qualities and potential for sound, and as a toddler begins to move throughout his or her environment, he or she can locate these objects in their natural context and have real experiences with them during natural routines. This interaction lays the foundation for the child's development of the ability to play with them in a more representational way.

Experiential learning—learning based on actual experiences in which the child engages in real-world activities—is the path to symbolic play or pretend play. Families can help lay the foundation for symbolic play by involving their child who is visually impaired in as many daily household activities as possible, fostering an understanding of the functional uses of many common household items and how they are employed in the real world. The toddler who has had many opportunities to go with her parents to the market, bring home the groceries, participate in putting them away,

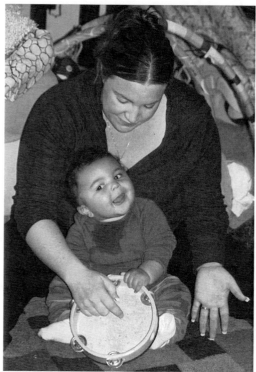 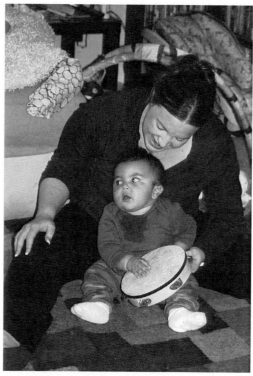

Lizbeth A. Barclay

This mother is demonstrating the sound the tambourine can make as the baby listens. Gradually, the baby reaches for the sound and discovers that he can produce it as well.

retrieve them for a snack, participate in preparing the snack, and of course enjoying the snack will have a rich background of fully developed concepts to bring to her ability to play symbolically.

Music and games can be used to elicit smiles and responses as infants begin to respond to predictable sound, developing their own repertoire of sound. Family members can use variation in pitch, inflection, and vocal pacing to encourage infants and toddlers to participate in the games and music that babies commonly enjoy. These variations play a significant role in the enjoyment of the following routine, for example: "How big is baby?" (Pause.) "So big!" (High pitch.) The deliberate use of vocal inflection also helps the infant to interpret meaning. For example, an upward inflection may signify a question or confusion; a loud, strident voice can signal caution or harm; and a higher-pitched voice may signify caring, nurturing, or time for play.

Parallel Play

Parallel play, when children play alongside each other using similar toys but not sharing them, typically begins occurring at around 18 months of age. For children who have vision, it is a time of observing what other children are doing in play and gaining important information that encourages them to imitate and begin to interact with other toddlers, sometimes in the most basic manner of taking from another child what interests them. Often during parallel play one child sees what another child is playing with, spurring interest in that toy or object. This process can be encouraged for children with visual impairments by ensuring that toys and objects are motivating and interesting to them because of the sound or action that they produce, and by making sure that they have been previously introduced to the toy in a deliberate way by a caregiver or other adult.

By the time of toddlerhood, family members, especially primary caregivers, have typically established a strong bond with their child, which is essential for progress in laying the foundation for communication and play skills. The strength of this bond, however, can have the potential to keep interaction with a parent more important to a child than interaction with his or her peers, delaying the transition to learning to play with others. Thus, it is necessary for families to provide support to help children move on to the next step of play involving others. Facilitated play, or supporting play (as described in Sidebar 2.7), allows the toddler with a visual impairment a greater level of predictability and control, which will encourage confidence and make enjoyment and learning possible during play with others. Shifting instances of turn taking and joint attention from the child's primary caregivers to others such as siblings and close family friends as the child becomes developmentally ready is important. The child's ability to listen and attach meaning to sound is very important in this process so he or she understands that different interactions are beginning to take place. (Sidebar 2.7 includes strategies to encourage and support parallel play with other toddlers.)

MOTOR DEVELOPMENT

Emerging listening skills relating to motor development include the following:

- ▶ bats at toys to hear something
- ▶ responds to music, making a physical response to rhythm
- ▶ makes a slight move toward a familiar sound
- ▶ orients to a sound source
- ▶ reaches toward a sound source in any direction
- ▶ reaches toward a sound source in the correct direction
- ▶ moves to obtain an object when given a sound cue

Two-year-old Matthew loves to go on walks with his mother, which they do almost every day. Blind as a result of Norrie's disease, he is learning about sound and its various qualities in different environments. Matthew's mother understands and appreciates Matthew's fascination with the sound of his footsteps as he walks; she has noticed that frequently while walking, he will simply stop and listen. For instance, when walking along a wall and coming up to an open doorway, he pauses, touching the edge of the doorway with his hand, and taps his foot while listening, first on one side of the threshold and then on the other, to hear the difference of sound on each side of the doorway. His mother quietly observes this learning process.

After Matthew finishes his exploration, his mother takes the opportunity to talk to him about his experience. Rather than talking with him while he is exploring, she allows him to have this listening experience; she then comments, "You noticed how it sounded different inside the courtyard and out on the sidewalk. Let's go now and explore inside the courtyard."

Babies enjoy movement, and they need to move. Movement is, in a sense, provided for them in utero before they are born when their mothers move throughout the day, and later as parents learn that their babies calm to movement and respond to the early movement games and activities that are provided for them. The first two years of a child's developmental life is called the sensorimotor period because it is a time when the child's learning is guided by the integration of sensory and motor experiences (Wood et al., 2001).

For many infants and toddlers who are visually impaired without additional disabilities, motor skills may develop at a slightly slower rate than for children without significant visual impairment, and some skills develop in a different sequence (Ferrell, 1998; Warren, 1994). However, the process of developing these skills proceeds for children who are visually impaired just as it does for children who have typical vision: beginning with large motor control and proceeding to fine motor control. As a baby matures, the development of motor control leads to each next step of learning, and movement helps a baby learn about his or her body in space and learn to develop motor control.

An understanding of environmental space develops when an infant has learned to move; yet in order to want to move with intentionality, infants need to first achieve some understanding of the concept of space. Vision and hearing play an important role in the development of purposeful movement. While studies have been conducted with infants who are sighted as well as infants who are blind regarding the developmental milestone of reaching to sound, the findings of the studies of both populations are very mixed; it is hard to draw conclusions about sound alone as a motivating factor for motor development (Warren, 1994).

What we do know is that the repetition of meaningful experiences that pair sound with touch greatly facilitates a child's budding understanding of object permanence, which provides reason to move, touch, and grasp an object (Ferrell, 2011). For example, a baby learns to reach out for a sound-making toy after hearing it, knowing that it will be where it was. While this pairing occurs through natural routines, it can also be nurtured more deliberately during play routines with toys and real objects, as described earlier in this chapter.

Some babies who are visually impaired are very selective about touching various textures, which is sometimes described as "tactile defensiveness" or "tactile sensitivity," and this sensitivity or aversion presents challenges for caregivers when trying to pair sound and touch. Nevertheless, it is important to discover a baby's tactile preferences and begin there, slowly introducing more objects and textures gradually as the child is ready, describing the objects while facilitating touch. It is also very important to tell a baby what she is touching, smelling, tasting, hearing, and, if she has some vision, what she is seeing and to keep trying exposures over time with gentle persistence. Sidebar 2.8 presents some guidelines for encouraging hand use while enhancing listening skills to help ensure that families and educators are sensitive to what is currently regarded as an optimal approach to teaching and guiding touch.

Learning to *localize*, or turn in the correct direction of a sound source, is another listening-specific skill that is crucial to learning about space and movement, as

Guidelines for Encouraging Touch and Hand Use

- Honor the child's hands. Do not grab or hold the child's hands any more than is absolutely necessary. Build trust between you and the child so that she is inclined to trust you not to try to control what she does with her hands.

- Watch what the child does with his hands. When we look at what the child does with his hands, we can have a better understanding of what the child might know about the world.

- Use a hand-under-hand approach in guiding the child or modeling actions with your hands. This also means offering objects to the child by bringing them up underneath her hand rather than taking the child's hand to the objects.

- Give the child objects that encourage the development of skills. For example, if you want the child to develop finger isolation, give him many different objects that encourage that skill, such as wire whisks, loose-knit fabric, rings or sections of tubing, containers with holes in them, and so forth. Expand skills horizontally (letting him practice this skill with many different objects) before trying to achieve higher-level skills.

- Provide the child with many opportunities each day to explore a wide variety of objects on her own. These should have different textures, weights, temperatures, shapes, flexibility, and hardness.

- Make your hands available to the child for him to be able to tell you something or show you something. A nice way to do this is to simply hold your hands out to the child with the palms facing up. Let the child take your hand and guide it where he wants.

- Model hand-use for the child as you do things. This is typically done using a hand-under-hand approach as you complete everyday activities such as opening, closing, twisting, rubbing, reading braille, signing, and so forth. The child can learn a great deal about hands from "watching" what you do with your hands.

- Let the child know you are experiencing the object she is experiencing. Co-actively touching objects that the child is touching is the equivalent of using a pointing gesture to reference an object that the child is looking at. This allows the child to share information with you about the object.

- Play hand games with the child. Begin by imitating what the child does with his hands. As time goes on and the child begins to attend to what your hands are doing, introduce new actions or movements. Clap, wiggle fingers, shake hands, rub them on a surface; any interaction the child is interested in will work.

- Provide more time for the child to explore objects within activities. What we can quickly take in with our vision requires more time to learn with our tactile sense.

Source: Adapted from K. Moss, "Some Things to Learn from *Learning through Touch*," *See/Hear* (Spring 2005), pp. 51–53.

discussed earlier in this chapter. Ultimately sound localization allows a traveler who is visually impaired to locate objects and travel safely within the environment (Lawson & Wiener, 2010). It enables the listener to interpret spatial questions such as "What is close and what is far away?" and, eventually, "How can I get to my destination?" (Sound localization is discussed more completely in Chapter 6.) Listening strategies and activities to promote the development of motor skills are found in Sidebar 2.9, as well as in Chapter 6.

((SIDEBAR 2.9
Listening Strategies and Activities to Promote Motor Skills

Movement and the development of motor skills can be enhanced by the following listening strategies:

ENCOURAGING REACHING TO SOUND

- Learning to reach and touch begins when parents or caregivers provide their face or hand for their infant to touch. Pairing touch while softly talking to the baby helps the child to learn to pair sound with pleasurable touch.
- When first teaching a baby to move to a sound source, it is important that the sound source remain stationary. In initial experiences, it is helpful to move the baby's hands to the sound source to teach its location.
- Infants can be encouraged to reach for motivating and sound-producing objects at midline. They will find it easier, at first, to reach for objects that they have already touched that are then moved slightly away.
- Provide motivation and orient babies to forward space and movement by providing encouragement and providing enticing objects (such as sound-producing toys) in front of them, rather than only from behind.
- To encourage infants to reach for sound-producing objects to the left or right of midline, present the objects first slightly to each side of midline. Begin with the familiar sound of the caregiver's voice and then move to the sound-producing object, bringing the infant's hands to the sound source to help her pair the auditory impression with the tactile one.
- To heighten the child's awareness of the environment, a wind chime can be hung by the entrance of a room or home and touched to produce sound as people enter, signaling to the toddler where they are and encouraging attending or reaching behavior if this is modeled.

USING SOUND TO ENCOURAGE MOVEMENT

- To encourage a baby to discover cause and effect with his feet and legs, secure a sound-producing soft toy at his feet to kick against.

- A bolster with bells will provide some babies enjoyment as they are encouraged to pat it and roll it to produce sound. It can also be used to practice moving from sitting to standing or to produce sound while crawling after it.
- Weighted push toys that produce sound as they are moved provide motivation and support for new walkers.

USING MUSIC TO ENCOURAGE MOVEMENT

- Musical mobiles can be hung above the infant's crib.
- Singing has long been used to calm, gain the attention of, and entertain infants and toddlers. Young children enjoy the many nursery songs that are sung to them, such as "Old MacDonald" or "This Is the Way," while bathing or dressing, especially those that are repetitive and predictable in nature, gradually giving them an opportunity to respond or join in.
- To encourage movement, rock young infants as you sing to them, or bounce them on your knees as you sing a movement song.
- Because an infant's earliest rhythmic experience begins in the womb, listening to the mother's heartbeat, listening to a regular consistent drumbeat can be calming and can help a toddler organize behavior.
- Using a steady drumbeat to provide toddlers with a consistent transition signal can help them prepare and move more easily to their next activity.
- Babies and toddlers enjoy "dancing" with their caregivers to a variety of types of music, and while providing them with a fun source of vestibular stimulation it also helps them begin to feel movement to sound. Bouncing to a Latin beat feels very different from gliding to a Brahms waltz or lullaby.
- Hand rhymes such as pat-a-cake and "Itsy Bitsy Spider" help infants and toddlers learn imitation skills, rhythm, and timing. Fade physical support and prompts as children learn the motions and begin to initiate the motions themselves.
- Toddlers may enjoy marching around the room to the beat of a drum or a song. They also enjoy learning and participating in songs that involve identifying and moving body parts such as "Head, Shoulders, Knees, and Toes." Provide support and modeling during these activities as needed, and fade the support as children have gained the skills to be independent.
- Percussion instruments such as xylophones, wrist bells, and drums are often highly motivating toys for toddlers and encourage interaction with objects and provide motivation for movement.

CONCLUSION

Deliberate guidance in the development of listening skills is essential for infants and toddlers with visual impairments. As children begin to demonstrate that what they hear is meaningful to them by the quality of their abilities to communicate, interact, and move with purpose throughout their environment, they are gaining the foundation for further development of listening skills. For each child the progress is individual and based on their own developmental course and temperament. Giving attention to creating the environment and opportunities for listening and to nurturing the development of listening skills to facilitate social, cognitive, play, and movement skills provides the groundwork for the next steps of learning to listen as youngsters transition from their home environment to their first experiences in playgroups and preschool. By providing a rich, experience-based foundation in listening skills, professionals can help infants and toddlers who are visually impaired obtain the tools they need to continue to develop meaningful listening skills in their new and more complex environments.

REFERENCES

Anthony, T., & Lowry, S. S. (2004). Sensory development. In T. Anthony, S. S. Lowry, C. Brown, & D. Hatton (Eds.), *Developmentally appropriate orientation and mobility* (pp. 125–240). Chapel Hill: Early Intervention Training Center for Infants and Toddlers with Visual Impairments, FPG Child Development Institute, University of North Carolina at Chapel Hill.

Anthony, T. L., Shier Lowry, S., Brown, C. J., & Hatton, D. D. (2004). *Developmentally appropriate orientation and mobility.* Chapel Hill: University of North Carolina at Chapel Hill.

Audiology Foundation of America. (1999). Facts: Audiology at a glance. Retrieved July 1, 2010, from www.audfound.org/index.cfm?pageID=50.

Bigelow, A. (1986). The development of reaching in blind children. *British Journal of Developmental Psychology, 4,* 355–366.

Bigelow, A. (2003). The development of joint attention in blind infants. *Development and Psychopathology, 15,* 259–272.

Bigelow, A., MacLean, K., & Proctor, J. (2004). The role of joint attention in the development of infants' play with objects. *Developmental Science, 7*(5), 518, 525.

Brazelton, T. B. (1983). *Infants and mothers: Differences in development.* New York: Dell Publishing.

Brazelton, T. B. (2006). *Touchpoints: Birth to three.* Cambridge, MA: Da Capo Press.

Bruner, J. S. (1981). The social context of language acquisition. *Language & Communication, 1*(2–3), 155–178.

Chen, D. (1999). *Essential elements in early intervention: Visual impairment and multiple disabilities.* New York: AFB Press.

Coggins, T. E., & Carpenter, R. L. (1981). The communication intention inventory: A system for observing and coding children's early intentional communication. *Applied Psycholinguistics, 2,* 235–251.

Dore, J. (1974). A pragmatic description of early language development. *Journal of Psycholinguistic Research, 3,* 343–350.

Durkel, J. (Spring 2000). What a concept! *See/Hear*, p. 2.

Ferrell, K. A. (2011). *Reach out and teach: Helping your child who is visually impaired learn and grow* (2nd ed.). New York: AFB Press.

Ferrell, K. A., with Shaw, A. R., & Deitz, S. J. (1998). *Project PRISM: Longitudinal study of developmental patterns of children who are blind or visually impaired. Final report.* Grant H023C10188, U.S. Department of Education, Field-initiated research, CFA 84.023. Greeley: University of Northern Colorado. Available at www.unco.edu/ncssd/research /PRISM/FinalPart1.pdf.

Fraiberg, S. (1977). *Insights from the blind*. New York: Meridian.

It's important to have your baby's hearing screened. (May 2011). NIH Publication No. 11-4968. Bethesda, MD: National Institute of Deafness and Other Communication Disorders. Retrieved May 25, 2011, from www.nidcd.nih.gov/health/hearing/screened.html.

Johnson, C. D., Benson, P. V., & Seaton, J. B. (1997). *Educational audiology handbook*. San Diego, CA: Singular Publishing Group.

Johnson-Martin, N., Attermeier, S., & Hacker, B. (2004). *Carolina curriculum* (3rd ed.). Baltimore, MD: Paul Brooks Publishing.

Lawson, G. D., & Wiener, W. R. (2010). Audition for the students with vision loss. In W. R. Wiener, W. L. Welsh, & B. B. Blasch (Eds.), *Foundations of orientation and mobility* (3rd ed.), Vol. 1, *History and theory*. New York: AFB Press.

Liefert, F. (2003). Introduction to visual impairment. In S. Goodman & S. Wittenstein (Eds.), *Collaborative assessment: Working with students who are blind or visually impaired, including those with additional disabilities*. New York: AFB Press.

Locke, J. L. (1995). *The child's path to spoken language*. Cambridge, MA: Harvard University Press. (Original work published 1993.)

Lueck, A., Chen, D., Kekelis, L., & Hartmann, E. (2008). *Developmental guidelines for infants with visual impairment: A guidebook for early intervention* (2nd ed.). Louisville, KY: American Printing House for the Blind.

Moss, K. (Spring 2005). Some things to learn from *Learning through Touch. See/Hear*, pp. 43–55.

Pesavento, M. E. (1986). *Getting there: A look at the early mobility skills of four young blind children*. San Francisco, CA: Blind Babies Foundation.

Pogrund, R., & Fazzi, D. (2002). *Early focus: Working with young children who are blind or visually impaired and their families* (2nd ed.). New York: AFB Press.

Ratey, J. J. (2001). *A user's guide to the brain: Perception, attention and the four theaters of the brain*. New York: Vintage.

Roth, F., & Spekman, N. (1984). Assessing the pragmatic abilities of children: Part 1. Organizational framework and assessment parameters. *Journal of Speech and Hearing Disorders, 49*, 2–11.

Rowland, C. (1984). Preverbal communication of blind infants and their mothers. *Journal of Visual Impairment & Blindness, 78*(7), 297–302.

Sacks, S. Z. (2006). Theoretical perspectives on the early years. In S. Sacks & K. Wolffe (Eds.), *Teaching social skills to students with visual impairments: From theory to practice*. New York: AFB Press.

Warren, D. H. (1994). *Blindness and children: An individual differences approach.* New York: Cambridge University Press.

Wood, K. C., Smith, H., & Grossniklaus, D. (2001). Piaget's stages of cognitive development. In M. Orey (Ed.), *Emerging perspectives on learning, teaching, and technology.* Retrieved July 2, 2010, from http://projects.coe.uga.edu/epltt/.

Chapter 3

Preschool and Kindergarten: Early Skill Development

Kathleen A. Byrnes

When I was 3, I realized with definite certainty that I was different . . . I knew that I had to hold hands with someone who I was walking with, and that I couldn't see pictures in books like my friends did. But one day our neighbor came in to return a comic book she had borrowed from my brother. My mom instructed her to put the book on top of the fridge. I was astonished. I remember feeling almost alarmed and unsettled. I did not know that there was a top to the refrigerator. I loved opening the door, feeling the cold air whooshing out, and how I enjoyed the little whap when I closed the door. I sat still. I said nothing. But in that instant, when life just moved on around me, I knew that I was blind. It was clear to me at that moment that I was missing many things. I was changed.

—Karen Karsh,
Colorado musician, May 2006

CHAPTER PREVIEW

▶ Listening and the Preschool Child

▶ Listening in the Home: Auditory Discrimination

▶ Attaching Meaning to What Is Heard: Experience and Description

▶ Learning to Listen: Concepts and Communication

- ▸ Social Communication
- ▸ The Transition to Preschool
- ▸ Acquiring Information in the Kindergarten Classroom
- ▸ Using Technology to Stimulate Listening

Karen Karsh's eloquent recollection at the opening of this chapter of her early realization of her visual impairment points out the vivid experiences young children undergo as they begin to understand the world around them and attach meaning to sound. Although Karen's story of her dawning awareness is both dramatic and moving, Luke's experience with his grandmother and the way in which he gradually attaches meaning to sounds is an equally profound illustration of how knowledge and language development evolve.

LISTENING AND THE PRESCHOOL CHILD

Luke, who is 3 years old, is blind. As he sits in his grandmother's lap, his grandma softly sings a little song: "Hello, hello, hello, and how are you? I'm fine, I'm fine, I hope that you are too." As she sings, she puts Luke's hand on his chest or on her own to indicate whose turn it is to sing. She repeats this process until all she has to do is become silent for Luke's part so he can fill in the words, and the song has become a musical conversation.

The world of 3- to 5-year-old children is centered primarily at home with family and caregivers, who provide the stability that allows young children to absorb information. In these familiar environments, where family routines form the constancy of daily life, children with visual impairments need to gain awareness of distinct environmental noises, sounds, and voices, associate them with corresponding actions, learn that sounds convey information, and attach meaning and understanding to what they hear. Many children go on to experience the new environments of day care and preschool before attending kindergarten, and these environments provide new opportunities and challenges for children in gaining the necessary skills of learning through listening. As preschool- and kindergarten-age children with visual impairments gain exposure in these new places, they also continue to spend most of their time with their parents and caregivers in the home, community settings, and perhaps playgroups.

During the preschool and kindergarten years of children who are visually impaired, parents, caregivers, and professionals need to collaborate to ensure that everyone involved pays attention to the development of listening skills as an active process of learning at home and in new environments. In so doing, they will nurture understanding and support the development of communication, movement, pre-academic, and social skills for children with visual impairments.

LISTENING IN THE HOME: AUDITORY DISCRIMINATION

Emerging listening skills related to the development of auditory discrimination in the home include the following:

- responds in different ways depending on the situation
- shows awareness and association of sounds with objects, persons, and actions
- recognizes musical sounds
- recognizes sounds in context
- recognizes cause and effect with sounds
- follows one- or two-step directions

Four-year-old Buddy, who is visually impaired because of retinopathy of prematurity, has a visual acuity of 20/600 with limited visual fields. His family tries very hard to identify and make sure he understands all of the environmental sounds he hears. However, they have not noticed yet that the competing sounds of the radio and TV make it hard for Buddy to appreciate and predict the sounds of natural family routines and to distinguish them from the electronic media sounds of cartoons or the ball game.

For the most part, home constitutes the young child's world, and, ideally, it represents security, emotional stability, and predictability. The very safety of this environment can be conducive to a child's actively learning the sounds of the home, the family, and neighborhood voices, listening for them, and attaching meaning to them. It is also within the home that connections are made through which the child begins to develop a sense of self. When children have been given an opportunity to learn the recurring sounds of their home, make predictions, and act on them, they become active participants in family routines and gain the chance to develop social interactions and meaningful relationships. Communication bonds forged at home between family members and the preschool child—like those formed between family members and the infant and toddler—are the base on which the child builds all lifelong learning patterns and emotions. Because of their inability or decreased ability to use vision to attach meaning to sounds, children who are visually impaired need to have clear descriptions and meanings provided to them by the family members who share their home environment, through explanations—often repeated—paired with other sensory, hands-on experiences. As it is during infancy, the pairing of language and experience is essential to building conceptual knowledge and language acquisition, all of which provide the foundation for the development of literacy skills and social relationships. As stated by the developers of the Perkins Panda Early Literacy Program, "In our primarily visual world, many experiences and the meaning of those experiences can be lost to children with visual impairments without special efforts on the part of parents and other caregivers to expose and interpret those experiences for them. Understanding these experiences and connecting words or symbols to them, however, is essential to the development of literacy" (Perkins School for the Blind, 2002, p. 7).

Natural Environments and Experiences

As a child with a visual impairment improves his or her ability to listen to, decipher, and apply information, the child's communication abilities can be reinforced as adults in his or her environment become attentive listeners to and interact with the child. Part C, Early Intervention, of the Individuals with Disabilities Education Act (IDEA) supports the concept that the home or community settings in which children without disabilities participate is the "natural environment" for the preschool-age child with a visual impairment. Practitioners may translate this concept of *natural environment* to mean the location where the child spends the majority of his or her time. It is where the child lives, plays, and spends time with family and caregivers, and includes the preschool setting. In general, people are the most important element of the child's natural environment at this age: parents, caregivers, family and friends, and playmates.

Within these settings and natural contexts, it is essential that young learners with visual impairments learn about their environment with real, meaningful objects and stimuli (Chen, 1999; Chen & Dote-Kwan, 1995; Dote-Kwan & Chen, 1995; Ferrell & Muir, 1996). For instance, it is important to take children to the grocery store to touch and talk about the foods that are located in different sections of the store. Fruits and vegetables found in the produce section can be brought home or back to school to fully explore and eventually make into an enjoyable snack or meal.

Not only is the home the most common natural environment for young children and the place where most listening skill development takes place, but it is usually the environment that is the easiest to control. A key factor in promoting early listening skills is the reduction of extraneous noise in order to create an optimal learning environment. When the environment is simplified in this way, children can learn more easily to differentiate background sounds from essential sounds that require response and reaction. In general, children need to be allowed to listen in environments free of competing sounds when they are expected to attend by listening. It is important that caregivers develop the habit of turning off the television or radio and create a quiet place for children like Buddy (in the previous vignette) to learn. In earlier writing about listening, Swallow and Conner (1982) wrote that "training children to attend auditorially to significant sounds in their environment and not be distracted by field noise is the real educational goal" (p. 121). By eliminating unnecessary noise whenever possible, adults can help children to focus on what is significant.

Opportunities to Listen

Another aspect of moderating the listening environment at home and in other natural environments is providing children with the opportunity to listen without interruption. Many well-intentioned caregivers and teachers often provide too little time for a child to listen and process environmental sounds. One good habit caregivers can develop is to wait an additional three to ten seconds before presenting other stimuli or responding to a child following a sound stimulus. During this time, they may wait for a nod or even the slightest change in facial expression or body position as among those signals that indicate the child is reacting to or processing information. At these times the child is quiet for a reason; he or she is using his or her senses, especially hearing, to take in and process information and assess where the information fits into what the child already knows. In such circumstances, most children respond to sound, given the appropriate time and expectation. When a child's concentration is interrupted prematurely by a well-intentioned adult who gives additional information or asks questions to evoke a response, the child's mental processing is interrupted, opportunities for problem solving may be thwarted, and cognitive development and personal confidence possibly waylaid temporarily. While it is important to give information, have a discussion, and ask questions, it is equally important to give a child enough time to respond to an inquiry and to make his or her own observations known. It is important that children interact with attentive listeners who provide them with enough time to respond.

Nevertheless, providing opportunities for listening experiences and enough time for processing auditory information needs to be balanced with providing oral information to young children with visual impairments. For all children, one of the stronger modalities for early learning is listening. Prereaders learn much through oral language. Before learning to read, they have learned about the world to a great extent by what they have been told and taught by parents, caregivers, and teachers. They listen to words and information about what they are experiencing, and they learn about the nuance of emotion, emphasis, phrasing, and pauses that give language meaning. Swallow and Conner (1982) termed this type of listening skill development *auding*, which they described as a cognitive-orientation skill, stating, "Auditory perception and linguistic competence are both developmental and learned aspects of auding. Therefore, it should be quite apparent to the teacher of any visually handicapped child that, from the very onset of both infant stimulation and preschool programs, special attention and training are required for the development of auding skills" (p. 120).

Listening is often easier when it is coupled with predictability. Beginning at home, children with visual impairments benefit from hearing simple explanations about new and unfamiliar sounds. When identifying information is given in the sequence in which the action of a sound occurs, the child can learn the pattern of family routines and becomes better able to predict and anticipate future sequences, thereby gaining awareness and command of the home environment. Commentary on familiar routines such as Dad's arrival at home—his car entering the driveway, which explains that the next sounds to be heard will be the garage door opening, Dad's car door closing, his keys jangling as he opens the door, and his steps coming into the home—provides the child with a chance to develop an understanding of auditory sequences, a necessary skill in learning to read. The activities and strategies provided in Sidebar 3.1 facilitate listening skill development at home, which prepares children for listening in preschool and kindergarten.

((SIDEBAR 3.1
Listening Activities and Strategies at Home

The following suggestions will help parents and professionals encourage and support the development of listening skills in the home environment:

CREATING AN ENVIRONMENT FOR LISTENING
- Provide a quiet place in the home for those times when the child becomes overstimulated by noise, people, and the general busyness of family activities that can result in acoustic overload. Providing the child with some quiet gives the child a chance to recover receptivity for listening.

EXPLORING THE SOUND ENVIRONMENT
- Acquire the habit of telling the child who is in the room, and have family members and friends identify themselves as they enter and say good-bye when they leave.
- Wear squeaky shoes or jangly bracelets or keep keys in a pocket to provide auditory support for orientation and movement in space, body image, and laterality. This will assist a child to localize and associate sound as to where it is coming from, what part of the body could be involved, in this case wrists and ankles, and a beginning sense of whether it is to the left or right.

- Identify environmental sounds for the child. When possible, guide the child to touch the source. Develop a routine of anticipating sounds (mail delivery, beeps of household machines) and identify the incidental sounds throughout the day.
- Teach the child about categories of sounds, such as kitchen, car, and grocery store sounds.
- Create games around identifying the sounds in an environment, such as the following:
    - "What do you hear?" Begin by saying, "Toby, Toby [substitute child's name], what do you hear? I hear a dishwasher washing here." Let the child go up to each sound source and explore it.
    - After sounds have been identified in an environment for the child, go on a "sound hunt"; for example, "Let's find something that goes 'ring, ring, ring'"; "Let's find something that goes 'whish, whish, whish.'"
    - Describe a familiar sound sequence or routine and have the child indicate what sound will come next. Say, "I am opening the refrigerator. I am getting the milk. Now I'm getting a glass and setting it on the table. What will you hear next?" (Pouring the milk.)
    - Play "I hear" the same way that you play the game "I spy." For example, say to the child: "I hear a buzzing sound high above us. What do you think it is? Yes, it's a plane!" Having the child point to the object once it is identified also encourages sound localization and positional concepts.

PLAYING WITH SOUND-PRODUCING TOYS

- Play with different sound-producing toys so the child can learn the variations of sound, as well as begin auditory localization.
- Play with balls that have a bell or sound source inside. Roll the ball and have the child point to it as it moves to practice auditory tracking.

COMMUNICATING AND INTERACTING

- Encourage conversation to facilitate language and social skills. In the kitchen say, "What do you want to eat?" In the bedroom, "It is cold today, what would you like to wear?" "How are you feeling?" Use open-ended statements that invite conversation, such as "Tell me about your favorite toy."
- Call attention to a family member's voice. Walk with the child to the person and let the child discover an identifying feature such as a beard or ring. Encourage the child to look at the person or turn his or her face toward the person's voice.
- With the child in your lap during story time, use different voices for the various characters, allowing the child to experience the rhythm and vibration of breath and voice. Pause to observe the child's attention and ability to absorb the story experience.
- Imitate the child's sounds and words. Encourage reciprocal imitation to begin phonemic awareness; for example, "The cat wore a hat as she sat on a mat. What do you think of that?"
- Teach emotion with your voice, for example, by saying "hello," using happy, sad, excited, surprised, frustrated, and fatigued intonations.

(Continued)

((Sidebar 3.1 *(Continued)*

- Encourage the child to make up a story about a trip, activity, or favorite pet. This will help the child's auditory memory and imagination.

FOLLOWING DIRECTIONS

- Teach safety by encouraging the child to respond to a spoken "stop." A good way to start is with a freeze dance to music. When the music plays, have the child perform an action such as dancing or walking. When it stops, say "stop," and teach the child to stop. It may be necessary to provide physical modeling to teach this concept. Encourage the child to stomp each foot when he or she stops, for the kinesthetic feedback.
- Encourage following one- to two-step directions through games, such as "Run to the tree, and then come back and give me a hug." It also is important to teach following functional directions, such as "Get your cap and meet me at the door." Have the child repeat the directions while you hold up one finger for each step; for example, "What did I say first? [Hold up one finger.] Good. [Hold up second finger.] What did I say next? Good." This process encourages auditory sequencing and memory.

USING MUSIC

- Try singing directions to the child. For example, using the tune from "Here We Go Round the Mulberry Bush" (or "This Is the Way"), give specific directions, such as "Now it's time to get your backpack, get your backpack, get your backpack."
- Make up and sing songs about transitions in the day for the child, for example, "It's a great time to take a nap."
- Help the child learn to imitate patterns and rhythm by having him or her clap hands or tap sticks.
- Dancing to music with an adult can help establish rhythm. Try having the child stand on your feet.
- Provide scarves for the child to wave in different patterns while dancing to music. Waving the scarves encourages bilateral and large muscle movement. Vary the movements with different tempos: marching, hopping, and walking forward, backward, and to the side.
- When singing familiar songs, play pretend games using the voice of a bear, a cat, or a mosquito for fun and engagement.
- Provide hands-on access to as many musical instruments as possible.

ATTACHING MEANING TO WHAT IS HEARD: EXPERIENCE AND DESCRIPTION

Emerging listening skills related to the development of maintaining auditory attention during routine experiences include the following:

- quiets to listen to adult during caregiving routine
- responds to people or objects in the environment through actions or sounds
- listens in a quiet environment

Maya loves to go to the grocery store with her father. He makes their trips to the market very meaningful by systematically describing the sounds of the store to Maya, who has very little vision in only one eye. He talks about the hiss of the spray mister above the produce and the whir heard at the frozen food section. Maya giggles as Dad chats with the butcher. She anticipates this routine, knows what's coming in the sequence, and eagerly awaits their turn at the checkout stand so she can say "hi" to the checker.

By the time they are preschoolers, children with visual impairments typically have already learned to listen to the voices and activities of family and friends in the safety of their home (California Department of Education, 2003; Huisingh, Barrett, Zachman, Orman, & Blagden, 1993). They are able to attend for longer periods. They are able to listen in quiet or noisy environments and love especially to listen to stories (Huisingh et al., 1993). Sounds that once were noticed in isolation now string together to make patterns and words, directions to follow, and listening images (California Department of Education, 2003; Johnson-Martin, Attermeier, & Hacker, 2004; Pestor, 1972). A jingle of keys at school can now be understood to mean that the custodian or principal is making the rounds through the school hallways, and at home it can mean a parent is emptying a pocket or purse of the day's contents. Many preschool children demonstrate their newly acquired skill of auditory localization when they turn their heads to the speaker when their name is called. Children like Maya are able to remember an auditory sequence, anticipate what's next, and use the information to communicate effectively.

At this stage, many children with visual impairments are beginning to increase their auditory attention, learning social skills through explicit instruction, preparing for reading, and gaining more conceptual understanding of the nature of objects, places, and events. They can learn from descriptions and experiences using all their sensory modalities when lessons and activities are thoughtfully prepared to build on their prior experiences and contribute to new learning. While playing next to each other in parallel or cooperative play, 3- to 5-year-old children may hear and listen to the same sounds but not acknowledge or communicate with one another about their shared experience. To become social listeners and communicators, they need to be taught, among other abilities, to look at or face their partner when talking to one another. Many children of this age love to receive comfort and curl up in a parent's lap to listen to a story, especially after hearing a startling, overly loud, or frightening noise.

Generalizing Learning

Perhaps one of the more profound developments in the acquisition of listening skills is the transfer of acquired knowledge to new settings and situations. Taking in the sounds or speech of the moment during an activity, remembering them, and generalizing them for future reference is a hallmark of developmental progress. An example of this kind of transfer can be seen when a child has learned to respond physically to a spoken "stop," perhaps through a game-like activity in school, and is able to do so when told to stop when nearing a street corner. Children at this age begin to generalize and can tuck that "stop" experience away and bring it to bear in future experiences in different neighborhoods with different caregivers. This reapplication of learned meaning is possible for the preschool child who has had rich experiences with listening and doing.

Learning from Experiences

For children with visual impairments, an important aspect of learning to attach meaning through listening is the development of the ability to attend to and interpret description. The sighted child can see the cartoon figures shown on the TV screen, while the child who is blind depends on someone else to describe them. Considering how much information a sighted child obtains visually at every turn, the amount of description required for a child without sight can be extensive. All preschool children are acquiring concepts, but description presented to a child who is visually impaired might be meaningless, and too abstract, if related tangible experiences have not been connected to the description. As Santin and Simmons (1977) wrote of the perils of too much description, it is important that what we portray for these children is within their realm of the already experienced. If it is not, we need to be prepared to provide them the tangible activities to support the concepts.

It is most helpful for young children with visual impairments to have repeated opportunities for hands-on experiences that include simultaneous description with well-chosen vocabulary. For instance, hear-

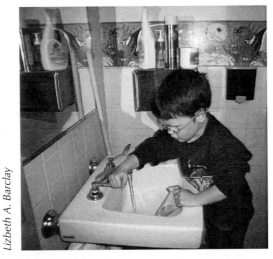

Lizbeth A. Barclay

Daily routines such as washing hands provide opportunities for listening skill development by pairing hands-on activities with language and sensory experience.

ing the words "put the plate *on* the table *in front* of the chair" and "put a napkin *on each* plate" while regularly helping a caregiver set the table and being guided through that experience until it becomes an independent activity gradually helps build understanding of those language concepts. Sidebar 3.2 highlights strategies and activities that combine sound and active learning through experience.

The preschool years are a time to pair the senses and combine sensory input on behalf of learning. When vision is greatly reduced or absent, it is important to determine which sensory system provides the child with the most accurate information and pair other sensory experiences with that system. Placing the hands on a musical instrument as it is played, singing songs about muffins while they are cooking in the oven, and exploring a book while someone is reading are examples of ways to enhance the development of sensory skills. When a child learns to use all the senses, the child's parents and teachers can discover the sensory modality that provides the

---

(((SIDEBAR 3.2

Combining Sound and Active Learning through Experience

The following activities combine sound and active learning through experience:

- Describe sounds the child is hearing so that child can begin to associate a sound to its source. Include practical and functional sounds, such as the sound of the toaster as the toast pops up, as well as background noises such as the hum of the refrigerator. Do this indoors and outdoors in both familiar and unfamiliar settings.

- Experiment with sounds together. Hold a large plastic, metal, or wooden bowl or pan in front of your face, then the child's while making various sounds. This will help the child to understand that reflected sound can be different, depending on the surface. Modulate the sounds, as it is also a good time for learning loud, soft, high, low, etc. This is also a good activity for fostering turn taking.

- Get a play microphone or karaoke machine, and imitate each other.

- Form a kitchen band! Use wooden, plastic, and metal spoons to tap on anything you can find. Funnels and paper-towel tubes are fun to make noises through.

- Make sound shakers by filling plastic bottles with different materials, such as beans, pebbles, and sand.

- Use a digital recorder to have fun discovering body sounds. Demonstrate, then encourage the child to snore, sniff, laugh, cry, sneeze, yawn, hum, sing, click his or her tongue, kiss, clap, cough, hiccup, whistle, sigh, whisper, shout, tap feet, and snap fingers.

- When teaching and reinforcing concepts, provide the description of the activity from the child's perspective; for example, "Let's put your foot into your sock; now let's pull up your sock."

greatest information to the child. This discovery leads to the determination of whether the child is primarily a tactile learner (using objects and braille), a visual learner (using pictures and large print), or an auditory learner (using primarily auditory modes of learning). The child may also rely on a combination of senses, depending on the specific task at hand.

The Importance of Music

As the vignette about Luke suggests, music can play a vital role in the acquisition of listening skills at the preschool age, and recent research indicates that music may be an important support of intellectual development (Schlaug et al., 2005). According to Rauscher et al. (1997), early music training can stimulate the development of the brain, especially with spatial abilities. "Music provides an additional framework into which you fit content, rhythm, rhyme and reason. Children who listen to nursery rhymes use music as it engages their attention to words and phrases that they associate with sound. That content finds its place into a different part of their memory" (Jerry Kuns, Technology Specialist, California School for the Blind, personal communication, December 2005).

Music can become a lasting and reinforcing memory and can support communication when it is paired with social activity. When rhythms are simple and words and phrases repeated often, it may be easier for a child to remember the sequences and to add simple movements during activities that engage peers. Besides, music is enjoyable for children and adults alike. Family members and teachers therefore may want to take particular care to expose children to music and involve them in listening games or awareness during playtime. Sidebar 3.1 includes specific suggestions for the use of singing to teach concepts, give directions, and even make transitions.

LEARNING TO LISTEN: CONCEPTS AND COMMUNICATION

Emerging listening skills related to the development of auditory memory for concepts, directions, and sequence include the following:

- points to ten body parts when directed
- points to top, bottom, front, and back on self or objects when directed
- demonstrates positional concepts such as *high, low, over, under, above, below, inside, through,* and *away from*
- responds to a spoken "stop"

- follows three-step directions in sequence involving two or three different objects
- repeats sound patterns of voice, clapping, or tapping
- recounts experiences in a logical sequence
- remembers parts of rhymes or songs
- relates an experience or creative story in a logical sequence
- remember objects in the order they were presented

At snack time, 5-year-old Zahir hears another child take some of his food. Later that morning, the children sit at circle time and play duck, duck, goose. When it is Zahir's turn to be the goose and go around the circle to choose someone, he listens for that child, localizes where he is sitting, and as he walks around the circle, gives him more than a tap to tell him he's the new goose.

Concept Development

In the scenario just described, Zahir demonstrated his knowledge of the concept *around* when he walked around the circle, enabling him to choose his new goose quickly. *Concepts* are a child's understanding or mental representation of people, places, objects, and events. Children without a working knowledge of the concepts related to their body awareness, movement, and position and of object concepts such as quantities, shapes, sizes, and textures have difficulty learning at the same pace as their peers. In addition, the knowledge of concepts forms a foundation for receptive language, or what is understood, and expressive language, or what is expressed or spoken.

Vision plays a major role in the formation of concepts, and when visual functioning is disrupted, learning often needs to be channeled through the other senses. As Pogrund and Fazzi (2002, p. 128) have stated, "Children with visual impairments must find alternate or supplemental means for learning about the world." Karen Karsh's story at the beginning of this chapter illustrates this need. Karen knew enough about the spatial concept of *top* to be bewildered then awakened to the understanding that the box shape of the object *refrigerator* has a top. All children learn best as they experience something in its entirety. Hearing can play an essential role in helping children who are visually impaired develop concepts and knowledge about what they may see only partially or imperfectly. However, children with visual impairments often need to learn concepts from part to whole (Pogrund & Fazzi, 2002), touching, using, or seeing only part of something.

During the preschool and kindergarten years, as children gain skills that help them move, listen, touch, and explore, they learn more about the world through home and school routines and are introduced to more and more information. Concepts and mental images are formed as they learn to organize, recall, and apply this information to new situations and in new ways. Concepts provide the foundation for all learning and give meaning to the language that a child hears, speaks, reads, and writes (Wright & Stratton, 2007). This foundation is constantly expanding as children learn more about the world through experience.

As explained in Chapters 1 and 2, listening, unlike hearing, is an active process and plays an essential role in concept development; the ability to listen effectively needs to be developed and supported. Concepts are formed by children with visual impairments through a combination of what they hear and touch and listen to. The sound of the dryer as the clothes revolve in the drum combined with the feeling of warmth and vibration as clothes are being dried provides important information through experience that enhances a child's understanding. Careful description ("Let's open the dryer door") paired with the opportunity to touch—in this case, opening the door and feeling the warm towels ("Pull out the towels; they're warm and dry") as they are pulled from the dryer—provide more information. Repeated opportunities to perform this sequence help the child consolidate the experiences and form thoughts about the object, *dryer*, its function, and its basic attributes, which will serve as concept building blocks for future learning. This combination of experience paired with sound and description builds concepts. Listening is an essential component, and, when paired with touch, it is a powerful ingredient in concept formation.

Description and Concept Formation

In promoting children's abilities to listen, formulate meaning, and establish concepts, the key is not so much to tell the children about the world around them as to provide the children with experiences that allow them to create concepts. Words can be used to describe what a child is experiencing but are not fully understood without the experience itself (Durkel, 2000). The combination of listening to *water* as it is turned on and the sensation of wetness and possibly warmth help a child understand various aspects of *water* as the word is spoken.

The content and complexity of descriptive language and the child's ability to attend to description are important aspects of the process of concept formation. For children of preschool age who are beginning to learn to listen in order to acquire information, words need to have a practical and experiential base. To maximize the use of description during experiences, the following guidelines are suggested to enhance concept development:

▶ Use the child's name during instruction.

▶ Use short, simple sentences with easily understood information about what is happening, such as "Pull out the towels. They're warm and dry."

▶ Build on the child's prior knowledge, using concepts that have been mastered; for example, when introducing the child to the concept of seeds during a unit about things that grow, present a variety of seeds that the student may have already encountered for comparison.

▶ Think carefully about the literal meaning of commonly used phrases and slang, minimizing ambiguous words or phrases. For example, one might call a restless child a "wiggly worm." This comment would best be followed by a description of a worm, or better yet, holding a worm for the child to understand the reference.

▶ Minimize extraneous noise in the environment, including background noise, talk, and music.

In preschool and kindergarten, children are presented with new objects and ideas, both within their daily experiences and during curricular activities that are outside of their daily routines. Families and professionals who wish to help children with visual impairments gain understanding of these new concepts may find it helpful to employ strategies based on an understanding of how concepts are formed. Because the formation of concepts is so important for all learning, knowledge of the hierarchy of concept formation is useful. The hierarchy of concept formation as described by Lyndon and McGraw (1982), consists of a series of the following steps:

▶ sensory exploration
▶ identifying same and different
▶ identification of characteristics
▶ identification of defining characteristic
▶ systematic analysis
▶ comparison with nonexamples
▶ abstract common element

Sidebar 3.3 provides an example of how to use the hierarchy of concept formation. In addition, the activities in Sidebar 3.4 are effective in enhancing concept development and communication.

((SIDEBAR 3.3
Example of the Hierarchy of Concept Formation: Pumpkins

By keeping the sequence of steps in the hierarchy of concept formation in mind, parents, teachers, and related specialists can incorporate activities that provide experiences for children with visual impairments that lead to true understanding of concepts and development of their listening skills. With each experience, such as the example of exploration of a pumpkin outlined here, the child should be given time to explore and time to respond to inquiry and comment.

Sensory exploration: Explore and discuss the sensory aspects and attributes of the pumpkin, both whole and in its parts when cut open.

Identifying same and different: Ask how a pumpkin is the same and different from other types of food. Give a wide variety of examples for comparison, such as an apple, a slice of bread, a banana, and milk.

Identification of characteristics: Describe the pumpkin: It has smooth skin with ridges and a rough stem that was attached to a plant in the ground.

Identification of defining characteristics: Explain that when the pumpkin is whole it is smooth and dry, and when it is cut open, it is wet and cold inside, with many smooth seeds and a web of connecting fibers.

Systematic analysis: Teach that pumpkins come in many sizes, that they are plants, and that they grow from soil in the ground.

Comparison with nonexamples: Ask how a pumpkin is the same as and different from other types of vegetables.

Abstract common elements: Pumpkins are a source of food and decoration. Most pumpkins are round.

Source: Adapted with permission from information presented by K. Zebehazy at the Getting in Touch with Literacy Conference, Costa Mesa, California, November 12–15, 2009.

SOCIAL COMMUNICATION

Emerging listening skills related to the development of listening and social communication include the following:

▶ shows concern when others are unhappy or upset

▶ attends to other children's behavior

▶ responds to adult guidance in negotiating conflict

▶ follows rules given by adults for new activities or simple games

▶ follows rules when participating in routine activities

((‹ SIDEBAR 3.4

Strategies and Activities to Enhance
Concept Development and Communication

The following activities can help preschool-age children learn concepts and develop communication skills:

CONCEPT DEVELOPMENT

- Sing songs about everything to reinforce concepts you are teaching. For example, select a simple tune and sing about putting clothing on and off, washing body parts in the bathtub, moving the body, to experience concepts, and following directions. One example might be to the tune of "Row, Row, Row Your Boat": "Go, go get your coat, as quickly as you can; merrily, merrily, merrily, off to school again."
- Teach a concept in as many ways as you can. For example, to teach the concept of *corner*, teach the child that *corner* can mean the corner of a table, book, or room, and also where two streets meet. Provide hands-on experiences in the construction of corners from cardboard, wood pieces, or blocks; make picture frames and play tents from boxes.

COMMUNICATION

- Role-play and practice situations that the child may encounter at the park or in preschool, such as when one child's block castle is accidentally bumped over by another. Make a sand or block castle for the child to knock over "by accident," and model the language and conversation associated with repairing this social interaction. Reverse roles and practice.
- Use toy telephones to teach conversation skills, beginning with a typical script for answering a telephone and identifying oneself. Teach the child how to answer a telephone, role-playing having a conversation and taking messages. Encourage turn taking during conversation.
- Make up little plays, incorporating dress-up to help make them enjoyable, to help model interactive dialogue.

▸ localizes and looks at, or faces, speaker when listening
▸ participates in a conversation without monopolizing it

Micah is 3 years old and very curious about activities the other children are doing in his preschool. He has to get so close to see what they are doing because of his low vision due to congenital nystagmus, however, that he often knocks over their carefully arranged toys or curricular materials, upsetting the other children. When this happens, Micah is left silent, not knowing what to say or do.

Social communication (known in linguistics as *pragmatics*) requires that individuals learn and understand how to use language for different purposes when interacting with others. In addition to understanding that language is used for different occasions and functions, such as for greeting or apologizing, children need to know how to change language according to the needs of the listener or situation (for example, speaking one way in the classroom and another way on the playground) and how to follow the rules of conversation (for example, taking turns) (American Speech Language Hearing Association, n.d.). This will require opportunities for modeling social language and practice, within social exchanges as well as during one-to-one instruction. For instance, when children are playing together with toys, model language that can be used to share a specific toy, such as "Can I have a turn with the drum?" or "It's your turn." Learning to express one's thoughts appropriately and respond to peers and adults is the basis for social communication. Knowing how to listen in a social situation, to interpret who is speaking, to follow the subject, to decipher the emotion behind the words spoken, and to respond in a useful manner to the speaker is a complex set of skills; they are not developed automatically. Listening skills for social interaction need to be taught and also need to be considered to be a part of the process in all learning situations.

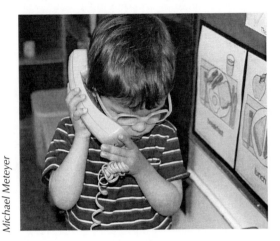

Michael Meteyer

This little boy is practicing both listening and social skills while pretending to talk on the phone with his friend.

All students learn social communication skills through modeling and by observing personal interactions taking place around them, but students with visual impairments have additional challenges that necessitate more deliberate instruction. Much of this instruction involves learning to listen. For example, without visual cues, such as eye contact, children who are visually impaired may not know when they are being spoken to by another child, or they may lack the body language of looking at or facing someone when conversing. In general, ongoing assistance and in-the-moment intervention with an adult modeling the appropriate language for the children involved in an interaction may be important in helping a child build skills in listening in a social situation. For example, in the scenario mentioned earlier, if Micah accidentally knocked something over and the other child loudly summoned the teacher, both children could be led through a script of the appropriate language; for example, "What made you knock over the blocks?" and "I didn't mean to. Can I help you build it again?"

It is important to teach a young child who is visually impaired about simple greetings. A prompted response of "I am fine, Kate. How are you?" while turning to the speaker who greeted the child is an important kind of social communication that needs to be taught. Likewise, it is important to model a handshake and remind the student about smiling. Young students with visual impairments are not automatically aware of these social rules, but their sighted classmates in all likelihood will be more willing to befriend them if social graces are initiated and returned.

Thus, preschool children with visual impairments, unable to visually observe how people react and interact, need to be deliberately taught about social interaction, unlike their sighted peers, who are beginning to incidentally pay attention and respond more naturally to one another. In Micah's situation, he needed a trusted and nurturing adult to lead him through the pragmatic language required to negotiate this typical preschool scenario and to foster his sense of others.

THE TRANSITION TO PRESCHOOL

Emerging listening skills related to the development of early skills for learning and reading readiness include the following:

- repeats new words to self
- gains information from listening to books about real things
- engages in a conversation about a book
- participates in rhymes, songs, and games that play with sounds of language
- recalls one or two elements from a story
- enjoys following along in books being read
- makes rhymes to simple words
- after hearing the meaning of a new word, uses it in speech
- listens to a story and retells it in own words

Chrissy has just started in her new preschool class. She has a severe visual impairment and will probably be a braille reader. Chrissy is fearful of the class and the children. During the first week, many of the children come up to her and talk, and then they run away. Chrissy has no idea of who they are or what their names are.

The Move from Home to School

Going to school can initially be difficult for many 3-year-olds with visual impairments, as the shift to a more complex environment is undertaken. Family and caregivers are no longer the sole participants in and interpreters of the listening environment. With this transition, day-care professionals, preschool teachers, and other children suddenly fill the world with familiar and unfamiliar sounds, speech patterns, and descriptions. For some children with visual impairments, home environments, rich with conversation, possibly songs, and a myriad of familiar activities with relatives and friends may have provided opportunities to build skills important in the child's next steps and future experiences in listening. The child now begins to apply these skills in a wider environment, refine them, and build others.

The transition to preschool is a big leap with regard to the listening environment. Structured group activities such as circle time are vital in the development of learning how to listen and learn within a social setting. According to the *Desired Results Developmental Profile*, published by the California Department of Education (2003), preschool program experiences can provide opportunities to help children develop those listening skills. In addition to preschool, other natural environments such as playgroups, kindergym, classes available from local parks and recreation departments, and play dates with other children and family contribute to the widening base of experiences for children at this age. Skills of attending to sounds, discriminating among them, and remembering the differences gain a solid base as children begin to generalize and apply their knowledge of the sounds heard in these new environments. Children with visual impairments now need to expand their listening skills to begin to be able to focus their attention on instruction and to develop the auditory figure-ground perception essential for successful school experiences. In preschool, it is time to learn to categorize and generalize sounds and communication skills. For example, the child needs to focus on the teacher's voice, even though there are many distracting sounds, both inside and outside of the classroom.

Supportive Measures

Transitions can be difficult for many children, but for some children with visual impairments, transitions can be very confusing without guidance and explanation. As they did when they were younger, preschool children need to listen to the sounds around them within their daily routines in order to establish a sense of predictability and trust. As children make the transition from home to the school environment, simple description and hands-on experiences are needed to support them and provide explanations for the sounds present in these new situations. For instance, during preparation for snack time, a parent, if present in school, can say, "Oh, they're getting the plates out for snack just like we get them at home when we eat." Or if a child hears everyone running outside during a kindergym class, he or she will know why only if prior explanation is given about what will happen. An explanation can be paired with a sound signal, such as a small bell that is consistently rung when it is time to go. These types of listening cues help the child with a visual impairment put some auditory consistency and predictability into the day. They are supports that help the child begin to develop an awareness of auditory sequencing, or the ability to remember, order, or reconstruct information that is heard, which will begin to develop at this age. Sidebar 3.5 presents additional strategies that can be used to help children with the transition to preschool.

Key for a successful transition into a preschool environment is for families and the vision and early intervention specialists in a child's life to provide information to preschool teachers and staff about the child's visual impairment and learning and listening needs and requirements. It is most beneficial when children who are visually impaired participate in, or listen to, this information and advocacy efforts, so that they can begin developing their own understanding of their vision and learning needs.

It is a common best practice for teachers of students with visual impairments to provide workshops and in-service training for teachers and school staff, sometimes for an entire teaching staff, and for the classmates themselves when a student with visual impairment enrolls in a school. Common and useful topics include structure of the eye and vision functioning, braille reading and writing, human guide instruction, orientation and mobility, and the use of the white cane.

In-service presentations need to be geared to the needs of the student and the staff. Listening can be part of the focus. Depending on the circumstances, topics can include the importance and development of listening skills in young children and young children with visual impairments, the auditory and listening environment

(« Sidebar 3.5
Making the Transition to Preschool

The following strategies and activities can be used to help a child with a visual impairment with the transition to the new preschool environment and can be enjoyed during either one-to-one teaching or group instruction:

- Before a routine has become familiar, tell the child what is going to happen. For example, before going into the preschool classroom for the first time, talk about greeting the teacher and other children and discuss some of the activities that may occur.

- Teach about sound landmarks, such as a generator or air conditioner that is always on. It is fun at this time to teach about sound reflection; that is, if you make noise with your feet by marching under an overhang, it will sound different than it would when marching under an open sky.

- Reinforce time and sequence concepts by using a digital recorder to record with the child her or his schedule for the day. For example, "First I'll get dressed, then I'll have breakfast, and then I'll go to play at Katie's house and Dad will pick me up." This could be followed up by a story at bedtime about the day's activities.

- It will be helpful to the child's transition to preschool to become familiar with some of the activities and songs commonly utilized. Teach the words and actions to activities such as Simon Says; Duck, Duck, Goose; The Wheels on the Bus; and so on.

- Because teachers in a school setting will be using description, it will be helpful to teach and model the language of description. For example, "Tell me about your kitty. Is she soft or scratchy, smooth or fluffy, sleepy or busy? How many legs does she have? Let's count them. How many legs do you have?"

- Read a book with a prominent pattern of repeated sounds, such as one by Dr. Seuss, several times to the child until it becomes very familiar. Then read it leaving out a word or line and let the child complete it. For example:

    Adult: I do not like green eggs and ham; I do not like them . . .

    Child: Sam I am!

- Create a sound diary by recording and categorizing the sounds at home, of family members, pets, or inside or outside noises, or in the community, of the grocery store, a park, or a local pool.

of the classroom and school, and tips for voice pitch, volume, pacing, intonation, and proximity. Strategies that can be used to design in-service sessions for teachers and classmates to help them learn about visual impairment are included in Sidebar 3.6.

Providing In-Service Training to Teachers and Classmates

The following suggestions can be helpful in creating an informational session for teachers and classmates of a student who is visually impaired to help them learn about visual impairment.

Decide on the focus of the training, and budget from 50 to 90 minutes. The training outlined here focuses on the skills of listening the student needs to learn and how teachers can optimize the learning environment. At other times, in-service training might focus on orientation and mobility (O&M) skills, human guide training, peer interaction, or braille reading and writing.

PRIOR TO THE IN-SERVICE TRAINING

- First, discuss the in-service training with the parents of the child with a visual impairment. They may have pertinent information and insight about their child that may be helpful.

- Discuss the training with the child at the child's developmental level, including the reason why a teacher of students with visual impairments comes to work with him or her. Give the student an active role in the in-service session as appropriate.

- Schedule the time, place, and anticipated duration of the training session, and notify the participants.

INTRODUCTION TO THE IN-SERVICE TRAINING

- Describe the role of a teacher of students with visual impairments and the support this teacher provides to students who are visually impaired.

- Provide a brief and simplified description of the child's visual functioning to support teachers in their understanding of the student; this may be a good time for the student to tell a little about what he or she knows about his or her visual functioning.

- Discuss the specific adaptive strategies the child uses (such as braille, white cane, assistive technology equipment, and other adaptive tools). The child with a visual impairment can share his or her special skills at this point.

- Discuss briefly the challenges a student with visual impairments encounters and the skills the student needs to acquire to become successful in school. For example, the student
  - ▸ misses visual incidental learning
  - ▸ needs hands-on experiences
  - ▸ needs cues, landmarks, and O&M skills to travel independently
  - ▸ needs to navigate open space without vision
  - ▸ needs to use listening skills instead of vision

(Continued)

((Sidebar 3.6 *(Continued)*

GROUP ACTIVITIES

After presenting the information outlined here, introduce a group listening activity such as the following:

- Have the group listen quietly for about 20 seconds and ask the group what they have heard. Ask the group if they all have a mental picture of how each of those objects producing the sounds looks and functions.
- Have the group do a task without using their vision by listening to instructions, such as following a five-step paper-folding lesson, or constructing a box using scotch tape or a stapler, or placing paper in a three-ring binder. Ask what worked well and what they would want to do differently next time, and discuss how visual memory aided the process.

FOCUS ON LISTENING SKILLS AND CREATING A FAVORABLE LISTENING ENVIRONMENT

- Discuss strategies that need to be practiced during each encounter with the child, such as identifying oneself when approaching the child and, especially, saying that one is leaving before walking away.
- Explain that the child with a visual impairment needs to sit close to the teacher to see his or her best, use his or her hands to feel, and increase his or her ability to attend and listen. Demonstrate how close proximity to the teacher's voice, movements, and instructional objects gives the child a more direct experience, aides in attention, and reduces distraction from incidental classroom noises.
- Suggest that the teacher read a book such as *Blueberry Eyes* (Beatty, 1996) or *Listen for the Bus* (McMahon, 1996) to the class.
- Teach the importance of allowing time for the child to respond to questions and commands. Demonstrate a 3-, 5-, and 20-second wait period.
- Demonstrate the importance of giving precise directions (e.g., "Go three steps forward to your friend") and avoiding vague terms ("Go over there"). Tell teachers they will become better teachers for all their students by using precise and positional language and their own senses more keenly.

ACQUIRING INFORMATION IN THE KINDERGARTEN CLASSROOM

Emerging listening skills that children will need in order to acquire information in the kindergarten classroom include the following:

▸ attends in small group

▸ attends within large-group setting, such as a class

▸ listens to a story and retells it in own words

▸ repeats/points to all letters

- ▸ listens and waits for turn when talking with others
- ▸ listens to an adult's direction when walking in a noisy environment
- ▸ participates in a conversation without monopolizing it

Tara attends a kindergarten with sighted classmates. One day during circle time, as Mr. Moe, her teacher, is emphasizing the sound of T *in tiger, a fire engine can be heard a distance away. As he continues to teach the children, he notices that Tara is not paying any attention to him. She has become very quiet as she focuses on the siren. Mr. Moe astutely says, "Tara, I can tell that you hear a fire engine, just like we heard one last week. Let's get back to learning our letters now."*

Essential Classroom Skills

For some children with visual impairments who do not use vision as a primary modality for learning, if at all, the auditory channel can be dominant for accessing information. These children hear everything that is going on, which can lead to some difficulty in filtering out the content of a lesson from background sounds. The classroom teacher attuned to this possibility and the child's learning characteristics can acknowledge this reality, identify the competing sounds, and redirect the child's attention toward the lesson. It is important that the teacher in such circumstances cultivate the child's ability to distinguish figure from ground by helping the child focus on what is being taught, as Tara was redirected to learning the alphabet.

By kindergarten, it is important that most of the basic auditory perception and discrimination skills be in place for children, as academics are beginning in earnest. Students are required to maintain attention when in a one-on-one session with an adult, when working in a small group, or when receiving instruction with the entire class. They need to be able to listen to an adult or another child when others are talking, or in a noisy outdoor environment. We teach and expect children at this age to match sounds, follow one- and two-step directions, and recognize cause and effect with sound. For example, if they hear someone insert a key into a lock, the next sounds to anticipate would be the opening and closing of the door, footsteps, and so on. Children develop and utilize their auditory memory when they are instructed to repeat patterns, numbers, and the alphabet, and even humorous things they have heard. They are learning their body parts and many positional, time, and measurement concepts and can respond to questions about color, size, and shape. At this point, most children need to be able to "close" and infer auditorily, meaning that when they hear part of a familiar message, they can figure out the rest of it. The strategies and activities in Sidebar 3.7 will facilitate children's ability to listen in the classroom.

((Sidebar 3.7

Encouraging Listening in the Kindergarten Classroom

The following strategies and activities will provide support for listening for students beginning kindergarten:

- Prepare the child for the different types of sounds he or she will hear at school. Tell the child what to expect and what to do, and address the student's curiosity about an action or event. Ask questions such as "What do you do when you hear the school bell?" or tell the child, "Yes, that's the principal's voice giving daily announcements" and "Today everyone will learn about being safe and what to do when you hear the fire drill alarm. Let's practice what you will do later today."

- Encourage the classroom teacher to make an audio recording of the circle time so that the child with visual impairment can share it at home and practice the activities in the daily routine.

- Teach the child to operate a digital player, touch screen tablet, or CD player. Listening to recorded stories at this age will introduce and prepare the child for more academic learning that will require the use of audio formats.

- Encourage the child to join with the other children in the listening center (a designated area in the classroom in which children can listen to recorded literature while they follow along with the book), and make sure the classroom has the books in an accessible format (braille or color large print).

- Teach the child to respond to *who, what, where, how, why,* and *when* questions about his or her daily activities so that the child is ready for these types of comprehension questions in the language arts lessons.

- Use technology. Many websites, interactive/audible books, and children's programs are available to provide listening enjoyment while enhancing early concept and literacy skill development through listening. (See the Resources section at the end of this book for suggestions.)

Strategies for Circle Time

Listening and social interactions among children become more refined throughout the kindergarten year as students engage each other in conversations. An excellent structure for this interactive process in most kindergarten classes is circle time. Although primarily a teacher-directed classroom activity, circle time can be the part of the day when children with visual impairments excel in their interactions because so much of what happens during circle time is aural learning and sharing. When materials are accessible, proximity to the teacher and materials is established, and dialogue and discussion provide the structure of routine, much listening, language development, and social growth can take place for a child who is visually impaired.

Skillful listening is required during this instructional period because the activities of circle time provide the child with an opportunity to learn a variety of social-cognitive skills, including listening to classmates, turn taking, and collaborative problem solving. Circle time provides a predictable routine during which concepts such as the following can be learned:

- seasons
- holidays
- months of the year
- days of the week
- counting days on a calendar
- oral counting to 100
- weather
- attendance
- early literacy skills such as the alphabet and sounds

For the student with a visual impairment, it is particularly important for teachers to provide support that will make it possible for the child to listen and respond in order to successfully learn alongside other students. Support that can help a child make the most of the listening opportunities during circle-time activities can be provided by using the strategies in Sidebar 3.8.

Listening and Early Literacy Skills

Listening to stories as they are read aloud, pairing objects with first-letter names and sounds, such as a key with the letter "k," and reciting the letters of the alphabet are common activities in preschool and kindergarten classrooms. During these years children participate in many activities that promote early literacy skills. The most recent findings of the National Early Literacy Panel (2009)—a government group mandated to review research on the development of early literacy skills in children from birth to age 5 to develop educational policy and best practices for supporting early language and literacy development—place great emphasis on instruction that promotes knowledge of the alphabet, phonological awareness and memory, rapid automatic naming of letters and objects, and the writing of letters. Listening plays an essential role in the development of these and many other early literacy skills. As stated in Chapter 1, reading, writing, listening, and speaking are components of an integrated language process; they are not isolated components of language (Rex, Koenig, Wormsley, & Baker, 1994).

Strategies for Circle Time

STRATEGIES FOR TEACHERS OF STUDENTS WITH VISUAL IMPAIRMENTS

- Provide ample time for children to inspect any objects presented for exploration. This may be time spent in addition to circle time, either before or after, describing the salient features of the object as the student manually explores it.

- Before students participate in circle time, provide orientation to instructional materials that are regularly used, such as calendars, name charts, counting objects, and pointers. Children also benefit from opportunities to practice with the materials so that when it is their turn to put the new number on the calendar, for example, they have a greater level of comfort and familiarity.

- Provide opportunities to practice the movements that accompany the songs that are regularly sung, explaining, when necessary, why they accompany the words in the song. For instance, when singing "I'm a Little Teapot," one hand is held up like a teapot spout, while the other is hand is placed on the hip, as if forming a handle. A real teapot can be shown to the child as a model during description and practice.

- Encourage youngsters with visual impairments to listen for the voice of their teacher or the person who is speaking during activities. Teach them to turn their bodies so that they face the speaker while seated. This will take practice until it becomes natural.

- Teach children how to raise their hands in response to and when asking questions during circle-time instruction. This, too, will take practice.

STRATEGIES FOR CLASSROOM TEACHERS

- Choose a circle-time seating arrangement that places the student with visual impairment in close proximity to instructional materials and actions. In this way the child will experience the activity more fully, and teacher support will be nearby when necessary.

- Use the names of children consistently so that the student with visual impairment will know who is called on or involved in an activity.

- Use precise positional terminology during instruction. For example with a math lesson, "Put the counting bear in the cup on the right."

- Encourage the child with visual impairment to participate during circle-time activities by calling on him or her regularly, with the expectation that the child can participate fully. In the beginning it will support the child if he or she knows in advance that he or she will be asked to tell the name of the day, for example. Prepare the child for what to expect.

- When presenting new ideas and concepts, link them to the child's prior experiences and knowledge.

For children with visual impairments, strong emphasis needs to be placed on ensuring not only that they receive the same early literacy experiences and opportunities as their sighted classmates, but also that listening skills are well supported during literacy instruction. This focus requires professionals to know and understand the skills and activities that children will be learning and to analyze the aspects of listening that need to be supported and developed. The early literacy skills that the National Early Literacy Panel (2009) found to be most important for the later development of literacy skills such as decoding, oral reading fluency, reading comprehension, writing, and spelling are listed in Sidebar 3.9.

Many of the skills listed entail learning the code of reading (which may be braille or large print for the student with a visual impairment) and sound-symbol relationships (sounds that each letter makes). Listening plays an important role in this aspect of early literacy learning because of the importance of phonological

---

((◗ SIDEBAR 3.9
Early Predictors of Later Literacy Skills

The following early literacy skills were found by the National Early Literacy Panel to be most important for predicting the development of later literacy skills such as decoding, oral reading fluency, reading comprehension, writing, and spelling:

STRONG AND CONSISTENT PREDICTORS
- knowing the names of printed letters
  - ‣ being able to label letters correctly, for example, that *F* is the letter called "eff"
- knowing the sounds associated with printed letters
  - ‣ understanding and correlating sounds with letters—that the sound /f/ goes with the letter *F*
  - ‣ or knowing that the letters *at* at the end of words are pronounced "aah-tuh"
- being able to manipulate the sounds of spoken language—breaking words apart into smaller sound units such as syllables or phonemes, adding or deleting sound units
  - ‣ understanding syllables—that the word *bulldozer* is made up of three syllables, *bull*, *doz*, and *er*
  - ‣ or knowing how to change words by changing a few letters—that if you take away the /j/ sound from the word *change*, you get the word *chain*

(Continued)

- being able to rapidly name a sequence of letters, numbers, objects, or colors
  - ▸ when shown a set of numbers, being able to name numbers in order, quickly and easily
  - ▸ or being able to recognize patterns of objects or colors
- being able to write one's own name and isolated letters
  - ▸ being able to put one's name on a drawing
  - ▸ or being able to correctly write letters that are shown on a set of word cards
- being able to remember the content of spoken language for a short time
  - ▸ being able to remember simple, multistep instructions from the teacher about getting ready for outdoor time (for example, clean up table, put materials on shelf, stand in line at the door)
  - ▸ or being able to remember earlier parts of a story read aloud to make sense of later parts of the story

MODERATE PREDICTORS
- knowing some of the conventions of English print, including how to use a book or other printed materials
  - ▸ understanding that print is read and written from left to right and top to bottom
  - ▸ or knowing the difference between the front and back of a book and that books are read from front to back
- being able to recognize and identify environmental print
  - ▸ being able to decode or read common signs and logos
  - ▸ being able to identify product or company names for common products or establishments (for example, Apple, Coke, McDonald's)
- knowing how to put concepts, thoughts, and ideas into spoken words, and understanding other people when they talk
  - ▸ having the vocabulary to be able to talk about interesting topics such as insects, dinosaurs, or weather
  - ▸ or being able to have a conversation about past events and be understood because word order and verb agreement are in place (subject precedes verb)
- being able to see similarities and differences between visual symbols, in other words, visual processing
  - ▸ knowing that capital letters are different from small letters
  - ▸ or being able to pick out a picture of a stop sign from among a set of pictures including other road signs with other shapes

---

Source: Adapted from National Early Literacy Panel, *Early Beginnings: Early Literacy Knowledge and Instruction: A Guide for Early Childhood Administrators and Professional Development* (Washington, DC: National Institute for Literacy, 2009). Retrieved October 10, 2010, from http://lincs.ed.gov/publications/pdf/NELPEarlyBeginnings09.pdf.

awareness and phonics. Phonological awareness is the ability to recognize, manipulate, and use sounds in words, including the ability to hear and discriminate the sounds in language. This capacity includes the "general ability to attend to the sounds of language as distinct from its meaning, noticing similarities between words in their sounds, enjoying rhymes, and counting syllables" (Snow, Burns, & Griffin, 1998, p. 52). Phonological awareness involves the auditory and oral manipulation of sounds.

Phonics is the association of letters and sounds used to sound out written symbols (Snider, 1995); it is a system of reading instruction that builds on the alphabetic principle, a central component of which is the teaching of correspondences between letters or groups of letters and their pronunciations (Adams, 1990; Chard & Dickson, 1999). Phonemic awareness and phonics are an integral part of the preschool and kindergarten years. Phonics needs to be explicitly taught to students with visual impairments as they are learning to read and write. Sidebar 3.10 presents early literacy instructional activities suggested by the National Early Literacy Panel. Adaptations for students with visual impairments are included in italics when appropriate.

((‹ SIDEBAR 3.10

Early Literacy Listening Activities

The following are instructional activities to support early literacy suggested by the National Early Literacy Panel. Adaptations for students with visual impairments are included in italics when appropriate.

ACTIVITIES THAT HELP CHILDREN LEARN THE NAMES OF THE LETTER-SHAPES IN THE ALPHABET AND THE SOUNDS THE LETTERS MAKE

- Play games like Alphabet Bingo to teach letter names and shapes. *Games can be marked with braille and tactile markers, or provided in enlarged print with high contrast and simplified format for large-print learners.*

- Teach the sounds each letter can make as well as the name of the letter. *Provide letters in the student's primary learning medium that can be used to pair with letter sounds during activities.*

- Sing songs and recite rhymes that include the sounds associated with letters ("D" is for dog-/d/, /d/, /d/ . . . dog). *Make a recording of the teacher singing the songs with exaggeration in the voicing of the target sound. Make a recording with the student singing the songs, with clear pronunciation of the target sound, so that it can be played at home for practice and entertainment.*

(Continued)

ACTIVITIES THAT HELP MAKE CHILDREN AWARE OF SOUNDS IN LANGUAGE AND PROVIDE OPPORTUNITIES TO PRACTICE MANIPULATING SOUNDS

- Use rhymes, songs, and poems to help children hear repetitive sounds at the beginning and end of words. *Model and personally teach any movements that are used during songs to reinforce concepts.*
- Move from simpler sound activities to more complex operations. Start with combining sounds to make words (c/a/t=*cat*); move on to manipulating sound units that make up words, syllables (/ba/by), word parts (un/der), and word families (*bat, cat, mat*), and phonemes (letter combinations that make different sounds, for example, *st, ch*); and to breaking apart words (*cat*=c/a/t). *Magnetic braille or large-print letters and metal boards or cookie trays can be used for easy manipulation of letters and words during instruction.*

ACTIVITIES THAT HELP CHILDREN REMEMBER SPOKEN INFORMATION

- Ask children to follow simple, multistep directions in preparing for activities or carrying out classroom routines, such as getting ready for morning circle time, gathering materials and setting up for easel painting, cleaning up after snack, getting ready for lunch.

ACTIVITIES THAT SUPPORT ORAL LANGUAGE DEVELOPMENT

- Read books that expose children to varied and rich vocabulary through discussion of the pictures, text, and story development and sequence. *(See the section on reading aloud in this chapter.)*
- Pose questions that ask the children to tell about what is happening in the story and in the pictures.
- Talk with children.
  - ▸ Extend discussions so that the children actively practice new language skills.
  - ▸ Initiate interactive dialogues that use new vocabulary and concepts and work with sounds and letters.
  - ▸ Show children how to ask questions (using words such as *what, when, where, why, how,* and *who*).
  - ▸ Help children develop language for making comparisons ("The cotton feels soft, but the table feels hard").
- Go beyond building vocabulary to using vocabulary as a foundation for more complex skills such as grammatical knowledge, definitional vocabulary, and reading comprehension.
- Help the child develop a deep understanding of new vocabulary by selecting print *or braille* that uses the new vocabulary in context, providing different meanings for the same word, using the same word in different kinds of sentences, especially throughout the days following the introduction of the vocabulary.

Source: Adapted from National Early Literacy Panel. *Early Beginnings: Early Literacy Knowledge and Instruction: A Guide for Early Childhood Administrators and Professional Development* (Washington, DC: National Institute for Literacy, 2009. Retrieved June 1, 2010, from http://lincs.ed.gov/publications/pdf/NELPEarlyBeginnings09.pdf.

Reading Aloud

Reading aloud to children has been described as the single most important activity for reading success (Neuman, Copple, & Bredekamp, 2000). It demonstrates to the child the rewards of reading and helps develop his or her interest in books and desire to be a reader (Mooney, 1990). In most preschool and kindergarten classrooms, the "read aloud" occurs each day, as children listen while sitting on a rug around their teacher as he or she reads. At home, reading aloud may happen just before bed, when the child is snuggled in a nest of blankets. This treasured and shared listening activity is a powerful learning experience. Reading aloud to children promotes the following:

▸ awareness of print and the conventions of written language (National Early Literacy Panel, 2009; Wright & Stratton, 2007)

▸ phonemic awareness (Burgess, 2002; Wright & Stratton, 2007)

▸ oral language skills (National Early Literacy Panel, 2009; Wright & Stratton, 2007)

▸ development of a rich vocabulary (National Early Literacy Panel, 2009; Wright & Stratton, 2007)

▸ the ability to use strategies to increase listening and reading comprehension (Gold & Gibson, 2001; Wright & Stratton, 2007)

For all children, the experience of listening to a favorite story as it is shared by a parent or teacher is greatly enhanced when the reader uses an interactive style of reading that engages the child, increasing involvement with the story and keeping interest at a high level. This read-aloud technique is called "interactive reading" and is sometimes referred to as the "think aloud," modeling how fluent readers think about the text and problem solve as they read. Modeling encourages children to develop the way of thinking that proficient readers employ (Gold & Gibson, 2001).

In their article "Reading Aloud to Build Comprehension," Gold and Gibson (2001) wrote that:

> helping children find and make connections to stories and books requires them to relate the unfamiliar text to their relevant prior knowledge. There are several comprehension strategies that help children become knowledgeable readers. Three are:
>
> 1. Connecting the book to their own life experience
> 2. Connecting the book to other literature they have read
> 3. Connecting what they are reading to universal concepts (Keene & Zimmermann, 1997, p. 4)

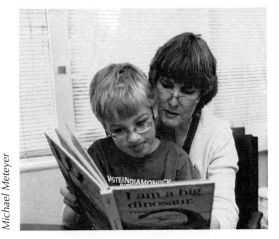

Michael Meteyer

Reading stories aloud and helping children make connections between the story and their prior knowledge enhances their literacy skills.

Parents and teachers can point out connections between prior experiences and the story, similarities between books, and any relationship between the books and a larger concept.

Interactive reading is particularly beneficial for children who are visually impaired because it provides many opportunities to pause during reading to comment and clarify concepts that may be confusing or unknown. Building on a child's prior experience and connecting new concepts and vocabulary help build listening comprehension. Interactive reading supports under-

---

((SIDEBAR 3.11
Read-Aloud Reminders

Every child should have a read-aloud story time that

- is fun and enjoyable
- is shared with a reader who also enjoys the story
- occurs every day or at a regular time
- encourages participation, such as
  ‣ holding toys related to the story
  ‣ imitating animal sounds
  ‣ saying the repeated parts
- appeals to personal interests or creates new ones
- encourages talking about the story with the reader
- allows time for talking about new or interesting words in the story
- relates to familiar experiences or suggests new experiences to try
- fits the level of understanding and attention span
- opens the door to the fun of communicating in print and braille
- creates a desire to read

Source: Reprinted with permission from S. Wright & J. M. Stratton, *On the Way to Literacy* (2nd ed.) (Louisville, KY: American Printing House for the Blind, 2007), p. 14.

standing during listening and increases attention by providing opportunities for fun and thoughtful engagement as the story is being read. Guidelines to promote listening during interactive reading are presented in Sidebar 3.11. Most important, read-aloud story time needs to be fun for both the listener and the reader.

USING TECHNOLOGY TO STIMULATE LISTENING

Technology is advancing and changing constantly, providing enhanced skill development and recreational opportunities for children at younger and younger ages. When used judiciously with preschoolers

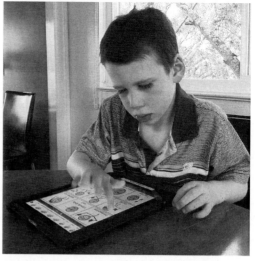

Michelle Cotton

Listening to his assistive communication program on a touch-screen tablet computer helps this student verbalize his feelings.

and kindergarteners with visual impairments, these highly motivating tools can stimulate and support the development of listening and literacy skills such as auditory attention, localization, cause and effect, comprehension, and following directions. Sidebar 3.12 provides some examples of how one type of technology, the touch-screen tablet computer, can be used to stimulate listening skills in preschool and kindergarten.

((SIDEBAR 3.12

Touch-Screen Tablet Computers

Touch-screen tablet computers are small, lightweight devices whose display allows a user to interact with the computer by touching areas on the screen. They can be held in the hand or easily positioned on a table, a wheelchair tray, or even a lap, creating easy access. Applications, or "apps"—programs for these devices—can be used to teach and reinforce many skills in fun and creative ways. For instance, the Voice Over application—a screen-reader program for Apple brand devices—provides highly motivating speech and sound.

The importance of reading aloud to a child with a visual impairment has already been illuminated in this chapter. And while these tablets are most easily accessed by children with some residual vision, they also provide a wonderful interactive portal into active listening to stories for those who are totally blind. For example, once a story has been set

(Continued)

((• SIDEBAR 3.12 *(Continued)*

up, the child can easily listen and then independently "turn" the page by flicking the tablet screen to advance it.

Following are example of the ways that these applications can be used to support the development of listening and literacy skills in young children who are visually impaired:

- To stimulate *auditory attention*, applications can be used that mimic speech and sounds. For example, an animated character repeats whatever sound or language the child says in a fun voice. This can be used for teaching body-image concepts when the tablet character repeats instructions (given by the teacher), such as "Touch your head," prompting the child to say "head" and touch his or her head.

- To reinforce *cause and effect* and *auditory localization*, another application shows a fireworks display, complete with the sound effects of explosions. As the child touches the screen, fireworks burst under his or her fingertips.

- *Auditory attention* and *cause and effect* are also stimulated with applications that allow for creating rhythm and music by tapping on the screen. A piano app displays keys on the tablet that can be played like a piano.

- Stories and books can be downloaded onto the tablet, and some applications prompt the child to turn the page by brushing the screen, enhancing attention.

- Listening can be encouraged by creating personal stories illustrated with photos and the recorded voice of a family member or teacher. The possibilities are endless.

- To provide an avenue of communication for students with expressive communication challenges, numerous applications provide a large vocabulary of words, represented by pictures and symbols, that students who can use vision can select and that are then voiced using synthetic speech.

- Touch-screen tablet computers can be particularly effective for use with some students who have cortical/cerebral visual impairment. Highly motivating visual and auditory information is paired and accessed when the screen is touched. (It may not be appropriate to use visual computer technology with students who experience seizures; in such cases, medical consultation and permission are advised.)

CONCLUSION

As children with visual impairments make the transition from preschool to elementary school, they continue to learn how to listen on a different level. Listening will serve them as a useful learning modality to support their acquisition of cognitive, social, and literacy skills. Their skill development depends on the provision of an abundance of experience-based learning opportunities, well-paced descriptions at their level of understanding, time for them to process information, and, where necessary, facilitated social interactions with peers. Experienced-based instruction leads children with visual impairments into becoming more active learners and better-skilled listeners who have gained the prerequisite knowledge to continue growth toward more complex concept development in the elementary years ahead. For children who are visually impaired, experience-based instruction can establish a foundation to facilitate strong listening habits necessary for social and academic success.

REFERENCES

Adams, M. J. (1990). *Beginning to read: Thinking and learning about print.* Cambridge, MA: MIT Press.

American Speech Language Hearing Association. (n.d.). Social language use (pragmatics). Retrieved July 9, 2009, from www.asha.org/public/speech/development/Pragmatics .htm.

Beatty, M. D. (1996). *Blueberry eyes.* Santa Fe, NM: Health Press.

Burgess, S. (March 2002). Shared reading correlates of early reading skills. *Reading Online, 5*(7). Available at: www.readingonline.org/articles/art_index.asp?HREF=burgess/index .html.

California Department of Education. (September 2003). Desired Results Developmental Profile instructions. *Child development: Contractor information.* Retrieved August 19, 2006, from California Department of Education website: www.cde.ca.gov/sp/cd/ci/desired results.asp.

Chard, D. J., & Dickson, S. V. (1999). Phonological awareness: instructional and assessment guidelines. Retrieved June 1, 2010, from www.ldonline.org/article/ Phonological_Awareness:_Instructional_and Assessment_Guidelines.

Chen, D. (1999). *Essential elements in early intervention: Visual impairment and multiple disabilities.* New York: AFB Press.

Chen, D., & Dote-Kwan, J. (1995). *Starting points: Instructional practices for young children whose multiple disabilities include visual impairment.* Santa Ana, CA: Blind Children's Learning Center.

Dote-Kwan, J., & Chen, D. (1995). Learners with visual impairments. In M. C. Wang & M. C. Reynolds (Eds.), *Handbook of special and remedial education: Research and practice* (2nd ed.) (pp. 205–228). Oxford: Elsevier Science.

Durkel, J. (Spring 2000). What a concept. *See/Hear.*

Ferrell, K. A., & Muir, D. W. (1996). A call to end vision stimulation training. *Journal of Visual Impairment & Blindness, 90*, 364–366.

Gold, J., & Gibson, A. (2001). Reading aloud to build comprehension. Retrieved May 20, 2010, from Reading Rockets website: www.readingrockets.org/article/343.

Huisingh, R., Barrett, M., Zachman, L., Orman, J., & Blagden, C. (1993). *The assessment companion: Communication checklists for SLPs, teachers, and parents.* East Moline, IL: LinguiSystems.

Johnson-Martin, N. M., Attermeier, S. M., & Hacker, B. (2004). *The Carolina curriculum for preschoolers with special needs* (2nd ed.). Baltimore, MD: Paul H. Brookes.

Keene, E. O., & Zimmermann, S. (1997). *Mosaic of thought: Teaching comprehension in a reader's workshop.* Portsmouth, NH: Heinemann.

Lyndon, W. T., & McGraw, M. L. (1982). *Concept development for visually handicapped children: A resource guide for teachers and other professionals working in educational settings* (rev. ed.). New York: AFB Press.

McMahon, P. (1996). *Listen for the bus.* Honesdale, PA: Boyds Mill Press.

Mooney, M. M. (1990). *Reading to, with, and by children.* Katonah, NY: Richard C. Owen.

National Early Literacy Panel. (2009). *Early beginnings: Early literacy knowledge and instruction: A guide for early childhood administrators and professional development.* Washington, DC: National Institute for Literacy. Retrieved June 1, 2010, from http://lincs.ed.gov/publications/pdf/NELPEarlyBeginnings09.pdf.

Neuman, S. B., Copple, C., & Bredekamp, S. (2000). *Learning to read and write: Developmentally appropriate practices for young children.* Washington, DC: National Association for the Education of Young Children.

Perkins School for the Blind. (2002). *Resource guide.* Perkins Panda Early Literacy Program. Watertown, MA: Perkins School for the Blind.

Pestor, E. (1972). *Listen and think.* Louisville, KY: American Printing House for the Blind, Inc.

Pogrund, R. L., & Fazzi, D. L. (2002). *Early focus: Working with young children who are blind or visually impaired and their families* (pp. 107–153). New York: AFB Press.

Rauscher, F. H., Shaw, G. L., Levin, L. J., Wright, E. L., Dennis, W. R., & Newcomb, R. (1997). Music training causes long-term enhancement of preschool children's spatial-temporal reasoning. *Neurological Research, 19,* 2–8.

Rex, E., Koenig, A., Wormsley, D., & Baker, R. (1994). *Foundations of braille literacy.* New York: AFB Press.

Santin, S., & Simmons, J. N. (December 1977). Problems in the construction of reality in congenitally blind children. *Journal of Visual Impairment & Blindness,* 425–427.

Schlaug, G., Norton, A., Overy, K., and Winner, E. (2005). Effects of music training on the child's brain and cognitive development. *Annals of the New York Academy of Sciences, 1060,* 219–230.

Snider, V. E. (1995). A primer on phonemic awareness: What it is, why it's important, and how to teach it. *School Psychology Review, 24,* 443–455.

Snow, C. E., Burns, M. S., & Griffin, P. (Eds.). (1998). *Preventing reading difficulties in young children.* Washington, DC: National Academy Press.

Swallow, R.-M., & Conner, A. (1982). Aural reading. In S. S. Mangold (Ed.), *A teachers' guide to the special educational needs of blind and visually handicapped children* (pp. 119–135). New York: American Foundation for the Blind.

Wright, S., & Stratton, J. M. (2007). *On the way to literacy* (2nd ed.). Louisville, KY: American Printing House for the Blind.

Chapter 4

Elementary School: Developing and Refining Listening Skills

Theresa Postello and Lizbeth A. Barclay

I have a very conscious memory as an 8-year-old, before going to the residential school, of lying in my bedroom at night, tuning up and down the band on the AM radio, finding so many far-away stations with so many kinds of music. Amidst the snapping static and crackling, I especially liked listening to the language usage, regional dialects, twang of the guitars, and whiny nasal sounds of country-western singers, all coupled with the long, mournful train whistle from the steam engine moving freight to some mysterious destination. I can remember being transported off to slumberland, carried away by the sounds of the receding train whistles and strains of music from remote radio stations.

—Jerry Kuns, Technology Specialist,
California School for the Blind

CHAPTER PREVIEW

- ▶ Listening and Learning
- ▶ Listening in the Classroom: Active Listening
- ▶ Listening in the Classroom: Critical Listening
- ▶ Listening Skills for Obtaining Information: Technology

- ▸ Listening and Social Skills
- ▸ Listening as Recreation

From our own first memories of school, most of us can recall certain experiences, stories, and information shared by our teachers. Our memories may contain snippets of detail, emotions, surprises, and revelations. The majority of these memories come from what we experienced, what we listened to, and what we now remember. The early memories that we have retained from elementary school are powerful, and they influence who we are today.

In the previous chapters the importance of the development of listening skills is described for infants, toddlers, and preschool-age children who are visually impaired. The secure world at home provides the first and most important base on which children build an experiential bank for the development of listening skills that they take with them to their first school experiences in preschool and kindergarten. In this chapter the focus is on children as they continue in elementary school, from the first through the fifth grade, when they need to transition from early childhood skills such as learning to distinguish different sounds and identify their sources to the more refined abilities of attaching meaning to sounds and interpreting their more subtle and complex implications.

As in previous chapters, the skills from the Listening Skills Continuum found in Appendix A that are relevant to each domain covered in this chapter are listed in the beginning of the corresponding section.

LISTENING AND LEARNING

The learning process requires that children learn to listen. Researchers have reported that sighted elementary school children spend a majority of their schooltime listening. Children spend as much time in school listening as they spend in activities of speaking, reading, and writing combined (Harley, Truan, & Sanford, 1997; Jalongo, 1991). It follows that in order to learn successfully, children need to learn to listen skillfully; that is, they need to listen to extract meaning from what they hear.

As children continue into elementary school and develop literacy skills, the skills of listening, speaking, reading, and writing are essentially and intrinsically integrated. Children who are visually impaired continue to require attention to the development of concepts to ensure listening comprehension—that is, to ensure that they are truly comprehending what they hear. Active participation in real

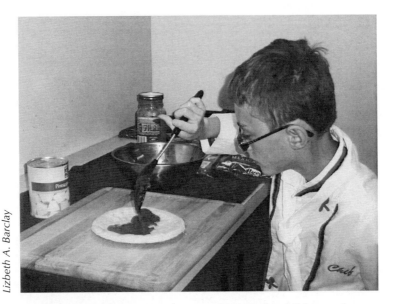

Lizbeth A. Barclay

Hands-on experiences, such as cooking, help children gain greater understanding of concepts that they hear about in the classroom and in literature.

experiences at home, in school, and in the community, providing opportunities for children to touch and manipulate real objects to give meaning to what they hear about, remain essential.

While the kindergarten curriculum usually provides many opportunities for active and experience-based learning, beginning in first grade the expectations for listening and learning in the classroom often require longer periods of sitting in groups and at desks, both listening to and participating in early literacy tasks involving beginning reading and writing. This change requires that families and educators of children who are visually impaired continue to find ways to adapt curricula and provide rich experiences that enhance listening comprehension (Koenig, 1996). Based upon their research of current (at that time) children's literature, Koenig and Farrenkopf (1997) listed the following experiences, which children typically gain through daily activities, that children who are visually impaired require in order to comprehend the literature that is read to them and that they will eventually learn to read:

- ▶ doing or making things (crafts, physical activity, cleaning up)
- ▶ experiences with friends—pretending (friends, games, competition, playing, party)
- ▶ working together, sharing, helping (helping, teams, sharing)

- ▸ looking for or finding something (mystery, treasure, finding something or someone)
- ▸ experiences in the community (community, cities, occupations, places in the community, parade, circus)
- ▸ experiences at home (parts of and objects in houses, clothes, cleaning up, sleeping)
- ▸ experiences with living creatures (animals, pets, birds, frogs, penguins, bears, buffalo, whales)
- ▸ experiencing emotions and a sense of well-being (feelings, sick, growing, freedom, imagination, jealous)
- ▸ exploring nature, plants, insects (things in the sky, outdoors, insects, water bodies, flowers, plants, forest)
- ▸ traveling or visiting others (traveling to visit relatives, friends, or places)
- ▸ experiences with books (fairy tales, legends, reading, writing, books)
- ▸ getting into trouble (breaking things, fighting, teasing, tricks)
- ▸ experiences with family and family traditions (family members, birthday, presents, special days)
- ▸ experiences with weather (weather, flooding, climate, storms)
- ▸ experiences with eating (food, meals, cooking, eating, fruits and vegetables)
- ▸ going to a farm (farm, fishing, hunting)
- ▸ learning about people who are different (blindness, braille, deafness, disability)
- ▸ exploring the arts (dancing, singing, instruments, music)
- ▸ school experiences (school, rules, practicing, alphabet, classroom, drawing)
- ▸ using different forms of transportation (transportation, flying, train, ships)

Continuing to allow the necessary time to provide deliberate explanation and hands-on experiences during these types of activities enables children with visual impairments to gain greater understanding of the concepts that they hear about in classroom instruction and literature.

Listening and Literacy Skills

Listening skills related to literacy include the following:

▸ discriminates and identifies verbal and nonverbal sounds

▸ demonstrates understanding of spoken words, syllables, and sounds (phonemes)

▸ knows and applies grade-level phonics and word-analysis skills in decoding words

▸ asks and answers questions about key details in a text read aloud or information presented orally or through other media

▸ selects the main idea, summarizes, relates one idea to another, makes inferences

▸ recounts or describes key ideas or details from a text read aloud or information presented orally or through other media

▸ connects literary texts to personal experiences and previously encountered texts to enhance understanding and appreciation

Phonemic and Phonological Awareness

It is often said that the "business" of the early elementary years of school is learning to read and write. We know that while the development of literacy skills is taking place, literacy needs to be considered within a broad context of language skills, including listening and speaking skills. The integration of the skills of listening, speaking, reading, and writing (Rex, Koenig, Wormsley, & Baker, 1994) is evident within the literacy standards developed for the Common Core State Standards for English Language Arts (2010), part of a state-led initiative to create national standards for K–12 education based on the most effective models from states across the country. The Listening Skills Continuum in Appendix A provides a sample of listening skills that are pertinent to the development of literacy skills.

Within the language arts standards there is a strong emphasis on the development of an understanding of the relationship between sounds and their symbols or letters. This understanding begins with phonemic awareness, the ability to hear and manipulate sounds in words, which can be possible only if a child has prerequisite skills in the area of auditory discrimination. *Auditory discrimination* is the ability to hear and distinguish if words sound alike or different; for example, does the word *cat* rhyme with *bat* or *ball*? Phonemes are the smallest units composing spoken language. For example, the words *go* and *she* both consist of two sounds, or phonemes (/g/o/ and /sh/e/).

The skills of phonemic awareness are practiced in many playful and yet deliberate ways through the teaching of nursery rhymes and verbal play, usually beginning in preschool. Activities that promote the development of phonemic awareness can be found in Sidebar 4.1 as well as in Chapter 3, Sidebar 3.10. Sources for additional activities can be found in the Resources section.

(((SIDEBAR 4.1

Listening Activities to Support the Development of Phonemic Awareness

Most kindergarten and early elementary classrooms feature many activities that support the listening aspect of phonemic awareness. The examples of additional activities presented here can be included during early listening or literacy instruction by family members, teachers, and related specialists.

Techniques that target phoneme awareness most frequently involve direct instruction in segmenting words into component sounds, identifying sounds in various positions in words (for example, *fan*—initial: the sound made by the letter *f*; medial: the sound made by the letter *a*; final: the sound made by the letter *n*), identifying words that begin or end with the same sound, and manipulating sounds in a word, for example, saying a word without its beginning or end sound. The following oral and listening activities can be used to support the beginning development of phonemic awareness:

DISCRIMINATING AMONG RHYMING SOUNDS
- Read aloud poems, jingles, and nursery rhymes and discuss the words that rhyme.
- Ask children to stand up if they hear words pairs that rhyme, or clap when they hear words pairs that do not rhyme (for example, *bug/rug* versus *run/hop*).
- Make up rhyme riddles, such as the following:
  ‣ "I rhyme with *hall*. You play with me. What am I?"
  ‣ "My word is *sat*. Change one letter and get something that makes a purring sound" (*cat*).
- Complete rhymes by filling in the blank:
  ‣ "I got a new *guppy*, but I wanted a _____ " (*puppy*).
  ‣ "They will *talk* while they _____ " (*walk*).
  ‣ "It's something in your mouth and rhymes with *lung*" (*tongue*).
- Give students a word and ask them to find as many words as they can that rhyme with it (for example, *fish*: *wish/dish/squish*).
- Ask students to tell you the nonrhyming word in group of three words (for example, *red/said/wet*; *guess/go/yes*; *hide/ride/he*; *cook/box/book*).
- Say a word and ask students to say a rhyming word and do the corresponding action of that word (for example, *fun*: student *runs* a few steps; *pump*: student *jumps*; *joint*: student *points*; *rat*: student *pats* the desk).

(Continued)

((SIDEBAR 4.1 *(Continued)*

DIFFERENTIATING AMONG INITIAL CONSONANT SOUNDS

- Use real objects to represent words with the same initial sound (for example, words beginning with the sound of the letter *B* can be represented by a *ball, button, balloon, box*, and so on).
- For students with low vision, make sound books or collages of pictures cut out from magazines or digital photographs to illustrate words with the same initial sound (for example, words beginning with the sound of the letter *M* might appear with pictures of a *monkey, mouse, man, milk, moon*, and the like).
- Develop skill in hearing similarity and differences of initial sounds by saying three words, two with the same beginning sound and one that is different, such as *top/boat/ ton*; or *laughed/home/little*. Ask the student to name the two words with the same beginning sound or name the word with the different beginning sound.
- Review initial consonant sounds and make up riddles for different initial word sounds (for example, "I am thinking of something to put into your backpack that you read").
- Make categories and identify words with the same beginning sounds (for example, grocery store: *bananas, bread, bacon*; animals: *pony, puppy, pig*).
- Using tongue twisters (for example, "Peter Piper," "Sally Sells Seashells") and alliteration (for example, *sweet smell of success; jump for joy; howling, hooting, hissing witch*) is a fun way to reinforce same beginning sounds.

By kindergarten children are learning phonics, the sounds that letters make, to read or spell words. These foundations for learning to read and write that require listening are established in the early years of preschool and kindergarten. In elementary school the emphasis shifts strongly to being able to connect the skills of hearing and discriminating sounds to associating them with print and braille symbols.

During these early years, children learn to identify the sounds of words and word parts, to blend sounds (such as when hearing and understanding that the combined sounds /c/a/t/ make the word *cat*) and to segment sounds (conversely, knowing that the word *cat* is comprised of the sounds /c/a/t/) within words. They also begin to learn about the sounds made by the letters (symbols).

The oral and listening work that continues to be an important part of instruction in the early elementary years is almost always paired with pictures and print. Small- and large-group instruction takes place throughout each day, providing many opportunities for children to focus on skills of rhyme, rhythm, and alliteration, phonemic awareness, including blending and segmenting, and phonic knowledge. For children with visual impairments, access to all curricular materials in large print, in braille, and with objects is essential, and equally essential is the component of listening during the instructional process.

Most literacy activities have a very strong listening aspect, but particularly important during this time is the ability to hear and distinguish sound as it is paired with braille or print symbols. Memory plays an important role in this process. When it is suspected that a child is not gaining phonemic awareness skills at a rate commensurate with that of his or her peers, it is important to consult with educators and professionals who specialize in the assessment of auditory-based learning disabilities. Following are some signs that suggest a need for this type of assessment. The student

- ▶ may mispronounce words and repeat them as they are perceived
- ▶ may have difficulty learning sound-symbol associations
- ▶ may have difficulty with sound blending
- ▶ may have difficulty with word discrimination
- ▶ may have difficulty learning to read or spell

A more complete list of characteristics that may signal auditory-based learning disabilities appears in Chapter 9. Listening activities to support the development of phonemic awareness can be found in Sidebar 4.1.

Listening Comprehension and Reading Comprehension

Jorge, a second grader who has braille instruction at the beginning of each day in the resource room, spends the rest of the day in his mainstream class, with the support of his teacher of students with visual impairments, Ms. Wells, and a part-time instructional assistant. Jorge loves his braille books, which have been creatively enhanced by Ms. Wells. He knows that each time he opens a new book he will find a variety of tactile illustrations that will be described by his teacher the first time that they read the story together. In the story about a policeman, his badge is a foil-covered star, the path that he traveled is made with pipe cleaners, and a plastic whistle is included for blowing for attention.

Jorge's teacher of students with visual impairments has also illustrated many of the books that are read to Jorge with book boxes, which contain many of the objects or parts of objects that are described in the books. For example, the book If You Give a Mouse a Cookie, *by Laura Joffe Numeroff (1985), has a box containing a cookie, cup, milk carton, straw, mirror, scissors, dust broom, sponge, blanket, pillow, crayons, tape, and paper (Drissel, 1997). When Jorge goes back to his mainstream classroom, story time is one of his favorite activities with his classmates. Sometimes he shares his book box with his friends, who also enjoy the objects that go with their story.*

There is considerable correlation between listening comprehension and reading comprehension. *Listening comprehension* involves the ability to process auditory information in which spoken language is converted to meaning or understanding (Harley et al., 1997). *Reading comprehension* is the ability to apply meaning to what is read (Ellery, 2005). When listening to stories and information presented orally at home and in school, early listeners need to learn many of the same skills necessary for reading comprehension. The following listening skills are among the skills recommended as a foundation to reading:

- attends to and recalls events in a story (auditory memory skills)
- answers simple comprehension questions
- follows a sequence in a story
- follows simple directions
- discriminates sounds
- uses a listening vocabulary sufficient for concepts in stories
- detects similarities and differences in words (Harley et al., 1997; Spache & Spache, 1973)

In the classroom, there are many opportunities for listening that are linked to literacy. Listening to poetry, fiction, and nonfiction occurs throughout each day, with the level of language vocabulary and comprehension skills ever increasing as students progress each year. Knowledgeable teachers and parents read aloud to their students and children because they know that reading aloud has long been viewed as a critical factor in a child's becoming a successful reader. Routman (2000, p. 29–30) noted that:

Being read to helps a child:

- Enjoy reading
- Develop a sense of how stories work
- Predict
- Comprehend and know
- Understand literary language
- Acquire grammar
- Notice how authors write
- Listen better
- Read more

Reading aloud to children is a wonderful way to demonstrate the joy of a good book. When parents and teachers think aloud, while predicting and summarizing as they read, and facilitate understanding by explaining complex vocabulary and ideas, they help children experience literature that they cannot yet read. For children who are visually impaired, the daily "read aloud" is just as important as it is for their classmates. For it to provide equal value, however, attention needs to be given to ensuring that students who are visually impaired truly comprehend the literature that is being read.

During the first through the third grade, many of the books read to students are beautifully illustrated, providing children with much visual information upon which to build their understanding of story concepts and vocabulary. Because these helpful images may be unavailable to students who are visually impaired, to ensure that they build their conceptual understanding while listening, it is important for parents and teachers to follow these guidelines when reading to their children:

▸ Provide a "picture walk," describing the salient features of each picture, especially as they relate to new concepts or experiences in the story.

▸ Whenever possible, provide objects that are featured in the story and pictures.

▸ Relate the pictures and concepts to a child's own prior experiences.

▸ Provide opportunities for repeated listening, questioning, and probing for understanding.

▸ For students who can use vision to view pictures, provide them with their own copy of the book whenever possible, for personal picture viewing.

▸ When an extra copy of the book is not available, provide additional time for personal picture viewing, pointing out salient features of the pictures that may be misinterpreted as a result of the child's visual impairment.

In addition, commercially published books with sounds that are adapted with braille and tactile markers can increase interest, imagery and association with objects and living things, and comprehension of content.

Children with visual impairments can gain so much information during listening when they are given the time, attention, experience, and adapted materials required to learn about the ideas and concepts presented in visual materials used in the classroom to support listening comprehension.

LISTENING IN THE CLASSROOM: ACTIVE LISTENING

Listening skills related to active listening include the following:

▸ identifies and responds to nonverbal sounds, such as a school bell, telephone, running water, and the like

▸ identifies and responds to verbal sounds and voices in the environment

▸ demonstrates listener-speaker responsibility; focuses attention on the person who is speaking (attention and reception)

▸ participates in collaborative conversations with diverse partners about class topics and texts with peers and adults in small and large groups

▸ participates in collaborative conversations with diverse partners about class topics and texts, building on others' ideas and expressing his or her own clearly

Alyssa, who is 7 years old, attends her general education first-grade class for the majority of the day. She also attends her special day class for students with visual impairments each day because she is visually impaired due to retinopathy of prematurity. Alyssa has vision in one eye only, with visual acuity of 20/400.

Each day Alyssa quietly enters her first-grade classroom with curiosity and enthusiasm to be involved in activities and discussions. She follows two classroom schedules with ease, adapting when schedules change and making appropriate adjustments. Because she has been taught to actively listen, she is able to follow directions in both her mainstream program and her special day class, giving her a sense of security and belonging in both settings.

In the elementary classroom, students listen during small- and large-group instruction to a myriad of directions and to rich and complex concepts within language arts, mathematics, science, and social studies. They are often required to shift their focus of concentration in a variety of environments within the classroom, as they listen while seated at their desks; then gather as a group while sometimes seated on the floor during circle time, for example; or participate in activity centers for small-group instruction. The listening environments and the listening content are varied and demanding.

During such classroom activities, teachers expect their students to use *active listening*; in other words, to listen attentively with the intention of understanding. Listening in the real world is an everyday skill. Listening is not synonymous with hearing; rather, it is synonymous with thinking, feeling, and responding. Hearing is an inactive, involuntary process that occurs when the ears pick up sound waves being transmitted by vibration and then forward them to the brain. Listening is an active, voluntary process that includes recognizing, comprehending, and correctly interpreting messages received. Active listening in the classroom requires participation, attention, patience, energy, and the intention to "get it"—not just what the speaker said but what he or she intended to communicate (Kovalik & Olsen, 2002).

Just as a superb topic sentence hooks the reader, use of active listening strategies is a way to get students focused and to engage the brain. According to Kovalik and Olsen:

> To actively listen, the brain must be physiologically active. Not only must it perceive the sounds correctly but it must also compare words to emotional nuances for consistency, then convert words into images that can be analyzed, compared, and used to create new understandings, and then store them for future reference. This is an extremely active process, requiring neural wiring. (Kovalik & Olsen, 2002, p. 9.7)

Active listening is critical because it is the entryway to understanding and a foundation for academic success. It requires a quiet, orderly, and intellectually rich classroom environment. In this context active listening manifests itself in a number of different ways. For most students it requires that they be "quietly attentive," with eyes that are on the teacher or speaker and "voices off." There would be a minimum of fiddling with books, pencils, and papers. For students who are visually impaired, being "quietly attentive" may appear different; for instance, the head may be bent forward and the eyes closed rather than looking forward at the teacher. But the act of active listening and "getting it"—that is, fully understanding all the nuances and meanings of what is being heard—is very important for students who are visually impaired.

"Getting it" is an interpretive process in which the student takes in information auditorily and then has the appropriate response. Whether at school or with family and friends, when a student with a visual impairment is not attending to auditory information, he or she is unable to make an appropriate response; this can be problematic. There are academic, physical, behavioral, and social implications to "getting it." The child who is not able to respond to information heard in the classroom without constant individual support will fall behind in academic skills and often be regarded as not paying attention and following directions, leading to correction and reprimand. This singles out the student as being different from peers, sometimes leading to social isolation. However, when the first-grade teacher rings a chime and sings, "It's time to change language arts centers," the youngster who is visually impaired may initially need more extensive verbal guidance and description to ensure he or she "gets it"—that is, knows where to go and what to do next. If it is suspected that the student has a particular challenge with maintaining attention in curricular or social situations, this may be caused by auditory-based learning disability, discussed thoroughly in Chapter 9.

The skill of active listening is very important in elementary school for children who are visually impaired. The following environmental and instructional strategies are necessary accommodations that facilitate the ability to accurately acquire information and respond appropriately:

▶ use of accurate and precise positional language when giving directions, for example, "Put your homework in the basket on the second shelf from the top" rather than "Put it over there"

▶ providing placement near the teacher or speaker to maximize access to instructional materials and help with attention maintenance

▶ providing direct instruction and explanation regarding how to interpret gestures, face the speaker, use eye or face contact, and signal attention, for example, by raising the hand to reply to the speaker's questions or to ask questions

▶ providing hands-on opportunities to explore materials being used, such as pictures, illustrations, diagrams, and models

Sidebar 4.2 provides additional strategies to enhance active listening skills.

((SIDEBAR 4.2
Strategies for Developing and Promoting Active Listening

FOR TEACHERS

The following strategies are often used by elementary classroom teachers to promote active listening:

• Create a comfortable listening environment by establishing classroom rules such as the following: raise a hand to contribute or speak, show respect for the person speaking, wait patiently to take a turn in a discussion, and interrupt the speaker (adult or classmate) only for emergency reasons.

• Use a calm voice and a kind tone. Through example and direct reminders, encourage students to use proper volume. Often teachers collaboratively create with their students rules for acceptable noise levels during various instructional activities (for example, a "three-inch voice" means a whisper, whereas when giving a presentation the student may use a "loud-and-proud voice").

- Consider possible sources of distractions and strive to eliminate or at least minimize them; spend time discussing how *distractions* can interfere with listening ability (define *distraction*, *concentration*, *paying attention*, and *wandering thoughts*).

- Vary instructional locations within the classroom to promote concentration. Establish listening stations with earphones for children who need sound, and quiet study areas for those who work better in silence.

- Use calming sound cues such as a chime, bell, or clicker to signal that students need to "stop" whatever they are doing; do not proceed until getting everyone's attention.

- Gently touch a student's shoulder to signal active listening.

- In kindergarten and first grade, recapture focus using a kinesthetic approach, by having students use "hook-up" arms: crossing their arms at the chest and holding each other's hands as they form a circle. This allows students to feel their heart rate and center themselves.

- Periodically throughout the day, between lessons or after sitting for some time, do sensory motor activities such as Brain Gym, an integrated sensory approach to learning through movement based on brain function research developed by Paul E. Dennison and Gail E. Dennison (1989).

- Use lots of "target talk" to remind students that active listening means listening with your eyes and ears and giving your undivided attention. Target talk is an instructional tool, appropriate for kindergarten through second grade, that labels a behavior with *who*, *what* was demonstrated, and *how* it was used; for example, "Alyssa, you were using active listening when you faced the speaker, looked interested, and were able to tell in your own words what the speaker meant."

- Establish patterns and anticipation with rhymes, songs, and sounds, such as the following:
  - Say "One and a-two, we know what to do; three and a-four, sit quietly on the floor" (appropriate for kindergarten).
  - Say and clap the rhythm, "Bump, budda, bump, bump," and students respond with, "Bump, bump."

- Teach and use sign language (appropriate for students for whom it is visually accessible).
  - Cup one's ear with one's hand or make "coyote ears"/the "peace" sign with the first and second fingers extended; then wait quietly before beginning group instruction (appropriate for third grade).
  - For individual students, use the "respect" sign (middle finger crosses index finger and thumb holds down third and fourth finger) to indicate any off-task behavior, prompting the student to think about how to be more respectful (appropriate for fourth and fifth grade).
  - Use the "zero talking" sign with thumb and first finger, forming a circle, keeping the other three fingers straight.
  - Use the fingers in an L shape near the ear to demonstrate active listening.

(Continued)

- Use focusing phrases to regain attention, such as the following:
  - ▸ "If you can hear me, raise your hand."
  - ▸ "I will go on when everyone is listening to me." (Teacher stops talking until he or she has everyone's attention.)
  - ▸ "I really like the way _____ is paying attention."
- Create mental images during listening; for example, when listening to a story, provide a "picture walk" by describing all of the important details in story illustrations or pictures that are displayed during instruction.
- Model good listening habits; communicate that listening is valued through the teacher's own listening behavior; emphasize standards of courtesy.
- Teach children to listen to one another. Coach children who are visually impaired on how to participate in discussions, how to use verbal and nonverbal signals to let others know they are listening (for example, a nod or a low-key verbal acknowledgment such as "Uh-hum" or "Exactly!"), and how to use different ways to respond appropriately.
- Have students reflect on how good it feels when others listen to them with undivided attention.
- Set a focus for meaningful listening to sustain short attention spans; provide a purpose for children's listening; for example, "We will be making our masks today, and there are three things you must remember" (appropriate for first and second grade).
- Give clear directions, using short sentences, to avoid having to repeat them; encourage students to pay attention to what is said the first time.
- Check on listening comprehension by asking students to put instructions in their own words rather than merely repeating the message.

FOR STUDENTS

Some listening behaviors require direct instruction for the student who is blind:

- Look at or toward the speaker (although it should be understood that some students who are blind may be listening when not looking at or toward the speaker).
- Use open body posture/language or nonverbal signals (head nodding, smiles, giving the thumbs-up signal) to indicate understanding.
- Offer encouraging verbal responses ("Wow!" "Uh-hum," "Really?" "Excellent!").
- Understand that an auditory cue may be paired with a gesture. For example, when the chime rings, if taught to do so, students may know to immediately put their arms up like champions (in other words, hands above the head like a champion athlete at the completion of a good play) and silently count down with their fingers from five to zero before the teacher speaks.

Active Listening and Working with a Paraprofessional

An important result of visual impairment is reduced information. This means that core curriculum and social information may be limited because it is partial or misperceived. A paraprofessional is often assigned to work with students who are visually impaired to attempt to fill some of these gaps. The responsibility of the paraprofessional is to work with the teacher in giving students with visual impairments access to accurate, rich, and meaningfully organized information about their learning environments. Sidebar 4.3 provides a list of guidelines to follow when working with paraprofessionals to this end.

All children need to listen actively as they go about everyday living and learning in elementary classrooms. By the time students with visual impairments start school, they have begun to develop a foundation of listening skills and rely heavily on their auditory abilities to participate in the classroom. Active listening is a complex task that demands that we "listen" with our eyes and ears, with our undivided attention, and with the intention to receive the intended message.

((SIDEBAR 4.3

Guidelines for Promoting Active Listening when Working with a Paraeducator

Paraeducators may play a specific supporting role for students with visual impairments, for example, preparing and ensuring that the student has access to curriculum materials, giving specific verbal directions and descriptions during instruction, and providing support for the development of social skills. Promoting independence always needs to be a priority, whether or not a student is supported by a paraeducator. To ensure that students with visual impairments gain maximum independence in listening when support is provided by a paraeducator, the following guidelines need to be observed:

- The student needs to be encouraged to listen primarily to the classroom teacher. This means that students need to be taught that whenever classroom instruction is being delivered, all conversation with others needs to stop and attention needs to be directed to the teacher.

- Let the classroom teacher serve as a clearinghouse for all questions and needs. The classroom teacher can then decide to (a) respond to the student, (b) delegate other adults or students to help, or (c) ask the student to try to work it out independently.

- Have students discreetly ask their classmates for information (for example, what page they are on, what is the school lunch, who the teacher is talking to, and so forth). Coach them to do this from home on the telephone in the evening as well as during school hours.

If a student is not learning sufficient independence when working with a paraeducator, try the following suggestions:

(Continued)

(« SIDEBAR 4.3 *(Continued)*

- Have paraeducators maintain as much distance from the student as possible. If they have been within arm's reach, have them sit just within earshot. If they have been sitting just within earshot, have them sit across the room.
- Keep a tally of the number of times in a lesson students appropriately go to their classroom teachers instead of other adults. This data will illustrate growth in listening independence or a need to develop strategies to work toward greater independence, such as setting up a system that rewards students for asking their classroom teacher questions of clarification or answering a question posed to the class.
- Tell other adults in the classroom that the paraprofessional is going to "step back" and ask them to remind the paraprofessional when this needs to be done.
- Phase out cues, such as physical and verbal prompts, so that students can take more responsibility for active listening.
- Let students make mistakes and get into trouble. It's part of the human experience!

Source: Adapted with permission from L. J. Hudson, *Classroom Collaboration* (Watertown, MA: Perkins School for the Blind, 1997).

LISTENING IN THE CLASSROOM: CRITICAL LISTENING

Listening skills that relate to critical listening include the following:

- ▶ asks and answers questions about what a speaker says in order to clarify comprehension, gather additional information, or deepen understanding of a topic or issue
- ▶ determines the purpose or purposes of listening (for example, to obtain information, to solve problems, for enjoyment)
- ▶ paraphrases information that has been shared orally by others
- ▶ connects and relates prior experiences, insights, and ideas to those of a speaker
- ▶ retells, paraphrases, and explains what has been said by the speaker
- ▶ asks thoughtful questions and responds to relevant questions with appropriate elaboration
- ▶ summarizes major ideas and supporting evidence presented in spoken messages and formal presentations

▸ listens to follow instructions that provide information about a task or assignment

▸ listens to identify essentials for note taking

As children continue into their late elementary years, the requirements of listening comprehension quickly become increasingly analytical in nature. Students are required to take the leap from the concrete to the abstract. The analysis required while listening in the classroom builds in complexity and becomes very apparent in about the second grade, as listening comprehension requirements and literacy skills shift from topics about a child's experience, such as birthday parties and getting along with friends, to content areas for students going into grade three, such as science and the metamorphosis of a caterpillar to a butterfly. By the second grade, students are learning to "ask and answer questions about what a speaker says in order to clarify comprehension, gather additional information, or deepen understanding of a topic or issue" (Common Core State Standards Initiative, 2010). The listening expectations increase because the listening requirements are more complex. Students in elementary school need to learn to interpret what has been heard, evaluate the information, and then respond to it. These are the critical listening skills that require a higher level of thinking. They begin with *sensing* (hearing) and *auditory perception* (ability to discriminate among sounds, to blend together and to hold sequences of sound in memory), which have been discussed previously. The act of *interpretation* is the same as listening comprehension. *Evaluation* combines the ability to make meaning of what has been heard and hold information in memory in order to construct both literal and inferential meaning. The highest level of listening occurs when the student can respond to what he or she has heard, because it is dependent on sensing, interpreting, and evaluating, therefore, combining *knowing* with *feeling* (Jalongo, 1991).

For the child who is visually impaired, learning to interpret the sounds in the environment is the first part of learning to listen critically. Chapter 6 specifically covers this topic. Grade school presents a complex sound environment that can be very predictable and at times unpredictable. Just as in preschool, children require the adults who are with them to explain and interpret novel sounds and experiences when they occur.

Following directions is a critical listening life skill that needs to be developed early. By improving the skill of following directions, one can make one's life easier in school (following a teacher's directions, instructions, tests, homework assignments), on the job (carrying out an employer's instructions), and in everyday life (following directions on product labels and recipes, using a manual, following directions for locating a destination). In elementary school, especially the primary grades, more extensive direct instruction may be needed in order for students to "get it" with regard to directions without the visual input.

Students who are visually impaired are required to learn how to listen critically during classroom discussion and during presentations at school and in the community. Critical listening skills are also required as they learn to access some of their curricular materials in audible formats, such as recorded textbooks. Sidebar 4.4 highlights some of the critical listening skills that are utilized when children listen to instruction as it is delivered orally by their teachers, during instructional activities, and when they listen to curriculum that is read or recorded.

((SIDEBAR 4.4
Critical Listening Skills

CRITICAL LISTENING SKILLS DURING ORAL CLASSROOM INSTRUCTION

The following skills reflect the increasing complexity of listening skills required during classroom instruction in the elementary grades:

- Determines the purpose for listening (for example, to obtain information, to solve problems, for enjoyment)
- Listens to and follows verbal directions
- Paraphrases information that has been shared orally by others
- Asks questions for clarification and responds to questions with appropriate elaboration
- Connects and relates prior experiences, insights, and ideas to those of a speaker
- Listens to acquire information about procedures and directions
- Summarizes major ideas and supporting evidence in spoken messages
- Interprets a speaker's messages, purposes, and perspectives
- Makes inferences or draws conclusions based on an oral report

**CRITICAL LISTENING SKILLS TO ACQUIRE INFORMATION
FROM FICTION AND NONFICTION**

These skills are necessary when students listen to curricular information that is read or presented during classroom instruction or performance, or that students may listen to through digital or audible recordings:

- Connects literary texts to previous life experiences to enhance understanding
- Selects the main idea, summarizes, connects ideas, and makes inferences
- Identifies elements of character, plot, and setting
- Asks for clarification and explanation of stories and ideas
- Listens to literary texts and performances to distinguish among a story, a poem, and a play
- Identifies elements of character, plot, and setting to understand the author's message or intent

Many critical listening skills are intrinsic to the specific areas of the core curriculum. For instance, in science based upon teacher presentation, a fourth grader is expected to identify and differentiate different types of minerals. For children with visual impairments, the ability to build critical listening skills depends on their cognitive ability, the foundation of experiential learning that has been carefully and deliberately provided, and access to all curricular materials throughout their education. A more comprehensive list of critical listening skills for elementary school students is included in The Listening Skills Continuum in Appendix A. Sidebar 4.5 suggests some activities that support the development of critical listening skills.

((• SIDEBAR 4.5

Strategies and Activities to Help Develop Critical Listening Skills

LEARNING TO INTERPRET SOUND

- Train students to learn to be aware of direction cues or signals that get someone's attention, such as a chime, siren, fire alarm, telephone, timer, recess bell, and the like. Discuss sounds that are important and talk about why they are.
- Discuss what sounds the children like or dislike and why.
- Pair listening to the sound of objects with the actual object (timer, hand dryer, running water in a sink, microwave, chime).
- Analyze sounds during "listening walks" on the school campus and within the community, making associations between the sound and the area of the school to which it belongs (playground noises, lunchroom, photocopy machine) or between the sound and what is occurring in the community (leaf blower, siren, honking horn, dog barking).
- Point out characteristics of the sound—shrillness, hissing, pulsating beat. Categorize sounds as loud, soft, near, far, high, low, harsh, or pleasant. Short phrases can trigger a child's creative thinking about sounds around them (for example, "As quiet as a _____ " or "The noisiest place I know is _____ .").
- Analyze and identify voices (parents, teachers, classmates).

FOLLOWING VERBAL DIRECTIONS

- State directions so that each step in a series is presented in the exact order in which it is to be performed (for example, "Take out your book. Turn to page 72. Read the first paragraph.").
- Use words within the child's listening vocabulary, being careful to determine what needs to be clarified. For example, if positional or ordinal concepts are used, such as *center*, *left corner*, or *fifth line*, explicitly teach these concepts before using them.
- Use sequencing words and specifics—*first, second, after that, then, finally*—that add clarity to directions.

(Continued)

- "Chunking" directions can be effective using the "praise-prompt-leave" approach (for example, "I like the way you have your first and last name on your paper. Now braille the date. I need to step away to help another student, but I will come back to you in just a minute.").
- Encourage the student who is visually impaired to ask questions about unclear points.
- In class activities, make a policy of not repeating instructions. Inform students that they will be asked to repeat instructions. If repetition is necessary, have the student first ask a peer to repeat what was stated.
- After listening to messages on the school's public address system, have the students summarize the announcements.
- Reading aloud directions for a new game is a fun and social way to reinforce this skill. Directions need to tell how many players can play, describe the equipment needed, explain the game in proper order, tell how to score, and indicate how the winner is decided.

RECALLING FACTS AND DETAILS
- Read aloud one-sentence statements, a short paragraph, and then a long paragraph. Each time, ask students to restate as many details as possible.
- Teach how to take simple listening notes. Play the familiar game, "I am going on a trip and I am taking with me a/an _____." (Students can write or braille each new item.)
- For upper grades, riddles and jokes present a great opportunity for detailed listening as well as for creative sharing in conversations. Listeners need to remember the details to deliver the humor in the punch line.

IDENTIFYING SEQUENTIAL ORDER
- Read aloud a paragraph in which students then recognize or restate, from a list of choices orally given, the order of three events or objects in a sequence or list given.
- Use tactile reinforcement by using the student's hand to sequence events in a story by touching each finger as you say *first, next, then, after that*, and *finally*.
- After listening to a biographical story, list facts on paper, cut the list of facts into strips, and have students put the strips in sequential order to make a timeline. Use tactile material such as Wikki Stix (waxed pipe cleaners that can be bent into various shape) to "draw" a long line from left to right across another paper, or add little vertical pieces of Wikki Stix for each fact, then glue brailled or large-print strips on the paper.

DETERMINING THE MAIN IDEA
- Create brief headlines for newspaper articles or after oral story sharing.
- Listen to brief paragraphs from informational sources, offer three or four possible statements of the main idea, and have the student select the best option.

- For upper elementary students, listen to a recorded speech section by section. Stop the player after each section, discuss what the main idea is, and write it down. If this procedure is repeated for each section, the result will be a listing of main ideas and the beginning of an outline form.

SUMMARIZING

- When children are absent from class, give those present the assignment of summarizing and orally sharing the instructions absentees missed.
- Build purpose into beginning note taking by following up with an oral sharing time. Students refer to their own notes in the follow-up summary discussion.
- Give a daily listening assignment in which students listen each night for 15 minutes to a selection of grade-level literature in audible format.
- Have students keep a listening journal, in which they summarize what they've heard by listing, in order, three events using their appropriate writing medium.

LISTENING SKILLS FOR OBTAINING INFORMATION: TECHNOLOGY

At 7 years of age, Sam writes out one of many stories from his very vivid imagination on his electronic braille notetaker (personal digital assistant). He uses this device daily in his second-grade classroom routine. Hundreds of children's books from the Internet, most from electronic book sources, have been downloaded for Sam. Some of these books have been embossed and bound into traditional paper braille books, while many are transferred to Sam's electronic braille notetaker via an external storage device. The teacher of students with visual impairment and Sam agreed that he is expected to read the device's refreshable braille display with his fingers for at least 20 minutes to reinforce braille reading skills. After that he also is allowed to use the voice output feature if he so desires. While reading with his fingers, if he discovers a word or braille contraction he does not understand, he can easily route the cursor to that location and have that word spoken, the braille symbols announced, and the word spelled out. Using his listening skills reinforces his braille reading development.

Success in school, home, community, employment, and life is directly influenced by one's ability to gain access to information. The so-called information age, sparked by the widespread availability of information through computers and the Internet, is expanding our knowledge base at an incredible rate. Use of technology plays a critical role in all our lives, and it offers enormous benefits to children as young as preschool age. By the time youngsters are in first or second grade they need to be able to engage in information processing with technology.

Specialized technology is required to enable students with visual impairments to have access to the same information content as their sighted classmates. The Individuals with Disabilities Education Act (IDEA), the federal law governing education for children with disabilities in the United States, includes the following definition:

> The term *assistive technology device* means any item, piece of equipment or product system, whether acquired commercially off the shelf, modified, or customized, that is used to increase, maintain, or improve functional capabilities of a child with a disability (Individuals with Disabilities Education Act Amendments of 1997, 20 U.S.C. Section 1401, sect. 602 [22]).

Just as listening skills are included in states' language arts content standards and the expanded core curriculum for students who are visually impaired, technology skills are also components of both of these curricula. In developing the basic subject components of the expanded core curriculum, Hatlen included technology because "it's a tool to unlock learning and expand horizons: it can be the great equalizer. . . . It enhances communication and learning and expands the world of blind and visually impaired persons in many significant ways" (Hatlen, 1996).

Many states and school districts recognize the importance of technology in elementary schools to enhance students' access to information as a resource for education and recreation. The International Society for Technology in Education (2007) is in the process of updating and revising the National Educational Technology Standards. It is common for students to become proficient in technology skills starting with the earliest grades in elementary school, as illustrated by the following examples from two California school curricula (Millbrae School District, 2010; San Mateo–Foster City School District, 2008):

▸ Kindergarteners learn proper handling of electronic storage media such as digital video disks (DVDs) when interacting with a program, educational game, or application using a mouse, keyboard commands, or touch screen. They also learn to create art work using software illustration programs.

▸ First graders focus on keyboarding skills.

▸ Second graders begin simple report writing using sentences with graphics from software illustration programs.

▸ Third graders are introduced to the Internet and begin to learn slide show presentation programs.

▸ Continued use of the Internet and slide show software for research projects and other writing assignments occurs in fourth grade.

▸ By the end of fifth grade, students create documents using word-processing applications incorporating text, graphics, and sound from the Internet.

Technology is firmly ensconced in our elementary schools, and sighted students are being introduced to computers and other electronic information systems at very young ages. Since most of the available curricular information is presented visually on the computer screen or whiteboard in text, color, and graphics, it is essential that students who are blind have access to equivalent information through auditory and tactile media. It is imperative that students with visual impairments develop the same, or parallel, skills as their sighted classmates to ensure that they will be able to keep pace with a rapidly changing, technology-rich educational environment.

One method of obtaining access to electronic information is to have a sighted person, such as a paraeducator, classmate, or teacher, verbalize what is on the screen by describing a scene, settings, or diagrammatic information. Students who are visually impaired need to develop the auditory interpretive skills to organize and classify such verbalized information. The ability to understand and absorb this information described verbally requires a high level of understanding, making the continued building of concepts that occurs during guided listening, paired with a wide range of experiences, as discussed earlier in this chapter, essential for students to successfully access and utilize assistive technology. Table 4.1 provides an overview of the technology processes that students learn in which listening is an important mode for learning and skill development in school and at home.

Assistive Technology Tools Featuring Listening to Enhance Literacy Skills

The role that assistive technology has increasingly played in enhancing literacy skills in recent years cannot be overstated. As the use of technology in public schools has marched forward for all students, the advancements and application of assistive technology for students with visual impairment continue to develop and improve, providing greater opportunities for literacy growth and access. Presley and D'Andrea (2009, p. 8) list three major ways in which technology supports literacy for students who are blind or visually impaired:

TABLE 4.1

Technology and Listening Skills

Skill	Grade Level	Comments and Precursor Skills
Listening to audio materials such as books, Internet, radio, and television	Preschool through high school	Children begin to listen to recorded books in preschool for pleasure. By early elementary grades (first grade), listening centers can be found in classrooms. In the upper elementary grades (fourth grade), students should have regular listening assignments to help prepare them for later curricular listening, for example, note-taking.
Listening to curriculum on an interactive audio/tactile learning system such as the SAL2 System.	Can begin in pre-kindergarten and be used as long as helpful	Listening plays an important role in literacy skill development when using speech-assisted learning devices.
Listening to an electronic braillewriter such as the Mountbatten Brailler	Can begin from preschool to first grade	This tool is useful for pre-braille learners so they can "doodle" around, starting to get auditory feedback between braille dots and the shape of the dots in a cell, and then associating the dots with character sound; this tool also helps students learn the braille code.
Listening to an accessible PDA (electronic notetaker) with braille or speech output or both	Can begin when the student understands the braille code and is an early reader; student must demonstrate responsibility for care of equipment	Children can begin learning to use an electronic braillewriter as soon as they can read and braille the alphabet. Learning new contractions is supported when students listen to their voiced braille output.
Listening and interacting with auditory games and keyboarding tutor programs on computer	Can begin playing cause-and-effect games as a preschooler; can begin keyboarding in first or second grade	Instruction in word processing typically begins when students are beginning readers and writers, having knowledge of the alphabet and word reading and writing.
Listening to labels on tactile maps, diagrams, drawings, or courseware	Begins in pre-kindergarten, continuing through elementary school	Children can learn tactile exploration skills when using interactive touch tablets with labeled graphic overlays such as those provided by the SAL2 System.

Skill	Grade Level	Comments and Precursor Skills
Listening to a screen reader while using the computer	Third grade	Students must have basic keyboarding skills.
Listening to audible literature on digital players or recorders, computers, electronic notetakers, and accessible PDAs	Third grade	Students should have plenty of regular exposure to and understanding of typical print and braille formats. Listening to audible literature and curricular material does not take the place of print and braille literacy skills.
Listening while using scanning programs	May begin in fourth or fifth grade or middle school	Listening plays an important role in learning to use this valuable skill that will lead to increased independence.
Listening while using GPS	Depends on student's skill level	Use of these devices is covered in Chapter 6: "Listening Skills for Orientation and Mobility: Hearing the Whole Picture."

▶ It enables students to access print and electronic text.

▶ It enables students to produce written communication.

▶ It enables students and the professionals who work with them to produce materials in accessible formats.

The use of technology also supports children as they are initially acquiring literacy skills. In addition to touch, listening is essential for many aspects of technology access and, reciprocally, the use of these tools reinforces and enhances listening and learning and the development of literacy skills. For example, a student who is learning to use her electronic braille notetaking device or personal digital assistant (PDA) (see Sidebar 4.6) can hear a letter, contraction, or word announced in synthetic speech as she brailles it and then again when she reads it back on the device's braille display, reinforcing the learning of the new braille concepts. Hearing new contractions voiced as she brailles them gives her important feedback about the accuracy of her newly learned braille concept. Or, for the student with low vision, who uses screen enlargement software, added voice output can provide reinforcement for literacy skills.

The next sections highlight modes and tools of assistive technology that both require and enhance listening skills during learning.

Specialized Hardware

Touch Screens and Touch Tablets

There are a number of reading and writing tools for students who are blind or have low vision, providing speech output or auditory feedback that enhances the development of literacy skills. Touch screens and touch tablets that have audio output are appropriate for early learners. These touch tablets are connected to computers. When a preprogrammed braille sheet is placed on the tablet, students are instructed, via voice commands from the computer, to read the braille sheets or complete an activity on the braille sheet. Students press the braille and receive immediate auditory feedback. For example, if a student does not know a word on the sheet, he or she can press the word and hear how it is pronounced, spelled, and contracted. With these tools, students get immediate auditory feedback and reinforcement as to what is being felt—character, word, or braille contraction. Also with these tools, diagrams, charts, graphs, maps, or simple pictorial representations may be enhanced with audio labels to support the audio tactile learning process.

Electronic Braillewriters and Accessible PDAs

In addition to accessible PDAs (see Sidebar 4.6), the electronic braillewriter is a writing tool that has the capacity to speak the words being input as one writes, thus reinforcing the learning process through auditory feedback. Electronic braillewriters

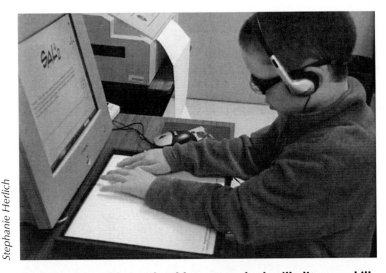

Stephanie Herlich

Students using this touch-tablet system for braille literacy skill development receive immediate auditory feedback when they place their fingers on the braille sheet.

Personal Digital Assistants

An accessible personal digital assistant (PDA)—previously known as an electronic notetaker—is a portable electronic device that functions in many ways like an accessible laptop computer. Input is accomplished through either a braille keyboard or a QWERTY keyboard. The output is through synthetic speech created by a text-to-speech software. Output may also be provided in refreshable braille—a row of plastic pins configured in the shape of braille cells that pop up and down to form the braille characters of the text being read.

When portable notetakers were first introduced in 1979 they had limited capabilities. Today, however, "PDAs with braille and/or speech access are commonly used technology tools by students with visual impairments. They are well-established as effective tools for students who need braille or speech access for personal productivity, communication, and access to information" (McNear & Kuns, 2006). PDAs commonly include "smart phones, palmtops, hand-helds and other portable information units with a suite of software for the Internet, calendar, address book, GPS, word processer and more. There are some commercial products which are partially or mostly accessible and several units tailored for people who are blind, with every feature and function being accessible through speech and/or braille" (Mike May, CEO, Sendero Group, personal communication, 2010). The many features available make *PDA* a more accurate description of these devices than just *notetaker*. PDAs expand the options students have to master literacy skills, especially listening to books and accessing the Internet.

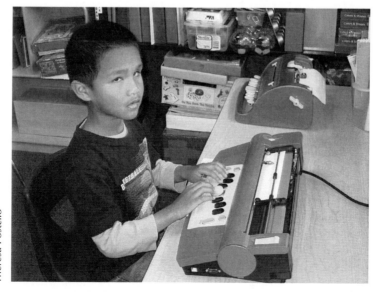

Theresa Postello

This electronic writing tool, the Mountbatten Brailler, has the capacity to speak characters and words as the student inputs them, thus reinforcing the learning process through auditory feedback.

require less finger strength than traditional mechanical braillewriters and have a variety of features in addition to speech, such as memory and correction features. Unlike PDAs, they emboss the brailled text, but they do not have the many other features of PDAs. Depending on the student's skill level, the electronic braillewriter with speech can be introduced in preschool or kindergarten, and an accessible PDA may be useful as soon as first or second grade when the child's basic literacy skills are sufficient.

The braille keyboards of these devices consist of six main keys, each corresponding to one of the dots of a braille cell, plus a space bar. Additional keys may be used to represent Dots 7 and 8, new line, back space, or other keyboard functions.

((SIDEBAR 4.7
Controlling Speech on Braille Devices

The speech features of most electronic braillewriters and accessible braille PDAs allow for echoing of characters, words, or both characters and words while writing in braille. For "character echo," every keystroke has a spoken label such as /d/-/e/-/ar sign/. For "echo words," the system is silent while the letters are input until the space bar is pressed at the end of the word, at which time the group of characters is voiced as a word—/dear/. In "spell mode" or "key-echo mode," a child learning braille can get audio verification of letters and numbers; in "word mode" the child can hear whole-word contractions, short-form words, initial or final contractions, and dot numbers. Spell mode is a feature available on many assistive technologies to speak the word, speak the braille characters, or spell the word. Key-echo mode is an input feature, whereas "spell mode" is a navigation or review feature. As students with visual impairment progress, they can get feedback on all braille symbols, which reinforces the finger-muscle memory through immediate auditory association.

The speech output on these devices can be controlled in a variety of ways. Initially, students learn to make adjustments to the speech preferences by customizing the volume, voice (for example, male, female, or child), pitch, and rate (speed) to suit their listening styles. When does listening to accelerated speech start to occur? Does it naturally happen that students change the rate setting on their devices to accelerate the speech heard as they become more used to hearing it? There is little objective data about how quickly and accurately younger students can understand by listening at accelerated rates or about the most suitable listening rates. Generally, good listeners adapt their rate to the purpose of listening. The rate used is determined by how much information is to be gleaned from the material as well as by the complexity of the auditory material. Just as in reading, there are different listening speeds. Using a faster listening rate may be equated to skimming in reading situations where the student is quickly listening for a particular fact, when the student needs to cover a large amount of material that is not important, or when the student is "pre-listening" before listening for details. It seems that the best pitch and rate for a particular listener depend on subjective preferences.

Early learners can explore keys, symbols, and other commands on the electronic braillewriter or PDA to get auditory feedback. For example, while writing a sentence such as "The kitty drank cream, ate food and slept" using a PDA with a braille display and speech output, a second grader might discover that pressing the Dot 2 key gives her new contraction information about the comma and /ea/ sign. Symbols such as the dollar sign are discovered by pressing /dropped d/ with the number sign. Pressing /e with spacebar/ may take the student to Exit or Escape. Sidebar 4.7 explains more about the kind of feedback provided by the speech features on these devices and how they can be controlled.

Computers and Specialized Software

Listening plays a very important role for students with visual impairments when they are learning how to type on a standard computer keyboard. Keyboarding skills can be developed rapidly and efficiently with interactive, auditory tutorials that provide instruction and reinforcement for correct key presses. It is critical to begin computer keyboarding and typing skills as early as possible. There are typing programs that speak while displaying lessons and games on the screen. Adjustments can be made for the student's skill level and visual impairment. The quality of the synthetic speech can reduce fatigue for audio users. It can also affect understandability of the utterances.

As soon as students become proficient with keyboard basics, they need to start learning keyboard commands for the Windows or Macintosh operating systems used on computers and other electronic devices. Students use keystrokes to perform equivalent functions to those of "clicking" and "dragging" with a mouse for managing features and functions of desired applications such as word processors, slideshow presentations, spreadsheets, Internet, e-mail, instant messaging, accessing media files, and so on. Learning keyboard commands is an essential skill for students with visual impairments if they are to be competitive with their sighted peers at school and in later employment. Students use a variety of assistive technology software to access information on the computer screen, such as talking word-processing programs, screen readers, screen magnification with speech, and scanners with optical character recognition. These programs all require keyboarding skills to control the application and access the information; however, a program with speech output voices what is on the screen, thus giving the user auditory feedback as keys are pressed.

Audiobooks

An audiobook is a live spoken recording of a book that may be an exact word-for-word version of the original printed work (unabridged) or a shortened or otherwise modified (abridged) version. An audiobook may be dramatized with multiple readers playing various parts and enhanced with music and sound effects.

Listening to live readers such as parents and caregivers, siblings, and teachers usually precedes listening to audiobooks. Discussion about listening comprehension and reading comprehension is found earlier in this chapter, as well as in Chapter 3. There is a sequence or continuum of learning to listen to recorded literature and curriculum materials; in other words, as a child learns to listen, simple sentence structures are expanded to include more complex content to correspond with the development of their more complex language and educational curricula.

A beginning first-grade student who is visually impaired most likely has already been listening to audiobooks for recreation and enjoyment. Language arts curriculum materials are the most suitable to supplement reading with listening at this level. Listening centers in first- and second-grade classrooms often use print/braille books—usually picture books with a plastic overlay on the pages containing a braille version of the text—in tandem with audiobooks to reinforce literacy and listening skills for students who are visually impaired.

Reading requirements increase by the beginning of fourth grade, but often students' reading rates in braille and large print have not increased to accommodate these curricular demands. Results of the Alphabetic Braille and Contracted Braille Study (ABC Braille Study) found that the fourth graders within the study had oral braille reading rates that were just half the oral print reading rates of their classmates without visual impairments (Emerson, Holbrook, & D'Andrea, 2009). As educators in the field of visual impairment continue to strive to increase their students' reading fluency, it is essential that students also learn to skillfully utilize listening skills to support and augment their literacy skills. If audiobooks are used to supplement text, students can listen to curricular materials that are at their comprehension level, helping to maintain grade-level proficiency.

Both sighted students and those with visual impairments have enjoyed commercially produced audiobooks on cassette tape and compact disc (CD) to enhance their education. Students who are blind or have low vision have been using specialized cassette tape players to listen to four-track talking books and other recorded material since the 1960s, primarily those recorded by the National Library Service for the Blind and Physically Handicapped and Recording for the Blind and Dyslexic (now Learning Ally). Audiobooks now being produced specifically for individuals who are visually impaired or have other print disabilities are in digital format, as discussed in the next section. However, cassettes and CDs are still in use, and older books are often in these formats.

The features of the players designed for these formats include controls for adjusting volume, speed, and pitch to provide a comfortable rate of listening. A feature for tape players known as *tone indexing* bookmarks locations in the recording with a series of beeps that can be heard while the user is fast-forwarding or rewinding the tape. Strategies for efficiently understanding and gathering information available on audiotape present challenges, as noted by one assistive technology specialist:

> Students must learn to listen and organize what they hear into a framework. All auditory information is linear in nature. One cannot hear more than one character or word at a time. This sequential presentation requires a different organizational process than is required tactilely or visually. When a person perceives a page of print, the eye may be able to take in a *gestalt*, an overview or framework in which the content is organized. With the use of attributes on a screen or print page, one's attention can be drawn to important content through the use of unit headings, bold, italicized or underlined passages and bullets. Whereas in hard-copy braille one can easily get some basic format elements such as centered, separations, titles, paragraphs, or columns, one cannot easily distinguish italics or underlined materials efficiently. For other attributes such as bold, highlighting or color print, an 8-dot electronic braille display can be set up to indicate the presence of such attributes under the braille characters.
>
> This is not possible auditorily. Tone-indexing or beeptone features are imprecise. One can assemble information into a framework but only if the content can be accessed by page, chapter, section, heading, subheading, paragraph, or phrase, yet still only at one character or word at a time. (Jerry Kuns, Technology Specialist, California School for the Blind, personal communication, 2010)

Although audiocassettes produced in analog format still exist as of this writing, the technology is rapidly being replaced by e-books and digital audiobooks, as already noted. Among their benefits, these digital books provide much more efficient navigation controls. Choices of all manner of information are far broader because of digital book access.

Digital Books

For the purposes of this book, the term *digital book* can refer to two types of media:

1. **Digital text or e-books**. E-books are text-based, computer-coded files that are listened to via synthesized speech or read with a refreshable braille display.

2. **Digital talking books that are recordings of live speech**. A digital voice recording is made by a live reader or narrator and may include sound effects and music. This digital recording requires some type of accessible

media player, such as a CD player, e-book reader, PDA, smart phone, or computer.

An electronic book—also known as an e-book or e-text—is coded text that can be made audible with text-to-speech software using a synthesized voice read on a computer, an accessible PDA, or a specialized device or with a refreshable braille display on one of these devices. Some sources of electronic children's books and textbooks that can be downloaded from the Internet are listed in the Resources section.

Specialized adapted players, other hardware devices, or software that installs on standard multimedia computers or accessible PDA with speech output are required to access digitally recorded books and e-text files.

Digitized text requires software and firmware (semipermanent programs within a computer or device) that converts computer text to synthesized speech output. This is commonly known as *text-to-speech* conversion software, which is a component of screen-reading and some text-enlarging software. Many modern adaptive devices can play both digitized speech and text-to-speech content.

Digital books including e-text and live recorded media are produced to a standard known as DAISY, or Digital Accessible Information System standard. (See Sidebar 4.8 for more information about DAISY.) This technology enables a student who is visually impaired to navigate through a book in a manner that is more comparable to the way a print book is used. For example, students can examine the book by page, section, or chapter or use a table of contents or an index. Students are able to interact with the material while listening by setting bookmarks and taking notes. Markers can be placed in the DAISY book to allow more efficient navigation (in other words, by paragraph, section, and page). In many devices, personal markers or electronic bookmarks can be inserted to flag special passages for study and further review; this applies to both e-text and live recorded media.

Audio-Assisted Reading

The ability to skillfully and efficiently gain access to all curricular materials is essential for all students with visual impairments. While learning to read and write is a primary goal, it is also the responsibility of educators to teach skills necessary to enable students to have choices of all types of learning media as curricular demands and volume increase. This includes the skills of listening to gain information.

Sometimes students choose to simply listen to literature that has been recorded, such as during recreational listening, but more often they use their audible curricular materials in tandem with braille or print textbooks. *Audio-assisted reading* was a term coined by Carol Evans in 1997 when designing a method for students with visual impairments and learning disabilities to use recorded books along with the correspond-

((Sidebar 4.8

DAISY, NIMAS, and NIMAC

The development of new tools for listening for people with visual impairments and other print disabilities started with the development of digital books and the founding of a new organization, known as the DAISY Consortium, committed to developing equitable access to information for people who have print disabilities. DAISY is an acronym that stands for Digital Accessible Information System and refers to a standard created by the consortium for producing accessible and navigable multimedia documents. In current practice, these documents are digital talking books, digital textbooks, or a combination of synchronized audio and text materials. DAISY is a globally recognized technical standard to facilitate the creation of accessible content. The standard was originally developed to benefit people who are unable to read print due to a disability such as visual impairment or learning disability, but it also has broad applications for improved access to text in the mainstream. The DAISY standard continues to evolve, and its features are now incorporated into the mainstream e-book format ePub3. For example, Google Books has downloadable public domain books in ePub3 format. (For further information, see www.daisy.org/about_us.)

A significant feature of the 2004 amendments to the Individuals with Disabilities Education Act (IDEA), the main federal program authorizing state and local aid for special education and related services for children with disabilities, was the addition of sections mandating the provision of textbooks and instructional materials in accessible formats for students who are blind, have low vision, or are print disabled, so they receive them at the same time students receive print materials. The mechanism created for doing so is the provision of the source files for print instructional materials by K–12 curriculum publishers in a standardized electronic format known as the National Instructional Materials Accessibility Standard, or NIMAS. NIMAS is a subset of DAISY.

These files are sent to the National Instructional Materials Access Center (NIMAC), a repository for the files established at the American Printing House for the Blind in Louisville, Kentucky. NIMAC receives and catalogs publishers' electronic files in a standard format: NIMAS. These standardized files enable authorized producers to create student-ready versions of textbooks and other core print instructional materials in braille, digital talking books, and large print for students across the country who are blind, visually impaired, or print disabled.

The combination of a standard format and a central repository significantly expedites the time frame in which instructional materials are delivered to students who need them in the classroom. Improved access and expanded learning opportunities for all students have resulted from DAISY, NIMAS, and NIMAC.

ing book in regular print, large print, magnified print, or braille. The method "allows the reader to use all available avenues of sensory input simultaneously to acquire and process information" (Evans, 2005). (The term *audio-supported reading* also is used.) While designed for use with students with additional learning challenges, the method has distinct advantages for many students who are learning to listen to recorded curricular materials on any of the great variety of listening tools described earlier. In many if not most digitized textbooks that consist of text extracted from the print files, visual materials such as illustrations, charts, graphs, and maps have not been described. In addition, format informs the reader/listener about the structure and hierarchy of the information presented that is not available by only listening. If the listener/reader is following along in the print or braille book, he or she is able to gain valuable information from examination of the illustrations.

Learning to utilize audible learning materials is a skill that needs to be deliberately taught. The curricular goals for these students are

▸ comprehension of information

▸ determining what information is important

▸ learning to listen for that information

Students can be prepared for listening for specific information by providing them with the prereading/listening strategies presented in Sidebar 4.9.

((SIDEBAR 4.9
Instructional Strategies for Audio-Assisted Reading

Learning to utilize audible learning materials is a skill that for many students needs to be deliberately taught. The curricular goals for these students are comprehension of information, determining what information is important, and learning to listen for that information. Students can be trained to listen for *who, what, when, where, how,* and *why* by providing them with prereading/listening questions.

Start by using materials of particular interest to the student. Examples of such high-interest materials include recordings of newspaper or magazine articles, Internet shows, audiobooks, and radio programs or podcasts from radio shows.

STAGE 1
- Using high-interest materials, locate or record three- to five-minute selections.
- Prepare simple *who, what, when,* and *where* questions (at least one per paragraph) in sequential order (that is, in the order in which the information occurs within the passage).
- Provide the questions in the student's preferred learning medium.
- Have the student read all questions before listening, or read them to the student and discuss them.

- Have the student reread the first question.
- Tell the student he or she can stop at any time and review the question.
- Tell the student to start listening and stop when he or she hears the answer to the first question (the teacher listens along with student).
- Have the student provide the answer (verbally, in print, or in braille) when he or she hears it.
- If the student does not provide the answer, ask the student leading questions in an effort to guide him or her to the answer.
- Repeat the preceding steps with different selections.
- Have the student practice using headphones without teacher support.

Follow the steps in Stage 1 of this process until the student achieves greater than 80 percent accuracy.

STAGE 2

- Increase listening time by using one question for every two paragraphs.
- Begin providing questions out of sequence.
- Return to one question per paragraph, but change the order of questions; for example, ask questions about paragraphs 2, 1, 3, 5, 4, 6, and so on.
- Ask the student, "What do the questions ask about?"
- Guide the student to understanding that the questions are asking *who, what, when,* and *where.*

Follow the steps in Stage 2 of this process until the student achieves greater than 80 percent accuracy.

STAGE 3

- Continue using high-interest materials.
- Record longer passages and stories.
- Use short articles from magazines.
- Return to sequential questions.
- Provide one question for about every two paragraphs.
- Start introducing some *how* and *why* questions.
- Introduce short chapters in books.

STAGE 4

- Do not provide the questions before reading.
- Ask the student to stop after several paragraphs.
- Ask two or three simple sequential questions about the content just heard.
- Once the student demonstrates proficiency, start asking nonsequential questions.

(Continued)

(« Sidebar 4.9 *(Continued)*

STAGE 5
- Continue using high-interest materials.
- Ask the student to read a selection at home.
- Discuss the content with the student without quizzing.

STAGE 6
- Begin using materials of less than high interest. (These materials can be found by consulting with a reading specialist. Ask for materials that have been recorded and have written questions.)
- Use the same strategies as with high-interest materials.

INTRODUCING TEXTBOOKS
Phase 1
- In order to ensure a successful first experience, begin with a chapter that has been previously covered in class.
- Use the same strategies as with high-interest materials.
- Ask sequential questions for each paragraph, page, or section. (The objective is for the student to have continued success, even though the content may be more complicated and of less interest.)

Phase 2
- Provide an outline of the chapter with headings and subheadings.
- Insert bulleted points or statements regarding important information, but leave blanks for some of the important words. Make it easy for the first few times until the student is performing at greater than 80 percent accuracy. Then make it a bit harder by requiring the student to fill in a short phrase or group of words.
- Leave adequate space for the student's answers.
- Ask at least one or two questions for each subsection of a chapter.
- Have the student fill in the outline with answers to questions and other important information.

Ike Presley
Project Manager
American Foundation for the Blind
Atlanta, Georgia

Additional Talking Technology

A variety of adaptive devices with audible output provide access to essential information for education, recreation, and daily living. State-of-the-art technology allows the user to hear words, numbers, and tones that provide qualitative and quantitative information, directions, measurements, and menu options. Students need to apply their listening skills to using these products as well. These products require the listener to make interpretive judgments such as near/far or left/right, follow step-by-step directions, and make quantitative comparisons. Each of these processes requires the development of listening skills for decision making.

There are a number of commercially available audible products, including the following:

▸ educational products: dictionaries, globes, maps, calculators, tape measures, puzzles, and dice

▸ recreation and orientation and mobility products: Global Position System (GPS), compasses, pedometers, balls, accessible pedestrian signals (APS)

▸ daily living/kitchen products: scales, thermometers, measuring cups, microwave ovens, pouring aids, light probes, color identifiers, watches, clocks, timers, glucose and blood pressure monitors, talking caller ID

Many off-the-shelf products have high-quality digital voice output, but others do not. All of these products can generally be understood and are useful. Having the opportunity to select tools from a well-stocked toolbox is essential in assisting students who are blind or visually impaired throughout their school years.

It is important to expose students to the range of assistive technology devices that allows them to access information electronically. Visit a conference exhibit hall where vendors and consumers who are visually impaired can provide hands-on demonstrations. Take a field trip to local agencies for individuals who are blind or visually impaired where students can examine and try out different technologies. Invite vendors to teacher staff meetings to showcase product lines. Ongoing specialized assessment regarding the technology needs of students who are visually impaired is required under the Individuals with Disabilities Education Act (Presley & D'Andrea, 2009). Formal assistive technology assessments are available through public and private sources to help identify the appropriateness of available technologies. Keep in mind that "a good assessor is one who is knowledgeable and proficient with computers, possesses expertise with the assistive technology devices used in the assessment, has knowledge of visual impairment, and is objective" (Anderson, 2003, p. 246).

Instruction in using listening skills early in the elementary grades takes on an important role in the preparation for reading digital books and textbooks in braille and large print supported with auditory feedback. Students who are blind or have low vision now have greater opportunities than ever before to acquire information through assistive technology tailored to their unique, individual needs. Even though technological advancements occur at rapid rates, the skill of listening retains its value.

LISTENING AND SOCIAL SKILLS

Listening skills related to social skills include the following:

> ▸ identifies tone of voice, such as humorous, sad, angry, silly
> ▸ builds on others' talk in conversations by responding to the comments of others through multiple exchanges
> ▸ follows agreed-on rules for discussion (for example, gaining the floor in respectful ways, listening to others with care, speaking one at a time about the topics and texts under discussion)
> ▸ demonstrates turn-taking ability in conversations and when playing with peers
> ▸ listens to locate and identify a specific peer and ask the student to play
> ▸ listens to join in a group that is playing or conversing

Many people would agree that a high quality of life correlates closely with the quality of our friendships. Indeed, the ability to make and maintain social connections is critical to life success for all young people, both with and without disabilities (Wolffe, 2006). Listening plays an important role in the development of social skills for children, and adults require listening skills in order to demonstrate interest in others and develop social connections. The ability to develop relationships with others, and to interact effectively with them, rests on being able to hear and listen to their statements and concerns, understand what is being conveyed, and be responsive in an appropriate way.

In the elementary school years children become more concerned about establishing and maintaining friendships, expecting their friends to demonstrate loyalty and trust. Children at this age are generally more tuned into and concerned about the opinions of their peers (Erin, 2006). The friendships of students with visual impairments, like those of their peers, are based on common interests and social roles (Rosenblum, 2000).

The social development of children who are visually impaired is dependent on a variety of experiences during their formative years and requires the support of parents, educators, and peers. Because their experiences outside of their immediate environment often can be limited, the social language of children who are blind may reflect more ego-centered experiences. This potential limitation is why the quantity and quality of experiences the child has with other children and adults is so vital (Sacks, 2006). To develop the understanding and ability to comfortably discuss common topics and interests, children who are visually impaired need to have the opportunity to fully participate in many age-appropriate experiences, such as those listed earlier in this chapter. Listening is essential to being able to respond to the ideas and interests of friends, so learning to listen during social interaction needs to be deliberately taught, modeled, and encouraged.

Initiating interactions with friends also requires good listening skills. Children who are visually impaired need to learn to listen carefully in order to locate and identify friends with whom they would like to play. In an environment marked by noisy activity such as a busy classroom or the playground, this task can be very challenging. Teachers can facilitate and support interaction by placing students who are visually impaired with children who have shown an interest in the students or whom the students seem to enjoy, in small-group learning opportunities.

Once students' preferences among the other children have been identified, strategies can be put in place to help students to find their friends more easily. For example, teachers can encourage their students to decide upon a prearranged meeting place with their friends, such as at the slide, during recess each day. Also, interesting activities, depending upon the student's interests, can be made available to draw friends to the student who is visually impaired. The specific activities will vary, depending on a child's interests and abilities; some children who are active will enjoy learning to play games with audible balls, while others may enjoy playing adapted board or card games. Digital recorders can provide much entertainment when children

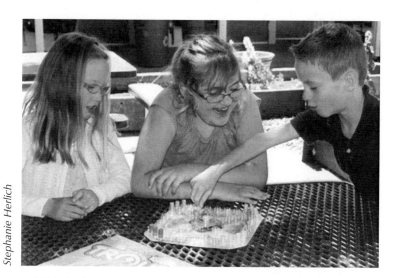

Stephanie Herlich

While playing a game and interacting with her friends, this student requires good listening skills to make her next move.

take turns recording messages, favorite songs, and sounds for each other. A digital recorder can also be used to record a treasure hunt on the playground for two buddies to follow.

Listening is an important aspect of conversation, which is essential to making and strengthening friendships. Nurturing the listening response with infants was described in Chapter 2, as parents and their babies learn to communicate through turn taking. In the preschool years, as described in Chapter 3, "the listening environment expands" and youngsters need to apply the early skills of engagement that they have learned with their family members to teachers and playmates in preschool and perhaps playgroup environments. As children enter the early elementary grades, turn taking in conversation happens quickly and sometimes incidentally during play and small-group instruction. Listening becomes essential in order to stay on topic, ask and respond to questions to keep the topic going, and use appropriate tone and volume in response.

In order to really get to know someone, students need to listen to understand and develop interest in others. Students who are visually impaired can learn that questions are useful tools that can help them to understand experiences that cannot be seen (Erin, 2006) and that provide a way to indicate interest in others. Children can learn to obtain information about their friends and show interest by learning to ask questions such as "What did you do over the weekend?"; "What is your favorite sport?"; or "Do you like to go horseback riding?" As children learn the nuances of careful listening, they acquire social behaviors that expand two-way understanding. This involves making certain that one understands what the other person has said or intended to say. It can be done by learning to restate the content, asking clarifying questions, and reflecting on the ideas of others, for example, "You mean you don't like it either when the horse makes those funny snorting noises?"

Much of what goes on in communication is nonverbal. Listening can be an important tool in learning to interpret the nonverbal cues of others. By learning to listen carefully to the tone of others' voices, children can learn a great deal. Does the speaker sound cheerful, humorous, cranky, or bored? The tone of voice is an important part of any verbal communication.

Body language is an important way that we show the speaker that we are listening. Facing the speaker lets him or her know that we are paying attention to what is being said, as do various actions such as nodding and smiling. Just as body language can indicate attention and interest, it can also show boredom or disinterest when the listener yawns repeatedly, turns his or her face and body away, taps a pencil, or begins rocking. These important social skills are often learned incidentally by most children, but they need to be deliberately taught to children who are visually impaired.

Sidebar 4.10 presents some activities to develop social listening skills. These lessons were designed to be taught in a social skills group consisting of both students

Lessons: Activities to Develop Social Listening Skills

TALKING WITH FRIENDS (KINDERGARTEN–SECOND GRADE)

Objective: Students will learn how to listen and take turns in a conversation.

Skills Addressed

- active listening
- staying on topic
- taking turns
- showing interest

Introduction: Explain to students that they are going to learn about listening and taking turns in a conversation.

Materials and Game Ideas: big ball, small ball, three-minute timer, blindfolds/low vision simulator optional

Activity

1. Choose one student to start talking about something that he or she did yesterday. Tell the student that no matter what you say, he or she should stay on topic. As the student talks, start talking over the student about something different. After a few minutes, stop and ask the group what was wrong with that conversation. Be sure to explain how neither participant was listening to the other or responding to what was being said.

2. Explain that students are going to practice listening to each other and responding to what is being said. Students will take turns sharing stories and asking questions about the stories. Each story will last for three minutes, as timed by the timer. The big ball is the "story ball" and the small ball is the "question ball." The teacher will begin telling a story while holding the story ball. A student will hold the question ball and when the story is over will get to ask a question. The question must be about the story. After the question is answered, the person with the question ball will hand the ball to a new student who will get to ask a new question. When the timer rings, the story ball will be handed to a new student and the game will start over with a new student telling a new story. (If a student cannot think of a story, the teacher can prompt with ideas.)

Note: Remind students to turn and face each other when talking.

PLAYING WITH FRIENDS (THIRD–FIFTH GRADE)

Objective: Students will learn how to ask a friend to play.

Skills Addressed

- choosing appropriate friends to ask to play
- finding friends
- using appropriate language starters for effectively making initial contact with peers
- listening skills

Introduction: Discuss what students like to do at recess. Ask students if they wanted to play one of their favorite games how they might get a friend to play with them. Discuss how students go about finding their friends.

(Continued)

Materials: jump ropes, hula hoops, large bouncy beep or bell ball, swings, jungle gym, low vision simulators, and blindfolds

Activity

1. Explain to the group that they will take turns playing three different games. Two people will play the game, and the rest will close their eyes and put on blindfolds or low vision simulators. The blindfolded group has to listen and guess what game is being played, such as Simon Says; Red Light, Green Light; and Duck, Duck, Goose.

2. Once the first game is guessed, ask blindfolded students to raise their hand if they would like to join the game. Choose one student and ask him or her how he or she would join the game. Tell the student to try his or her method.

3. Now there are three students playing the game. Again ask the group if someone else would like to join in the game. Have him or her explain how he or she will join and then let the new student try his or her method.

4. Recap and review how the students identified the game with their hearing and how they approached the game players and joined the game.

5. Repeat this sequence for one or two more games.

Note: Be sure to choose three activities that the student who is visually impaired is comfortable with and enjoys. Practice activities prior to doing this lesson.

MAKING CONVERSATION (THIRD–FIFTH GRADE)

Objective: Students will learn how to start a conversation that includes a group of people. Students will also learn the importance of posture and using group members' names to indicate with whom they are talking.

Skills Addressed

- body awareness
- conversation
- turn taking
- listening

Introduction: Discuss the importance of having good posture, looking at or facing everyone in the group, and using names to indicate with whom you are speaking when having a conversation. Discuss how easy it is to become confused when appropriate conversation skills are not used. For example, a person may not respond to a question because he or she may not realize the speaker is directing the question to him or her. The speaker's feelings may then be hurt.

Materials: KidTalk conversation cards, blindfolds, low vision simulators

Note: KidTalk cards are commercially available cards used to elicit conversation about a variety of topics.

Activity

1. Three students will be chosen to carry on a conversation. The students will sit with their backs to one another. They will carry on a short conversation but will not be allowed to use names. Choose one student to begin by saying, "Hi, how are you?" After two minutes, discuss with the whole group what made the conversation difficult or easy.

Note: Allow for pauses in the conversation and interject feedback only if absolutely necessary.

2. Next, select two more students who will be blindfolded or who will use low vision simulators. A third student will not be included, and that student will choose from the pile of KidTalk cards. He or she will start a conversation. All students must keep in mind that they must use good posture and state the name of the person with whom they are speaking. Make sure the KidTalk cards used are brailled or in large print so that all students can read the cards.

3. Repeat Step 2 with different students.

4. Discuss the difference between the different types of conversations. Was it difficult to not use each others' names? Why? Was it easier when your name was used in the conversation? Why? How did it feel to be blindfolded when carrying on a conversation? How did it feel to be the only sighted student in a conversation?

Source: Reprinted with permission from N. Crow & S. A. Herlich, *Getting to Know You: A Social Skills/Ability Awareness Curriculum for Students with Visual Impairments and Their Sighted Peers* (Louisville, KY: American Printing House for the Blind, forthcoming).

---

with visual impairments and their sighted peers. Teachers may choose to teach these lessons as outlined or adapt the lessons as necessary. The lessons provided highlight the importance of listening skills.

LISTENING AS RECREATION

Claire is in fourth grade at her neighborhood school, where she receives itinerant vision services. Her decreased vision is due to optic albinism. A television monitor is mounted high on one of the walls in her classroom. Using her monocular, Claire is able to comfortably view short videos; longer movies are problematic because the height of the screen causes neck, arm, and eye fatigue.

When weather is inclement Claire and her classmates eat lunch and have recess in their classroom. To contribute to the classroom teacher's arsenal of indoor activities during the rainy season, Claire's teacher of students who are visually impaired provided the audio described video of Harry Potter and the Goblet of Fire. *The narrated descriptions of nonverbal cues and visual elements—scene changes, body language, sets, actions, and costumes—are woven into the pauses of the film's soundtrack. Claire is proud of having this accessible format available for people who have trouble seeing the screen because it makes her feel a part of the mainstream without having to rely on someone else to describe the visuals. Audio description not only provides enjoyment, but also has educational value in reinforcing the development of literacy skills through the use of enriched language and vocabulary. Claire's classmates and teacher are eager to see other described movies, as Harry Potter was such a hit!*

Listening provides all of us with countless aesthetic and practical possibilities for enjoyment. For many children who are visually impaired, listening presents an avenue for fun and recreation. Some children are naturally so tuned into sound that they learn to play with it, the way children with vision play with certain toys. These children naturally tune into sound in all aspects of their environment, and it plays an important role for them in terms of interest and enjoyment. One man who is blind casually referred to himself as a "hearing jock" as a young person and told a story about being able to differentiate and name each type of coin when dropped on a bed by hearing the amplitude caused by the mass of the coin landing on the surface of the bed. He also shared his continued interest in and ability to differentiate and name different types of cars from the sound of their engines.

Some children who are visually impaired do not naturally tune into sound for recreational purposes, but they can be taught to appreciate it. Children who are in elementary school have many avenues to enjoy sound through toys, music, recorded stories and nonfiction, and electronic games and devices. Some of the electronic devices described earlier in this chapter, while providing essential tools for the development of literacy skills, can also provide hours of listening enjoyment.

For children who may enjoy a finer differentiation of sounds they hear in the environment, possibilities for listening enjoyment are countless. They will enjoy noticing, naming, and sometimes imitating the sounds that they hear in nature, technology and machinery, voice tone and pitch, and music, to name a few. Children may find it fun to use a digital recorder to record sounds that they hear. They might also enjoy making digital recordings of their friends as they talk, or record "collages" of the sounds of places they go, just as some people make a scrapbook or photo album. Some children enjoy recording themselves reading for later listening. This can also be done with friends, taking turns while reading a story or the parts of a play.

Many children love to listen to music, and during the elementary school years, their taste in music begins to become more defined as they are exposed to a great variety of music at home and at school. Learning to independently operate music-playing equipment provides them with access to their music, and learning to organize their collection of music allows them to more consistently and fully enjoy their musical choices.

Students in the early elementary grades need to be signed up with the National Library Service, mentioned earlier in this chapter, to regularly receive the tremendous variety of literature available in braille and recorded materials for recreational reading and listening. This access to both braille and digital materials allows children the choice of media, and listening to both fiction and nonfiction for pleasure promotes the development of literacy-related listening skills while providing another mode of recreation and enjoyment. Not only are books available, but the National Library Service provides a number of periodicals that children can enjoy. (See the Resources section and the earlier section in this chapter for more information about listening to recorded materials.)

For many families, listening to their favorite sports teams on the radio or watching them compete on television is a regular ritual, and this is something that can be shared with their children who are visually impaired. Again, however, this is a culture that needs to be deliberately taught and explained. Not all children will naturally pick up the family interest in baseball, but with gradual explanation and exposure over time, many children will enjoy the tremendous excitement that is evident during a radio broadcast game, especially when they are sharing that experience with other family members or friends.

Listening to movies or television shows can be a fun activity to share with family or friends that can be made even more enjoyable for children who are visually impaired with the addition of audio or video description. Audio or video description is a service that makes television programs, films, and other visual media more accessible by including audio description of the key visual elements in a program, such as the actions, costumes, gestures, and scene changes. Audio-described programs, which can be very satisfying for listeners, are available on some television stations and in some movie theaters and live theatrical performances.

Many other recreational activities are enhanced by good listening skills. Joining youth groups; playing goal ball or beep baseball; tandem biking, canoeing; or kayaking; and taking dancing lessons are just a few of the fun activities that children may enjoy that involve active listening.

CONCLUSION

Children who are in elementary school are both learning to listen and listening to learn. The skills of listening, speaking, reading, and writing are integrated throughout each day, facilitating the development of literacy skills and access to the core curriculum. Students who are visually impaired need to learn to become active listeners in order to gain information from the increasingly complex listening environment. The listening aspect of assistive technology enables them to successfully gain access to all areas of the core curriculum and leads to the development of critical and analytical listening skills as they make the transition to middle and high school.

REFERENCES

American Foundation for the Blind. (n.d.). National instructional materials accessibility standard (NIMAS). Retrieved December 7, 2006, from www.afb.org/Section.asp ?SectionID=58&TopicID=255.

Anderson, J. (2003). Expanded core curriculum: Technology. In S. A. Goodman & S. H. Wittenstein (Eds.), *Collaborative assessment: Working with students who are blind or visually impaired including those with additional disabilities.* New York: AFB Press.

Common Core State Standards Initiative. (2010). Common core state standards for English language arts and literacy in history/social studies, science, and technical subjects. Retrieved July 22, 2010, from www.corestandards.org/the-standards.

Crow, N., & Herlich, S. (Forthcoming). *Getting to know you: A social skills/ability awareness curriculum for students with visual impairments and their sighted peers.* Louisville, KY: American Printing House for the Blind.

The DAISY Consortium. (n.d.). About the DAISY consortium. Retrieved September 13, 2010, from www.daisy.org/about_us.

Dennison, P. E., & Dennison, G. E. (1989). *Brain gym.* Ventura, CA: Edu-Kinesthetics.

Drissel, N. M. (Summer 1997). What is a story box? *Awareness* (NAPVI newsletter), pp. 24, 25.

Ellery, V. (2005). *Creating strategic readers: Techniques for developing competency in phonemic awareness, phonics, fluency, vocabulary, and comprehension.* Newark, DE: International Reading Association.

Emerson, R. W., Holbrook, M. C., & D'Andrea, M. F. (October 2009). Acquisition of literacy skills by young children who are blind: Results from the ABC Braille study. *Journal of Visual Impairment & Blindness, 103*(10), 610–624.

Erin, J. (2006). Teaching social skills to elementary and middle school students who are visually impaired. In S. Z. Sacks & K. E. Wolffe (Eds.), *Teaching social skills to students with visual impairments: From theory to practice.* New York: AFB Press.

Evans, C. (2005). Changing channels—AudioAssisted reading: Access to curriculum for students with print disabilities. From *Instructional Resources*. Retrieved July 1, 2011, from www.tsbvi.edu/braille-resources/70-changing-channels-audioassisted-reading-access-to-curriculum-for-students-with-print-disabilities.

Harley, R. K., Truan, M. B., & Sanford, L. D. (1997). *Communication skills for visually impaired learners: Braille, print, and listening skills for students who are visually impaired* (2nd ed.). Springfield, IL: Charles C Thomas.

Hatlen, P. (1996). The core curriculum for blind and visually impaired students, including those with additional disabilities. *RE:view 28*(1), 25–32.

Hudson, L. J. (1997). *Classroom collaboration.* Watertown, MA: Perkins School for the Blind.

International Society for Technology in Education, National Educational Technology Standards (NETS). (2007). Retrieved June 15, 2010, from www.iste.org/standards/nets-for-students.aspx.

Jalongo, M. R. (1991). *Strategies for developing children's listening skills.* Bloomington, IN: Phi Delta Kappa Educational Foundation.

Koenig, A. J. (1996). Growing into literacy. In C. Holbrook (Ed.), *Children with visual impairment.* Bethesda, MD: Woodbine House.

Koenig, A. J., & Farrenkopf, C. (1997). Essential experiences to undergird the early development of literacy. *Journal of Visual Impairment & Blindness, 91*, 14–24.

Kovalik, S. J., & Olsen, K. D. (2002). *Exceeding expectations: A user's guide to implementing brain research in the classroom* (2nd ed.). Covington, WA: Susan Kovalick & Associates.

McNear, D., & Kuns, J. (2006). *Personal data assistants for students with visual impairments and additional learning challenges.* Paper contributed to the Annual CTEBVI Conference (47th), Anaheim, CA.

Millbrae School District. (2010). *Millbrae School District Technology Plan July 1, 2010–June 30, 2015* (pp. 60–65). Millbrae, CA. Retrieved September 6, 2010, from www.millbrae schooldistrict.org/Curriculum/2010_2015_Millbrae_Tech_Plan.pdf.

National Instructional Materials Access Center. Welcome to the NIMAC! Retrieved December 7, 2006, from www.nimac.us.

Numeroff, L. J. (1985). *If you give a mouse a cookie.* New York: Harper Collins.

Presley, I., & D'Andrea, F. M. (2009). *Assistive technology for students who are visually impaired: A guide to assessment.* New York: AFB Press.

Rex, E. J., Koenig, A. J., Wormsley, D. P., & Baker, R. L. (1994). *Foundations of braille literacy.* New York: AFB Press.

Rosenblum, L. P. (2000). Perceptions of the impact of a visual impairment on the lives of adolescents. *Journal of Visual Impairment & Blindness, 94*, 434–445.

Routman, R. (2000). *Conversations: Strategies for teaching, learning, and evaluating.* Portsmouth, NH: Heinemann.

Sacks, S. (2006). Theoretical perspectives on the early years of social development. In S. Z. Sacks & K. E. Wolffe (Eds.), *Teaching social skills to students with visual impairments: From theory to practice.* New York: AFB Press.

San Mateo–Foster City School District. (February 13, 2008). *Highlands Elementary School Overview of Computer Technology Curriculum.* San Mateo, CA.

Spache, G. D., & Spache, E. B. (1973). *Reading in the elementary school.* Rockleigh, NJ: Allyn.

Wolffe, K. (2006). Teaching adolescents and young adults. In S. Z. Sacks & K. E. Wolffe (Eds.), *Teaching social skills to students with visual impairments: From theory to practice.* New York: AFB Press.

Chapter 5

Middle School and High School: Advanced Skill Development

Stephanie Herlich

Just by listening, the world and the people in it come alive. If we learn to be patient and to focus our attention on what we hear, we grow to understand not just the words but the stories and feelings of others. Listening is the art of keeping silent so that we can fully engage with what and who is around us in a meaningful way.

—Elizabeth Phillips,
Graduate student at the University of Arizona

CHAPTER PREVIEW

- ▸ Learning by Listening
- ▸ Listening in the Classroom
- ▸ Listening Tools Used to Acquire Information
- ▸ Listening in Social Situations
- ▸ Recreational Listening

As students leave their elementary schools for middle school and then go on to high school, they are learning new skills and achieving new levels of independence at a seemingly exponential rate. Students who are visually impaired are undergoing these same experiences and expectations; however, these students will be presented with additional challenges. In middle school, students are changing teachers and classrooms many times throughout the day, often for the first time in their school experience. Each teacher will have different expectations and directions. Each classroom may have different students and configurations. Once students reach high school, they are used to the changing teachers, classrooms, and peers; however, new demands of independence and greater academic demands emerge. The student who is visually impaired needs to use all his or her resources to adapt to these changes.

In this chapter, readers will learn what specific listening skills students need to be successful adults. Middle school and high school can be thought of as the gateway to adulthood; therefore, listening skills are taken to a whole new level as students become more and more independent in their abilities. The following essential skills that students need before leaving high school are discussed throughout the chapter:

> ▸ *Ability to independently identify and evaluate spoken information.* As discussed in Chapter 4, students in elementary school begin to learn how to listen critically to oral classroom instruction. For example, teachers may ask students to predict what is coming next or relate a given topic to a personal experience. In middle school and high school, students need to be able to listen independently to information and extrapolate more abstract thoughts and concepts. After listening to a lecture about magnetism, for example, students might be asked to use the information to develop a demonstration explaining or showing the effects of magnetic forces.

> ▸ *Ability to independently organize spoken information, such as taking effective notes.* In elementary school students begin copying notes from a presentation surface, such as a white board or an electronically projected presentation. When students enter middle school and high school, they become much more responsible for the information being taught. Students at this level need to be able to take effective notes, organize their information, and know how to retrieve the information for later use. Teachers expect that students will be able to use their notes to study for upcoming exams.

> ▸ *Knowledge of listening technology that is available and appropriate.* In elementary school, students need to be introduced to a variety of technologies. Technology is constantly changing, and it will continue to do so as students mature and technology advances. Students need to continually be assessed and introduced to new devices if appropriate. For example, an elementary school student who reads braille may begin learning

braille with the assistance of a touch tablet and simple braille keyboard, but as the student's skills improve, he or she will need to be introduced to an accessible personal digital assistant (PDA).

▸ *Ability to work with sighted reader.* Middle school and high school are the gateways to adulthood. Students are preparing to become independent adults. In middle school, students with visual impairments may have assistance from a paraeducator. This person might help the student find needed information in a textbook or may even assist in reading a chapter. In high school, students need to begin learning how to find and use the assistance of a sighted reader independently.

▸ *Ability to be a good social listener.* Children begin to learn the listening skills needed to be successful socially even before they enter elementary school. These social listening skills must continue to be taught as children advance through elementary, middle, and high school. There are many age-appropriate activities that can both teach social listening and help students refine their social listening skills.

Table 5.1 helps to illustrate the differences in how listening skills are addressed as students advance from elementary school to high school. For example, in elementary school, students are not expected to take full responsibility for upcoming projects. Notes and e-mails may be sent home and parents or caregivers are expected to help their children remember future events. In middle school, students are often required to keep a log of assignments. Teachers guide students in how to do this, and students may be graded on how well they keep their assignment logs. By the time students reach high school, teachers expect that students can keep their own assignment calendars or logs. Teachers announce and post information, expecting that their students can record it independently.

LEARNING BY LISTENING

Throughout their school careers, "students are *learning to listen* so they can *learn by listening*" (Mangold, 1982, p. 126). The listening skills students learn throughout elementary, middle, and high school enable them to become learners through listening. It is important for educators to realize that listening is a skill that needs to be taught throughout a student's school career. As stressed throughout this book, being able to hear is not the same as having the ability to listen. Listening requires a great deal of mental effort (Ferrington, 1994). Special instruction in active listening can improve a person's analytical listening abilities. Being an active listener means that one is taking in information and immediately interpreting that information to determine

TABLE 5.1

Evolution of Listening Skills from Elementary School to High School

	Elementary School	Middle School	High School
Organizing information	The teacher sends home announcements of upcoming projects and tests.	The teacher requires students to maintain an organizer with upcoming projects and tests.	The teacher announces upcoming projects and tests and expects students to remember or record information independently.
Technology	The teacher presents student with digital recordings of trade books and closely monitors usage.	The teacher provides digital recordings of trade books and textbooks and assigns tasks for students to complete using technology.	The teacher presents the assignment and expects students to use appropriate technology to complete it.
Note taking	Students learn to take notes while information is dictated.	Students are given templates with main ideas and are expected to fill in supporting details.	Students are expected to take and organize their own notes.
Social skills	Students with visual impairments are taught to participate in conversations with peers by responding to what is already being discussed.	Students with visual impairments are taught how to find peers and initiate two-way conversation.	Students are expected to be able to find and initiate conversations with increasing independence.

how it should be used for either immediate or future use. A teacher cannot assume, for example, that a student can listen to an audiobook and then use that information to study for an exam or answer questions on a worksheet. Some students may not be able to synthesize what they hear into meaningful information. Students who take notes, ask questions about what was heard, and control the speed of audio materials do much better in listening than students who sit passively. Students who have been taught to use well-organized listening techniques have shown significant increases in their academic performance (Boyle et al., 2003; Harley, Truan, & Sanford, 1997).

As in elementary education, middle and secondary schools throughout the nation need to strive to adhere to the rigorous curriculum standards set forth by their states. As of this writing, 48 states plus the District of Columbia, the U.S. Virgin Islands, and four other territories have adopted the Common Core State Standards, a state-led effort "to provide a clear and consistent framework to prepare children for college and the workforce" (Common Core State Standards Initiative, 2010, "About the Standards"). In each state, curriculum requirements are tested each year as students progress through school. For instance, in the seventh grade, within the Speaking and Listening standards—part of the Common Core State Standards for English Language Arts and Literacy in History/Social Studies, Science, and Technical Subjects—students are required to "pose questions that elicit elaboration and respond to others' questions and comments with relevant observations and ideas that bring the discussion back on topic as needed." In eleventh and twelfth grade, students need to continue to show proficiency in the seventh-grade standards, as well as "come to discussions prepared, having read and researched material under study; explicitly draw on that preparation by referring to the evidence from texts and other research on the topic or issue to stimulate a thoughtful, well-reasoned exchange of ideas" (Common Core State Standards Initiative, 2010). By the end of high school, the listening skills required for all students are at an extremely sophisticated level, and students are expected to utilize their listening skills for comprehension, analysis, and evaluation each and every day.

These curricular expectations with regard to listening, as well as all other areas of the core curriculum, are the same for students who are visually impaired. Through specific instruction in listening skills as part of the expanded core curriculum (see Chapter 1), students who are visually impaired utilize listening as an essential compensatory mode that will continue to support their access to the core curriculum.

It is important to remember that the listening skills being discussed throughout this chapter, and elsewhere in this book, are not meant to replace reading skills or any other skills a student might use to gain information. The aim is for listening strategies to enhance students' repertoire of skills that they may utilize to gain needed information and independence.

As students advance through the school system, the focus begins to shift from the skills needed at the present moment to the skills a student needs as he or she looks forward to more independence, whether it is in the workplace or in future academic pursuits. This chapter focuses on activities and strategies that students who are in middle school and high school need for lifelong learning and involvement.

LISTENING IN THE CLASSROOM

Listening skills relating to listening in the classroom in middle school and high school include the following:

- ▸ listens critically to oral classroom discussion
- ▸ identifies the tone, mood, and emotion conveyed in the oral communication

▸ listens attentively, for an extended period of time, to a variety of texts read aloud and to oral presentations

▸ determines the speaker's attitude toward the subject

▸ initiates and participates effectively in a range of collaborative discussions (one-on-one, in groups, and teacher-led) with diverse partners on grade-nine and grade-ten topics, texts, and issues, building on others' ideas and expressing their own clearly and persuasively

▸ listens to and independently organizes spoken information by summarizing and taking notes about spoken ideas, literature, and curriculum

▸ reviews the key ideas expressed and demonstrates understanding of multiple perspectives through reflection and paraphrasing

▸ paraphrases a speaker's purpose and point of view and asks relevant questions concerning the speaker's delivery and purpose

▸ interprets information from media presentations such as news broadcasts and taped interviews

▸ synthesizes the information from different sources by combining or categorizing data and facts

▸ interprets information from media presentations such as documentary films, news broadcasts, and taped interviews

Sue is a sophomore in a public high school and is taking an advanced biology class. Sue reads braille and uses an electronic notetaker or accessible PDA, which she can take to each of her classes and take home at night. Sue has her biology textbook both in braille and in a digital format that she can listen to on a specialized electronic book player.

Sue is currently at home reading and listening to her biology book as she prepares for a lab that will take place the following day. As she listens to the recording, she is following along in her braille textbook so that she will not miss the spelling of new vocabulary words.

Tomorrow Sue will participate in a lab on mitosis and meiosis. Since this lab consists of observations of slides showing how cells divide, Sue knows she is going to need to listen very carefully to how her lab mates describe the slides. She plans to take notes on her accessible PDA and knows that she will need to ask questions to clarify her lab mates' descriptions. Since Sue likes the auditory feedback her notetaker provides, she will use an earphone during class to listen as she takes her notes.

Sue is a student who has "learned to listen." She uses her listening skills throughout her school day to accomplish all of the tasks that are required of her. Sue is a student with a visual impairment; therefore, good listening skills are crucial for her. Unlike her peers, who can look at the notes on the board to help them understand information, Sue needs to rely primarily on her listening skills. Throughout her school day, Sue needs to actively listen to her teachers' instructions and lectures; she needs to listen to her peers to know who is speaking, what they are speaking about, and from where they might be speaking; she listens to her assistive technology devices in order to record, access, and acquire information; and she needs to listen to her surroundings to assess her environment and changes that might be occurring around her.

This section focuses on listening in the classroom and highlights strategies that can be used when working with students with visual impairments so that they are successful in secondary school and beyond. The following is a sampling of the activities in which middle school and high school students find good listening skills to be essential:

- following instructions from a variety of teachers with a variety of expectations
- transitioning quickly between classroom activities, for example, from a lecture to a spelling test to writing down the instructions for an upcoming project
- working with partners in a science lab
- listening to classroom discussions, teacher lectures, group presentations, audio presentations, and the like
- quickly accessing information that was presented previously
- compiling information from a variety of sources, such as the Internet, digital books, notes, print books, and interviews, into a research paper
- listening to a digital book

Ferrington (1994) estimated that elementary and secondary students spend 50 percent of their time listening to teachers and others. In college, approximately 90 percent of their time is spent listening. Continuing to provide instruction in and opportunities for listening is critical for students to be successful in secondary school and beyond. Just as the foundation for effective listening is built in elementary school, there are many techniques and strategies that can be utilized to help increase a middle or high school student's listening skills.

Becoming an Efficient Listener

Listening to identify and evaluate needed information occurs throughout the school day, as can be seen from the extensive list of activities required of secondary students just presented. An efficient listener is one who can absorb spoken information and interact with it in the most appropriate manner according to the information. For example, in the previous scenario, Sue is planning to use her PDA during the science lab so that she can take notes on the information she will hear during the activity. Some students with visual impairments, like Sue, may enter the secondary grades with the ability to analyze spoken information the same way they analyze written information. For others, this task may be quite difficult. General education teachers spend a great deal of time teaching students how to analyze written information, for example, selecting facts and details, sequencing or putting information in a logical order, finding the main idea, summarizing, and making inferences. Teachers of students with visual impairments need to be sure that their students can analyze spoken information in the same way.

The listening skills described in Chapter 4 become increasingly important as students enter middle and high school. The state standards for secondary students (see, for example, the skills listed for middle and high school students in the areas of Active and Critical Listening in the Listening Skills Continuum in Appendix A) highlight the importance of students' being able to listen and participate in small groups, formulate judgments and questions based on information, and identify and evaluate types of spoken information. During the middle and high school years, the spoken word is of prime importance as a source of information, particularly as learning becomes based on more abstract concepts. In listening to speech, students have to extract critical information through concentration and selective listening (Best, 1991). To listen selectively, students need to be able to extract the essential and critical information. For some, extracting and evaluating critical information does not come easily. The strategies listed in the following sections may help secondary students become more efficient listeners in their classes.

Listening in Small Groups

As noted in the previous list of activities in which middle and high school students find listening skills to be essential, students have more and more opportunities to work in small groups as they get older. For example, students might be working with one partner during a science lab or in a small group when completing a project. When working in a small group, students will find themselves to be even more responsible for taking in information that is discovered or discussed. A student with a visual impairment needs to be an efficient listener during the small-group session since the classroom teacher will not know what each small group discussed; therefore, the student will not be able to go to the teacher to have the information repeated. Many of the listening skills taught in Chapter 4, such as *active* and *critical* listening, become essential in small-group situations.

Students with visual impairments need to be responsible for obtaining and retaining information independently when working in small groups. Middle and high school students need to be able to participate in small groups without a paraeducator. The dynamics of a small group change greatly when an adult is present. One of the reasons teachers require students to participate in small groups is so that they can learn to discuss, think, discover, and assimilate information without the presence of an adult. The following suggestions can help students who are visually impaired learn skills needed for working in small groups:

▸ Students who feel intimidated or shy working in small groups may benefit from role-playing in what they consider to be a safe setting or with very familiar people, such as in a resource classroom or during direct service time with a teacher of students who are visually impaired. Try choosing a topic of discussion or a fun project that can be done on the computer or in the library. Give students with visual impairments a very specific job during the role-play, for example, taking notes on the main idea and supporting facts.

▸ During small-group activities, a teacher of students with visual impairments or paraeducator can help facilitate without being directly involved by making sure each person in the group has a specific responsibility and understands his or her job. Some specific jobs may include note taker, reader, time manager, and a group leader who ensures that everyone is participating.

Formulating Judgments and Questions

The following suggestions can help students learn to formulate judgments and questions:

▸ Have students listen to short, interesting, and age-appropriate passages. These could come from magazines, digital books, newspapers, or the Internet. Throughout the reading, ask the students questions, and instruct students to ask the teacher questions. The questions should require the students to find the main idea, formulate an opinion, and focus on details and facts. For example, after listening to an article read from the

Internet, the students might be asked, "Do you think this author was influencing your thoughts on the subject?"; "What was the author's purpose in writing this article?"; and "What did you learn from this article?"

▶ To determine if students understand what they are listening to, have them write a short summary, including their opinion of what they heard. (Summarization is discussed in the section "Listening Tools Used to Acquire Information.")

▶ After listening to a passage, have students write two or three questions based on what they heard. The questions should seek out supporting details. If more than one student has read the passage, students need to exchange questions and then answer their partner's questions. After answering questions, students can work together to evaluate the accuracy of the answers.

▶ Have students listen to talk radio or a news program. After listening, discuss the show with students. Discuss the importance of evaluating information on accuracy, relevance, and the efficacy of the speaker. For example, "Was the information presented accurate?"; "Were there enough details to support the presenter's case?"; and "Do you believe the speaker? Why or why not?" Encourage greater discussion when evaluating information by making sure students can back up their opinions based on what was heard. It is not enough for students to say, "I do not think the information was truthful." The students need to explain why they feel that way.

Evaluating Types of Spoken Information

It is important that students be able to identify the different types of information that they are exposed to throughout the day. One activity that can help with this skill is the following:

▶ Assign students to listen to a morning news show, either in the classroom or at home for homework.

▶ Provide a checklist identifying different types of news stories that might be heard, for example, weather, world news, local news, entertainment, and personal interest. Have students check off each different segment heard throughout the broadcast.

Listening in Real Time

Matthew is sitting in his ninth-grade geometry class. Matthew has low vision and other orthopedic handicaps. Matthew has a paraeducator who assists him in his geometry class. The geometry teacher has just announced that all students need to open their books and turn to page 254. Matthew is physically able to do this. As all of the students reach into their backpacks and pull out their books, Matthew turns to the paraeducator and asks, "What page did he say?"

Students with visual impairments often have many helpers in their lives. These helpers may be parents, siblings, friends, teachers, and paraeducators. It is not unusual for students to begin relying on this extra assistance throughout their school day. It is important that teachers of students with visual impairments have the same expectations of students who are visually impaired as they would of any other student in their classroom. If students are expected to hear directions the first time they are spoken, students with visual impairments need to learn to listen like their peers. Too often, students turn to their paraeducators to hear the direction a second time or wait until their teacher of students with visual impairments repeats the instructions or information. Once a student reaches middle school and high school, he or she may not even realize the extent to which he or she is relying on someone else to repeat information. The following list provides some ideas to help a student begin listening in real time, not when the information is repeated a second time by a paraeducator, teacher, or parent:

▶ It is important that students with visual impairments understand a teacher's expectations of them. Talk to students and explain that they need to practice receiving information the first time it is spoken. Discuss a possible plan that would help students recognize when they are not listening in real time. For example, for two or three days, chart how many times a student needs to have information repeated. Do this with the student so that he or she begins to recognize his or her habits. Next, remind the student at the beginning of each class or lesson that he or she needs to listen to information the first time it is given. Continue to chart anytime requests are made to repeat the information. Challenge the student to decrease the number of requests he or she makes. After a week, tell the student you will no longer repeat information. He or she will need to ask the classroom teacher or a friend. Continue to monitor the student's listening to be sure he or she does not revert back to old habits.

▸ Be sure students are prepared to listen. Students need to be instructed that each time they enter a classroom, they need to automatically take out all of the materials needed for that class. Students with visual impairments often have a variety of materials they need to be independent and successful in their classrooms. For example, a student might need a monocular, an accessible PDA, bold-lined paper, and a bold pen. All of these materials need to be on the student's desk before class begins. Too often, precious time is lost and information is being presented while a student is searching for the materials needed.

▸ Often a student may not realize when or how often he or she is relying on a third party to repeat information. A way to highlight this is to quietly give the student a small token or ticket each time he or she asks for someone to repeat given information. If appropriate, use a chart or an incentive, such as a free homework pass or a chance to listen to a favorite song during class, to encourage the student each time he or she receives fewer tickets.

▸ Explain to all of the teachers and paraeducators who work with the student that the student is learning to listen in real time. Be sure that everyone involved understands that the expectations for a student with visual impairment should be the same as the expectations for his or her peers. If the student did not hear something the first time, direct him or her to ask the speaker to repeat the information.

LISTENING TOOLS USED TO ACQUIRE INFORMATION

Listening skills relating to using tools and technology to acquire information in middle school and high school include the following:

▸ listens to learn while using appropriate access technology
▸ selects and uses appropriate technology tools to accomplish a variety of tasks
▸ demonstrates advanced word-processing skills, such as cutting and pasting text, using a spell checker, and using formatting features
▸ demonstrates advanced use of screen-reading options
▸ demonstrates effective use of accessible PDAs using simple applications, such as word-processing file management, calendar, and calculator functions

  ▸ selects and applies technology tools for research, information gathering, problem solving, and decision making

  ▸ demonstrates advanced use of acccessible PDAs, such as advanced word processing

Jane is a junior at her local high school. She is visually impaired and uses braille as her primary learning medium. She is in the process of applying to a four-year university to attend after she graduates from high school. To complete her college applications, Jane has been using her computer with screen-reading software. She has also been using the Internet to research universities that have an undergraduate program that interests her. Jane has learned to use the screen-reading technology on her computer to acquire needed information. Throughout the college application process, she also found it very helpful to utilize a sighted reader. This person helped Jane sift through the piles of letters she started receiving from colleges and universities. Jane explained to her sighted reader that she wanted to know what programs each university offered. The reader was able to quickly scan for the information Jane wanted. Jane has learned how to use a variety of methods to acquire the information she wants in the most efficient manner.

Throughout the day, we listen to an extraordinary amount of auditory information. Some of what we hear becomes background noise; other sounds become a source for learning about our environment, for gaining knowledge, and for providing enjoyment. It is often thought that a person with a visual impairment has "better hearing" than people who are not visually impaired. People often reason that when one sense is compromised, the other senses begin to compensate. Researchers have found little scientific evidence to support this hypothesis (Goddard, Isaak, & Slawinski, 1998). As discussed in Chapter 6, the senses of individuals who acquire visual impairments do not automatically improve. Rather, individuals become more aware of the input received from other senses and learn how to maximize the usefulness of the input. It is imperative that individuals with visual impairments have a variety of tools at their disposal to help them sift through the abundance of auditory information they may be hearing and decide what method is best for receiving it.

One measure of success for students with visual impairments is that they can listen and learn independently; can tackle the same curriculum content as their peers; and have access to the tools that enable them to pursue their own education and professional dreams (RFB&D, 2007). Efficient listening enables students to

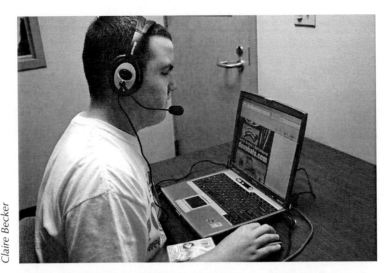

Claire Becker

This student, who has a visual impairment and limited use of his hands, is able to complete assignments independently using screen enlargement, voice recognition, and specialized word-processing software.

increase their learning efficiency through substitution for or supplementation of any of a variety of adapted materials, such as braille and large-print reading materials, or when using magnification devices. Other activities that enable a person to acquire information through listening include listening to digital books and magazines, listening to teachers, speakers, and friends, and listening to television, radio, computers (with speech output), the telephone, calculators, measurement instruments, and other electronic devices with speech output. The use of these tools is discussed in this section.

Note Taking and Listening

Miguel is in the ninth grade at his local high school. He has been blind since birth and receives services from an itinerant teacher of students with visual impairments. Miguel currently has a social studies class in which the teacher writes notes using an overhead projector while he lectures. Miguel did not even realize that these notes were visually available to all students until his teacher of students with visual impairments asked him if he was getting a copy of the notes. Miguel's grades significantly improved once he was given an advance copy of the notes in braille to compare to his own class notes. Miguel's teacher of students with visual impairments also noticed a significant improvement in the style of his note taking once he had the teacher's notes as a sample to refer to and learn from.

Students often do not fully realize the importance of note taking and listening. In addition, people are not intuitively good listeners. Research has shown that students typically recall only 50 percent of what they hear, and after 48 hours 20 to 30 percent of what is remembered is incorrect (Lee & Hatesohl, 1993). Taking notes is one of the main ways in which middle and high school students can be trained to develop effective listening skills. Note taking is often thought of as a means to record information; in addition, however, a skilled note taker is able to extrapolate main ideas and supporting details from the spoken information. A skilled note taker also has increased ability to pay attention throughout the presentation. By teaching students effective note-taking skills, teachers of students with visual impairments are preparing students to become effective listeners. The following are some key note-taking points to teach students.

- ▸ Take a minute to think about the importance of the material. Don't take notes just for the sake of writing something down.
- ▸ Don't write down everything that is heard. Listen for the main points.
- ▸ Notes should consist of key words or very short sentences.
- ▸ Shortly after taking notes, go back and review them. Add any missing information. Remember that information is quickly forgotten, so remind students to save time for this step.

Students with visual impairments often miss many visual cues and examples that sighted peers have access to on a daily basis. Providing students with as many examples as possible of good note taking helps them improve their own note-taking skills. Sidebar 5.1, adapted from a handout that is given to Dartmouth College students, presents helpful information and suggestions for taking notes on the college level. It also serves as an example of notes taken in outline form. Translating this example into large print or braille and then reviewing it with students provides an excellent sample and resource.

Another way to provide students with a good example of an outline is to ask the classroom teacher to provide students with visual impairments with an outline of his or her lecture. Having an example of a good outline helps to train students how to create their own effective outlines. Students can write directly on the outline (depending on his or her vision), or the outline can be put into an accessible braille PDA or computer

Taking Lecture Notes

I. There are many reasons for taking lecture notes.

   A. Making yourself take notes forces you to listen carefully and test your understanding of the material.

   B. When you are reviewing, notes provide a gauge to what is important in the text.

   C. Personal notes are usually easier to remember than the text.

   D. The writing down of important points helps you to remember them even before you have studied the material formally.

II. Instructors usually give clues to what is important to take down. Some of the more common clues are:

   A. Material written on the blackboard.

   B. Repetition

   C. Emphasis

      1. Emphasis can be judged by tone of voice and gesture.

      2. Emphasis can be judged by the amount of time the instructor spends on points and the number of examples he or she uses.

   D. Word signals (e.g., "There are **two points of view** on . . . "; "The **third** reason is . . . "; "In **conclusion** . . . ")

   E. Summaries given at the end of class.

   F. Reviews given at the beginning of class.

III. Each student should develop his or her own method of taking notes, but most students find the following suggestions helpful:

   A. Make your notes brief.

      1. Never use a sentence where you can use a phrase. Never use a phrase where you can use a word.

      2. Use abbreviations and symbols, but be consistent.

   B. Put most notes in your own words. However, the following should be noted exactly:

      1. Formulas

      2. Definitions

      3. Specific facts

   C. Use outline form and/or a numbering system. Indention helps you distinguish major from minor points.

   D. If you miss a statement, write key words, skip a few spaces, and get the information later.

E. Don't try to use every space on the page. Leave room for coordinating your notes with the text after the lecture. (You may want to list key terms in the margin or make a summary of the contents of the page.)

F. Date your notes.

F. Number the pages.

Source: Excerpted with permission from C. P. Thum, "Taking Lecture Notes" (Hanover, NH: Dartmouth College Academic Skills Center, 2001). Retrieved May 24, 2011, from www.dartmouth.edu/~acskills/docs /taking_notes.doc.

file. Practice with the student, discussing how to use the outline and add information to it prior to the actual lecture, as in the example in Sidebar 5.2. The student may need to be shown where to put appropriate information. If the student has never used an outline before, a more detailed outline may be necessary. Once the student understands how to add information to the outline, instruct the student to take notes during a lecture using the outlining method learned. As the student begins to understand individual components of the outline, such as main idea, headings, and subheadings,

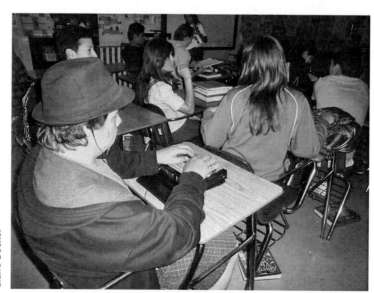

Claire Becker

In the often busy and chaotic atmosphere of the high school classroom, this student benefits from having the lecture outline on his accessible braille PDA, and it enhances his listening skills as he learns to take notes.

Teaching a Student to Use an Outline

The following sample is representative of a typical outline that a high school student who is visually impaired might receive from a teacher in a social studies classroom. The text in plain text was downloaded to the student's accessible PDA prior to the lecture. The text in italics was added by the student during class. The underlined text was added after class when the student and the teacher of students with visual impairments discussed the lecture.

Often students write down too much or too little information when listening to a lecture. Providing students with the beginning of an outline allows them to focus on the specific details of a lecture and add notes that directly relate to the most important information.

UNDERSTANDING THE THREE BRANCHES OF THE UNITED STATES GOVERNMENT

I. Legislative

    A. Defined by Article 1 of Constitution

    B. Has the authority to make laws

    C. Congress—*write, debate and pass bills*

        1. Includes Senate & House of Representatives

        2. Power to coin money, maintain military, declare war, regulate commerce. Controls taxes & spending

        3. Investigate and oversee executive branch

II. Executive

    A. Defined by Article 2 of Constitution

    B. Enforces law of the land

    C. President

        1. Commander in Chief of Armed Forces—cannot declare war

        2. Makes treaties with other nations, but Senate must approve treaties

        3. Approves laws passed by Congress—cannot write laws

        4. Power to veto laws

        5. Must be elected, must be U.S. citizen, must be 35 years old—can serve only two terms (8 years)

    D. Other parts of Executive Branch: Vice President, Departments, & Agencies

III. Judicial

    A. Defined by Article 3 of Constitution

    B. Supreme Court *(9 judges including chief judge) appointed for life*

        1. Power of judicial review—*decides if a law is constitutional (does a law support or violate the constitution of the U.S.)*

        2. Referee for all branches of government

the outline can become less detailed. Reviewing the student's outline with him or her will also help analyze and refine the student's listening abilities; the completeness and clarity of the student's notes will reflect the information he or she has gleaned from the lecture.

Another note-taking method is summing up what has been heard, or summarization. Teachers often mistakenly assume students know how to find a main idea or summarize information into its essential parts. Being able to summarize is just as important for listening comprehension as it is for reading comprehension (Tuncer & Altunay, 2006). Sidebar 5.3 presents a "summary" of teachers' experiences, expectations, and ideas when teaching summarization techniques.

People can absorb information at a faster rate than the rate at which information is typically conveyed. In their study of listening skills on normal, accelerated, and compressed speech, Bancroft and Bendinelli (1982) were able to support their hypothesis that the faster the speech rate, the greater the comprehension. Most Americans speak at a rate that is between 100–125 words per minute; however, people have the mental capacity to understand someone speaking at 400 words per minute (Lee & Hatesohl, 1993). Many individuals with visual impairments choose to increase the speech rate of audio materials to which they are listening, presumably helping them to absorb more information more quickly and helping to keep them engaged with the material. The discrepancy between listening rates and speaking rates is what allows a person's mind a chance to wander. The following suggestions will help students take advantage of their mental power and decrease the likelihood of daydreaming:

▸ Teach students to anticipate or predict the next point. Talk with students about the types of questions they can ask themselves while listening. Sometimes giving students examples of thought starters helps them think of the right questions. Make a list of thought starters and talk with students about how to turn these into complete questions. A thought-starter list might include:
  - What else . . . ?
  - When will . . . ?
  - Who were . . . ?
  - Who are . . . ?
  - Why are . . . ?
  - Where are . . . ?

Strategies for Summarization

The ability to review the key ideas expressed and demonstrate understanding of multiple perspectives through reflection and paraphrasing and synthesize the information from different sources by combining or categorizing data and facts, listed as standards for middle and high school students are key aspects of summarization. (See Listening Skills Continuum section "Listening to and Organizing Information" in Appendix A). When a student can effectively summarize information heard, he or she demonstrates the ability to maintain focus and listen for main ideas and supporting details. The following information was designed to help teachers effectively engage students with the content of their classes:

WHEN YOU ASK YOUR STUDENTS TO SUMMARIZE, WHAT USUALLY HAPPENS?

- They write down everything.
- They write down next to nothing.
- They give me complete sentences.
- They write way too much.
- They don't write enough.
- They copy word for word.

WHAT DID YOU *WANT* THEM TO DO?

- pull out main ideas
- focus on key details
- use key words and phrases
- break down the larger ideas
- write only enough to convey the gist
- take succinct but complete notes

HOW CAN I TEACH MY STUDENTS TO SUMMARIZE?

Here are a few ideas; try one . . . try them all. But keep plugging away at summarizing. This strategy is truly about equipping your students to be lifelong learners.

- Have students listen to a passage and take notes while listening. Next, students should create a summary paragraph of what they can remember of the key ideas in the piece. Students should look back at their notes only when they reach a point of being stumped. They can go back and forth between writing the summary and checking their notes several times until they have captured the important ideas in a single paragraph.

- Have students write successively shorter summaries, constantly refining and reducing their written piece until only the most essential and relevant information remains. They can start off with half a page, then try to get it down to two paragraphs, then one paragraph, then two or three sentences, and ultimately a single sentence.

- Teach students to go with the newspaper mantra: have them use the key words or phrases to identify *only* who, what, when, where, why, and how.
- Take articles from the newspaper and cut off their headlines. Have students practice writing headlines for (or matching the severed headlines to) the "headless" stories.
- When creating a summary, tell students each word costs 10 cents and give them a total amount they can spend. For example, if students have a total of $3.00, their summary can contain only 30 words. Challenge students to spend the least amount of money possible.

Source: Adapted with permission from R. Jones, "Strategies for Reading Comprehension: Summarizing" (ReadingQuest.org: Making Sense in Social Studies, 2007). Retrieved June 27, 2007, from www .readingquest.org/strat/summarize.html.

Have students practice using these thought starters as a short passage is read aloud. Instruct students to use a thought starter to formulate one question while listening to the passage. At the conclusion of the paragraph ask students to read the question and then decide if it was answered. Remind students that not all thought starters and questions will be answered but that using the technique will help keep them focused on what is being presented.

▸ Be certain that students can identify the main idea and supporting details of spoken information. Refer to Sidebar 4.5 in Chapter 4 for ideas on how to teach students to identify main ideas and supporting details.

▸ Teach students to mentally summarize what is being said throughout the presentation, not just at the end (see Sidebar 5.3).

▸ After a lecture, compare the student's lecture notes with notes from another student who takes efficient notes, an instructional assistant, or a teacher. Do this comparison with the student so that he or she begins to learn from a good example. It is also helpful to do this when the information is still fresh in the student's head so that he or she can edit his or her outline.

The note-taking suggestions provided here directly address the essential skills outlined in the state guidelines for middle and high school students found in the Listening Skills Continuum in Appendix A. The skills listed below are a summarization of several skills listed in the Middle and High School section of the continuum. These skills include the following abilities:

▸ evaluates the speaker and the information being spoken for accuracy and biases

▸ identifies the main idea and supporting information in a passage being heard

▸ restates and summarize a variety of spoken information

Learning to take notes addresses all of these skills and teaches students to become active, not passive, listeners.

Listening and the Use of Audio Materials

The use of digital books (please refer to definition of digital books found in Chapter 4) or audio books in the educational setting can be very beneficial for students with visual impairments. One of the main advantages is that a student's listening speed is often faster than his or her reading speed. Best (1991) noted that it is possible to understand spoken speech at a rate of approximately 250 words per minute, which is equivalent to a good silent-print-reading speed. Spoken speech is generally between 100–125 words per minute (Best, 1991). Students with visual impairments typically have a much slower reading rate compared to that of their sighted peers. In one study, for example, students with visual impairments reading large print and braille in grades 8 to 10 were 52 to 60 percent slower readers compared to students with unimpaired vision (Tellefson, 1999). Listening to a digital or audio book with adjustable speed can allow a student to access information at an increased rate and may enable students with visual impairments to complete some assignments as quickly as their sighted peers.

The technology for digital books is evolving rapidly, as described in detail in Chapter 4. Students are no longer limited to listening to two- or four-track tapes when listening to books. All books are now produced in a digital format. The technology used to access digital books includes personal computers, DAISY players, accessible PDAs, e-book readers, smart phones, tablets, and MP3 players. These devices have the ability to store many digital books, thus enabling a person to have an entire library of material available in one small device. The type of device used to access a digital book is dependent on the format of the electronic file being used, XML, mp3, wav, and so on. Table 5.2 lists a variety of file formats and how they can be used.

It is important that students be exposed to all of the tools and techniques that allow them to access materials in the most appropriate format. As discussed in Sidebar 4.8 in Chapter 4, mandates in the Individuals with Disabilities Educa-

TABLE 5.2

File Types Used in Assistive Technology

The following table outlines a variety of electronic files types and the common types of assistive technology in which they can be used.

File Extension	File Type	Where File Can Be Used
.txt	Text document	Optical character recognition on personal computer
		Braille translation program
.doc	Microsoft Word document	Personal digital assistant[a]
.docx	Microsoft Word document 2007 and later	Optical character recognition on personal computer
		Braille translation program
.brf	Braille-ready format	Personal digital assistant
	Embosser-ready file	Personal computer
		Personal computer with braille display
.dxb, .dxp	Duxbury[b] files	Personal digital assistant
		Duxbury to embosser
.abt	Edit-PC[c] or Braille2000[d] files	Braille 2000 to embosser
.meg	Megadots[e] files	Megadots to embosser
.html	Hypertext markup language (Web page)	Personal digital assistant
		Optical character recognition on personal computer
		Braille translation program
.rtf	Rich text format	Personal computer
		Personal digital assistant
.kes	Kurzweil[f]	Optical character recognition on personal computer
.ark	Open Book[g]	
.mp3	Sound file	Personal computer
		Personal digital assistant
		CD player
		MP3 player
.dtb, .dtd	DAISY[h] file format	DAISY player
		Personal computer with DAISY software
		Personal digital assistant
.xml	Extensible markup language (document and Web page)	Personal digital assistant
		Personal computer

Source: Adapted with permission from J. Kuns & A. Amandi, "Electronic Book Access," in *Proceedings from the 48th Annual Conference of the California Transcribers and Educators of the Visually Handicapped,* Santa Clara, CA, March 2007. Available on CSB website at www.csb-cde.ca.gov/technology.htm.

[a] Personal digital assistants are devices previously known as braille notetakers.
[b] Duxbury is commercially available braille translation software.
[c] Edit-PC is commercially available braille translation software.
[d] Braille 2000 is commercially available braille translation software.
[e] Megadots is commercially available braille translation software.
[f] Kurzweil is commercially available software that enables users to scan and listen to text on the computer.
[g] Open Book is commercially available software that enables users to scan and listen to text on the computer.
[h] DAISY stands for Digital Accessible Information System and is a standardized method of making content accessible to all users.

tion Act now require that files for textbooks for grades K–12 be made available to facilitate the creation of the books in accessible formats for students who are visually impaired. Publishers must send their files in the National Instructional Materials Accessibility Standard, or NIMAS, to a National Instructional Materials Access Center (NIMAC).

To obtain books so that students can have them at the same time as their classmates, teachers of students who are visually impaired need to compile a list of books students are using in their classes. This list should include both textbooks and literature books. When making this list, be sure to write down the title, author, publisher, publication date, and ISBN of each book. It is important to try to get the same edition as students have in print. When possible, teachers should obtain books in a digital format; however, since some teachers choose to use older versions of books some books are still only available in an audio format. Many states have a state instructional materials or resource center that acts as a central warehouse or depository for specialized media. Begin by contacting the state instructional materials center or equivalent entity to determine if the book is available and then begin searching for digital books using websites such as those listed in Table 5.3. Either order or download the digital books into the appropriate device.

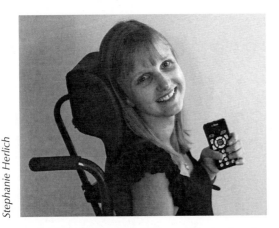

Stephanie Herlich

Listening to digital books, as this student is doing using a portable DAISY book player, not only provides access to textbooks but also can be enjoyable for students of all abilities.

As mentioned previously, publishers are required to provide NIMAS files for all textbooks; however, this does not include trade books, magazines, or other literature. Teachers will need to search other sources to find all of the books students will need. Digital books are available from a variety of sources on the Internet. Table 5.3 provides a list of some useful websites and information regarding books that can be downloaded from these websites. Some websites have subscription fees and some are free; some of the sources have electronic books that are properly formatted and easily downloaded to a computer, MP3 player, DAISY book player, and other reading devices; some sites are set up to only be read online.

In addition to the information in Chapter 4 about audiobooks and digital books, the following suggestions may help students with visual impairments incorporate listening to books into their routines:

TABLE 5.3

Online Sources and Formats of E-Books

Electronic books can be downloaded from a variety of websites. Use the table below to find a list of websites, including their fees, content, and available formats. (See Table 5.2 for explanations of file formats.) The devices that consumers can use to listen to and read books are changing rapidly. Smart phones and tablets are becoming more common place and many of the sources below are making their books available on these mainstream devices. Readers should be aware that websites change frequently and content and fee structures may have changed.

Source	Fee	Content Available	Formats Available
Sources of Books Formatted for People with Visual Impairments			
Web Braille (provides braille books, music, and magazines in an electronic format; part of National Library Service (NLS) for the Blind and Physically Handicapped) www.loc.gov/nls	Free to people who are visually impaired	Books, magazines, music	.brf (braille) electronic cassette customized for NLS players
BookShare (accessible books and periodicals for readers with print disabilities) www.bookshare.org	Free to people who are visually impaired	Books, periodicals	DAISY .brf
ManyBooks.net (electronic books) www.manybooks.net	Free	Books	.rtf .pdf .epub
The Online Books Page http://onlinebooks.library.upenn.edu/lists.html	Free	Books	.txt .html .pdf
APH Louis Database http://louis.aph.org	Free	Textbooks, books	.brf
Texas School for the Blind and Visually Impaired www.tsbvi.edu/instructional-resources/1978-braille-book-files	Free to people who are visually impaired	Books, braille	.brf .abt .dxb .meg
Project Gutenberg (electronic books) www.gutenberg.net or www.promo.net/pg/	Free	Books, speeches, videos, music, pictures	.txt .mp3 mpg (video)

(Continued)

TABLE 5.3
(Continued)

Source	Fee	Content Available	Formats Available
Learning Ally (formerly Recording for the Blind and Dyslexic) www.learningally.org/	Individual or group account	Textbooks, audiobooks	DAISY CD and downloads .dtb (DAISY) .wma
Sources of Mainstream E-Books			
Amazon.com www.amazon.com	Charge per download	Books	.dtp (desktop publishing file) .mp3
Barnes and Noble www.barnesandnoble.com/ebooks/index.asp	Charge per download	Books, magazines, newspapers	.pdb (used by specific devices) .epub (e-book file format) .pdf (viewable on any format)
Reader Store (Sony) ebookstore.sony.com/	Charge per download	Books	BBeB Book (LRF and LRX) .pdf
iTunes www.apple.com/itunes/	Charge per download	Books	.mp3 .epub
Public libraries	Free	Books (all varieties)	CD .mp3 .txt
Low Vision Classics www.classicbookshelf.com	Free	Books	Web presentation (good for individuals with low vision)
Audible.com www.audible.com	Charge per download or monthly membership charge	Books, magazines, radio shows, podcasts, other recorded entertainment and news	.mp3 CD Downloadable to most mainstream audio devices

Source: Adapted with permission from J. Kuns & A. Amandi, "Electronic Book Access," in *Proceedings from the 48th Annual Conference of the California Transcribers and Educators of the Visually Handicapped*, Santa Clara, CA, March 2007. Available on CSB website at www.csb-cde.ca.gov/technology.htm.

▸ If a student is new to digital books, begin with one format and device. For example, download a digital talking book into an e-book reader. Many of the digital talking books are formatted so that students can navigate or advance to a specific page or chapter of the book. Introduce students to the special features of digital talking books, such as navigation, variable reading speeds, and the ability to bookmark or save a specific location so that the reader can easily return to that same spot. Once the student is familiar with one type of device, then introduce another.

▸ Work with students on increasing speech rates. Instruct students to listen for something specific, such as the main points in a passage, while setting the speed higher than is normally comfortable (Best, 1991). Students should then restate what they heard. Have them listen again at a slower rate to find more information. Do these exercises a couple of times each week and chart the listening speeds. This exercise can be done using synthesized or human speech.

▸ Remind students that the listening rate may need to be adjusted according to the type of information to which they are listening. Work with students to find the fastest speed at which the student can still achieve full comprehension. Speeds may differ according to the type of reading materials; for example, a literature book may be listened to at a faster rate than a science textbook (Best, 1991).

Encourage students to listen to a digital book while following along in a braille or large-print copy. (See the discussion of audio-assisted reading in Chapter 4.) Not only can this help to improve reading speed, but it can also reduce distractions by helping students to focus both auditorily and visually or tactilely. The increased pace and the voice expression that comes with auditory material can greatly improve comprehension, and students with compromised reading speeds can keep pace with their peers and often participate in reading material that may be above their normal reading level (Evans, 1997). Following a braille or large-print text while listening is also important when new terminology, charts, or graphs are presented. Students who are following the text will be able to see the words or pictures being heard (Presley & D'Andrea, 2009).

Listening and Technology

As discussed in Chapter 4, technology has ensconced itself in our everyday lives at such a level that it is critical for all students to become proficient technology users.

The International Society for Technology in Education is in the process of updating and revising the National Educational Technology Standards. As with other curricular standards, there is not one specific set of standards followed by all states. The following standards from one school district are representative of what many states and districts are requiring all students to know in technology:

> ▶ Sixth graders are expected to type an average of at least 15 words per minute using touch typing.
>
> ▶ Seventh graders will be able to use a calculator for problem solving, statistics and probability, word problems, and percent.
>
> ▶ Eighth graders will create research papers using word-processing programs and an electronic data source such as the Internet. Students will be able to edit their work using an electronic spell check and the final project will include both text and graphics.
>
> ▶ Ninth through twelfth graders will be able to use an Excel spreadsheet and will be able to create a PowerPoint/Multi-Media presentation. (Manhattan Beach Unified School District, 2003, p. 17)

In order for students with visual impairments to achieve these types of technology goals, not only do they need to learn mainstream hardware and software, but in many cases they also need to become proficient with specialized hardware and software, typically referred to as *assistive technology*. The following description of Taylor illustrates how one student utilizes a variety of assistive technology devices to accomplish different tasks:

> *Taylor is a high school senior who has used braille as his primary learning medium since kindergarten. He is currently taking advanced courses in math and science in addition to his literature and social studies classes. Taylor has a braille PDA that he uses at school in addition to the computer he uses at home. He also keeps an e-book player in his backpack so that he can listen to assigned reading if he has time during his school day. This player currently contains all of his textbooks in addition to a variety of literature that he has enjoyed reading this past year. Taylor is currently listening to* Crime and Punishment. *He knows that he is going to have to write a paper on* Crime and Punishment; *however, he has not yet been given the exact assignment. In anticipation of the assignment, he is taking notes on his PDA while listening to the e-book. Taylor's notes will make the writing assignment easier to accomplish.*

Students today are fortunate to have access to a wide variety of technology. For example, students with low vision may be using video magnifiers (sometimes known as closed-circuit television systems or CCTVs), digital book players, and computers with screen-magnification software, which enlarges the print on the computer screen, and screen-reading software, which voices what is on the computer screen. Students who use braille may be using computers with screen-reading software, scanners with optical character recognition, PDAs with refreshable braille displays, audio calculators, and digital book players. Teachers today are often challenged to become familiar with this wide variety of technology. It is important not only that teachers instruct their students on how to use their technology, but also that they teach them when to use their technology and how to use their different devices in conjunction with each other.

Active listening is essential for students using assistive technology. Students who are using assistive technology need to become familiar and comfortable with a variety of speech output. Some technologies use human voices and some use synthetic speech. Synthesized voices have greatly improved over the past few years. Even though most students prefer human speech, students with visual impairments can learn to understand nonhuman speech with little difficulty. Learning to understand the speech emanating from a speech synthesizer has been compared to learning to understand someone with a significant accent (Kapperman & Sticken, 2000).

With the emergence of technology that utilizes speech synthesizers, it is important that students be exposed to speech synthesizers as soon as possible. Here are a few ideas to help increase students' comfort level with synthesized speech:

▸ There are several very good learn-to-type programs that teach keyboarding skills to students, such as TypeAbility (available from Yes Accessible, www.yesaccessible.com) and Talking Typer (available from the American Printing House for the Blind; see the Resources section). These programs often incorporate both synthesized speech and human speech. Not only are students learning how to use the computer; they are also learning how to listen to it.

▸ There are a variety of board games and computer games that students can play that require them to use their listening skills (a few sources of such games are included in the Resources section). Not only are these games fun, but they also teach children to listen.

▸ Download a popular book or magazine to a student's e-book reader that he or she can listen to just for fun. If the material is interesting and the student is motivated, he or she may not even realize the speech is synthesized.

Using technology with speech opens up many previously inaccessible aspects of our society. Using speech output and technology, students can now independently access the Internet, use cell phones, obtain money from an ATM machine, determine the color of an object, calculate complex mathematical equations, and even gain an enormous amount of information from a tactile map. Mastery of the appropriate assistive technology can enable students who are blind or visually impaired to gain access to the immense quantity of information available on the Internet and to transform that material independently into formats (such as braille, large print, or synthesized speech) with which they can deal effectively.

Secondary school is an optimal time to introduce students to a wide array of technology. The teacher of students with visual impairments plays a vital role in researching, introducing, assessing, and teaching students how to use their assistive devices. (See *Assistive Technology for Students Who Are Blind or Visually Impaired*, by Presley and D'Andrea [2009] for comprehensive information on preparing and conducting an assistive technology assessment.) Table 5.4 provides a helpful list of the wide variety of assistive technology—high-tech devices as well as mechanical tools and nonoptical low vision aids—that must be considered when working with students who are visually impaired. Most likely the teacher of students with visual impairments will need to work with an assistive technology team in order to evaluate the variety of devices that are available. The following are suggestions for exposing students to and teaching them about new technology:

▸ Ensure that students are using updated versions of software on their assistive technology devices. It may be helpful for teachers to create a spreadsheet like the one pictured in Figure 5.1 to keep track of the variety of technology students are using and the technology that a district or county owns.

▸ Let students know about upcoming technology workshops, exhibits, and seminars. If possible, take students on a field trip to such an event.

▸ Encourage students to join an electronic mailing list or user group that focuses on technology they are using or interested in obtaining.

▸ Contact a local vendor who can visit the school site and demonstrate appropriate new products to the student, teachers, and parents.

▸ When introducing new technology to students, be certain the device and software are working prior to the lesson. Nothing is more frustrating for a student than to have a new piece of technology and not have it work properly.

TABLE 5.4

Types of Assistive Technology for Students Who Are Blind or Visually Impaired

Types of Technology	Access Method		
	Visual Access	**Tactile Access**	**Auditory Access**
Technology for accessing print	Nonoptical devices • Large print • Reading stands • Acetate overlays • Lighting Optical devices • Handheld and stand magnifiers • Telescopes Video magnification systems Scanning and OCR systems Electronic whiteboards	Braille reading Tactile graphics Tactile math tools	Readers Audio recording • Digital talking books • Other audio formats Specialized scanning systems • Stand-alone electronic reading machines • Computer-based reading machines E-book readers Talking calculators Talking dictionaries

Technology for accessing electronic information	Computers
	• Screen-enlarging hardware
	  ‣ Large monitors
	  ‣ Adjustable monitor arms
	• Software options
	  ‣ Operating system display property adjustments
	  ‣ Computer accessibility features
	• Cursor-enlarging software
	• Screen magnification software
	Specialized scanning systems
	Accessible portable word processors
	Accessible PDAs
	E-book readers
	Large-print and online calculators
	Online dictionaries and thesauri
		Refreshable braille displays
		Computers
		Accessible PDAs
		Touch tablets
			Talking word-processor programs
			Text readers
			Self-voicing applications
			Screen-reading software
			Accessible PDAs
			Specialized scanning systems
			E-book readers
			Talking dictionaries
			Talking calculators
			Digital voice recorders

(Continued)

TABLE 5.4

(Continued)

Types of Technology	Access Method		
	Visual Access	**Tactile Access**	**Auditory Access**
Technology for producing written communications	Manual tools • Bold- or raised-line paper • Felt-tip pens and bold markers • Bold-lined graph paper for math Electronic tools • Dedicated word processors • Accessible PDAs • Imaging software • Drawing software • Talking word processor • Computer with word-processing and screen magnification software • Math software and spreadsheets • Laptop or notebook computers	Manual and mechanical braillewriting devices • Slate and stylus • Braillewriters Electronic braillewriting devices • Electric and electronic braillewriters • Computers with word-processing software • Accessible PDAs • Braille translation software • Braille embosser	Accessible computers with word-processing software Accessible PDAs
Technology for producing materials in alternate formats	Scanning and OCR system Computer with word-processing software Laser printer	Scanning and OCR system Computer with word-processing software Braille translation software Graphics software Braille embosser Equipment and materials for producing tactile graphics Materials for collage Manual devices for tooling graphics Fusers and capsule paper	Digital and analog audio recording devices Scanning and OCR system

Source: Reprinted from I. Presley & F. M. D'Andrea, *Assistive Technology for Students Who Are Visually Impaired* (New York: AFB Press, 2009), Table 1.1, pp. 9–10.

((FIGURE 5.1   **Sample Assistive Technology Spreadsheet**

Assistive Technology Tracking Form					
Software/ Hardware	Serial No.	School Site	Location/ID of Computer	Software Version	Notes
Digital book reader	32180	Bayview Elementary	Resource Room	3.31.35	Documentation in office
Speech synthesizer	54987	Wayside High	Room 501	7.30	District license

▶ Have students keep a detailed log of daily assignments, including the assignment, page numbers, and due date. This can be done using a computer spreadsheet or table, a mainstream task list, a calendar computer program, or an electronic device. Since a daily log of assignments needs to be created each day and often updated several times throughout the day, it is a great beginning skill with lots of opportunities for reinforcement and practice. Not only will this teach organization, but if the calendar is monitored, the teacher can determine if the student is actively listening to assignments given throughout the school day.

It is imperative that teachers make sure their students are using appropriate assistive technology and receive the proper training for the devices they have. Students who are comfortable with their technology have a significant advantage when pursuing postsecondary educational and vocational endeavors (Kapperman & Sticken, 2000).

Listening to a Live Reader

Another extremely efficient means of acquiring information is to listen to a live reader. Using a reader has several advantages for a person with a visual impairment. For example, a reader can visually scan a page of text for a specific item, a reader can be asked to repeat what was read or to skip ahead to the next section, and a reader can help organize materials. Adults who are visually impaired often hire readers to sort through mail, help pay bills, read instruction manuals, and help label new items of clothing or other similar personal items. Juniors and seniors in high school should be learning the skills necessary to achieve maximum independence once they have graduated, and one of these essential skills is learning how to find, interview, and hire a reader (Feeney & Trief, 2005). The ability to successfully employ and utilize a live reader creates independence because the individual with a visual impairment can control how, when, and where he or she acquires information. This control fosters independence. Teachers of students with visual impairments can begin teaching their students these essential skills during high school by:

▸ encouraging high school students to partner with a sighted friend for study purposes and group projects

▸ teaching students where and how to advertise for a reader

▸ discussing and researching options for employing and paying hired readers

▸ facilitating a connection with a rehabilitation counselor

The listening skills needed for effectively utilizing a hired reader are many of the same skills that have been discussed throughout this chapter. Individuals must be able to record the information they are hearing with an appropriate device; they must be able to organize the information being acquired; and they must be able to evaluate the information for its usefulness and efficacy. One crucial skill that has not been previously addressed and may be the most difficult for students to learn when using a live reader is directing the reader and explaining exactly what is needed. Throughout a student's school career, he or she is absorbing information and being directed through the learning process. It is not often that a student becomes the director. The following strategies help students understand and begin practicing the skills necessary to effectively employ a live reader:

▸ Teach students to develop a job description for a live reader. Ask students to think about what they would want their reader to do, their expectations of the reader, and qualifications the reader should have. Research job descriptions in help wanted advertisements either in the newspaper or on the Internet.

▸ Practice being the reader for students as often as possible. Pretend that the students' needs or wants are not known. At the beginning, prompt the students as often as needed, but gradually reduce the prompting so that the students begin to understand what it means to be the director. For example, during the reversal of roles, the student with the visual impairment will be asking the reader (the teacher) to assist in finding vocabulary words that need to be defined using the social studies text-book. The students will need to explain to the reader exactly how this should be done, that is, by using the glossary or looking for highlighted words in the text. The student cannot expect that the reader knows this process; the student with visual impairments can practice explaining these types of procedures.

▶ Discuss with students the importance of using time wisely. The student with a visual impairment needs to have all of his or her materials ready before the reader arrives and needs to know exactly what needs to be accomplished.

▶ Be sure students understand that when using a live reader, the end product must be the work of the student, not the reader.

The use of assistive technology and live readers helps students develop advanced listening skills. Being able to listen and learn independently, utilize a variety of technology appropriate to the task, and explain exactly what is needed to a live reader are essential skills students need as they prepare to leave high school and live and work independently as adults.

LISTENING IN SOCIAL SITUATIONS

Listening skills relating to listening in social situations include the following:

▶ utilizes effective listening strategies to engage in social interaction

▶ listens respectfully when others speak

▶ evaluates social situations to determine appropriate use of specific social behaviors

▶ converses with others on a range of interesting topics without dominating the conversation

Stacy is in fifth grade and is preparing to go to middle school. She has low vision and uses a CCTV, computer with speech, and electronic books in order to complete all of her schoolwork. Stacy recently took a tour of her new school in order to become oriented to the new campus. An eighth-grade student gave Stacy the tour and at the end asked if she had any questions. Stacy asked, "How many dances are there during the year?"

This question is typical of middle school students, but is it typical of middle school students who are visually impaired? Unfortunately it is not. Many students who are visually impaired are not socially active. Stacy is clearly a very social young lady. Has her visual impairment impacted her socially? What have her teachers done to help Stacy feel comfortable with her peers? Chapter 4 describes the importance of good listening skills in social situations and how to lay the groundwork for children in elementary school, such as by teaching students to obtain information about their friends by asking questions, learning how to show that they are paying attention by facing the speaker, and learning how to interpret tone of voice. Refining these skills to become a good social listener must continue throughout middle and high school.

It has often been demonstrated that placing a child who is visually impaired in a general education classroom does not mean that child will automatically make friends with and become part of the social network within the class (Hatlen, 2004; Hoben & Linstrom, 1980; MacCuspie, 1990; Rosenblum, 2006). One of the main reasons the expanded core curriculum was developed was that educators and parents recognized that students with visual impairments required instruction in areas other than academics (Hatlen, 1996; Hatlen & Curry, 1987; Huebner, Merk-Adam, Stryker, & Wolffe, 2004; Rosenblum, 2006). Goal 3 of the expanded core curriculum highlights the importance of specifically teaching social skills to students who are blind and visually impaired (Expanded Core Curriculum, 2007; Hatlen, 1996).

When students enter middle and high school, not only are their academic demands increasing, but so are the social expectations. Students are usually traveling between different classrooms and have several teachers throughout their school day. During lunch students are no longer required to sit with their class; they are allowed to sit and socialize with whomever and wherever they like. When a fully sighted teen was interviewed in 2003 and asked what it takes to "fit in" and what is considered "trendy," many of his responses involved being a good listener. This included being a good listener to what and whom other students are talking about; being able to instant message friends (today the criteria would undoubtedly include text messaging); listening to music, playing video games, going to movies; and participating in extracurricular activities (Wolffe, 2006, p. 96). Being a good listener in social situations is pivotal for students with visual impairments.

It is important for educators to remember that no matter a student's age or level of functioning, social skills are an essential part of the curriculum for students who are visually impaired (Crow & Herlich, forthcoming). Listening skills that relate directly to social skills include understanding the meaning of what is said, interpreting someone's spoken and unspoken intent and meaning, organizing an appropriate response, and listening to locate peer groups and social activities. The activities in Sidebar 5.4 provide ideas for helping students listen in social situations.

Activities for Practicing Listening in Social Situations

The following lessons, which highlight the importance of listening skills in social situations, were designed to be taught in a social skills group with both sighted students and students who are visually impaired. Teachers may choose to teach these lessons as outlined or may adapt the lessons as necessary. In addition to these activities, the Social Skills Board Games from Exceptional Teaching Aids include six games that involve players in discussing the solutions to socially challenging situations, encouraging all players to communicate, listen, and participate.

GETTING-TO-KNOW-YOU BINGO

Objective: Students will have an opportunity to learn about their peers through questions about likes, dislikes, and personal attributes.

Skills Addressed

- conversation
- listening

Introduction: Sighted people are able to gain much information through their vision and are therefore able to learn a lot about others and their environment. For example, sighted people are inundated with visual images of what might be appropriate and fashionable dress. A visually impaired person does not have visual access to this information. The following activity allows all the students to learn more about one another.

Materials: bingo cards (print/braille) and chips; bingo questions (listed at the end of this lesson); bingo callout sheet (sheet of numbers 1–75 used by the "caller" to announce the number players are to look for).

Activity

1. Explain to students that they are going to play bingo with a twist. Each student gets a print/braille bingo board and a set of bingo chips. Each student also gets a list of printed or embossed bingo questions. The teacher is the bingo caller. If needed, review the game rules of bingo with the students.

Bingo Game Rules

- A bingo card consists of five columns and five rows. A random selection of numbers is on each card. The *B* column contains numbers 1–15, the *I* column contains numbers 16–30, the *N* column contains numbers 31–45 (with a free space in the center), the *G* column contains numbers 46–60, and the *O* column contains numbers 61–75.
- The caller randomly selects a number from the callout sheet, and then calls out that number to the players. The caller marks that number off the callout sheet.
- The players check their cards to see if they have the matching number. If they do, they cover the number with a bingo chip.
- Play continues until someone achieves a "bingo," which is a straight horizontal, vertical, or diagonal line of bingo chips on the card.

(Continued)

2. In Getting-to-Know-You Bingo, when a student has a matching number, he or she identifies him- or herself to the group. Then the student looks at the list of questions and asks a designated student any one question from the list. The turn for answering questions passes around the circle to the left.

3. Students continue playing bingo until someone has a "bingo." If time permits, the game can be played more than once.

Note: Teachers should feel free to add or delete any questions that are or are not appropriate to their group of students.

Bingo Questions

1. What color are your eyes?
2. What color is your hair?
3. How tall are you?
4. What is your ethnicity?
5. Do you live in a one-story or two-story house or apartment?
6. What is your favorite type of book?
7. When is your birthday?
8. What is your sign?
9. Do you prefer pepperoni or cheese pizza?
10. Do you enjoy rap or hip-hop music?
11. Do you enjoy rock or country music?
12. Do you enjoy classical or jazz music?
13. Where were you born?
14. Do you like short or long hair?
15. Do you like tattoos?
16. Name one place you would like to go.
17. Do you prefer cold or warm weather?
18. Do you prefer math or English?
19. Which do you prefer, oceans or rivers?
20. What is your favorite movie?
21. What is your favorite ice cream flavor?
22. What is your favorite band?
23. Do you like wool or fleece jackets?
24. Do you prefer swimming or sunbathing?
25. Do you prefer running or hiking?
26. Do you prefer reading or eating?

27. What is your favorite cartoon?
28. Do you prefer a Mac or PC?
29. What is your favorite fast-food restaurant?
30. What is the latest you have ever stayed awake?

FINDING FRIENDS IN A CROWD

Objective: Students will develop an understanding of the difficulty of locating friends in a crowded area.

Skills Addressed

- listening
- mobility
- problem solving
- assertiveness

Introduction: Explain how people's voices can be difficult to discriminate in various settings. Large indoor spaces make it difficult to locate the direction of particular voices. Navigating through crowded, noisy rooms and open outdoor spaces presents additional challenges. For example, there are often extraneous sounds such as lawn mowers, airplanes, or construction noise.

Materials: blindfolds, low vision simulators, cane

Activity 1

1. The whole group goes outside.
2. Select one student to wear a blindfold. Other students stand at a specific spot outside and have a conversation using a normal tone of voice. Using a cane, the blindfolded student attempts to find the group.
3. Repeat with different students wearing the blindfold.

Activity 2

1. The whole group goes inside.
2. Select two students to put on blindfolds. Using a cane, these students try to locate nonblindfolded peers inside a crowded room (for example, cafeteria, recreation room).
3. Repeat with two new students.
4. Discuss experiences. Be sure to ask the group possible ways to make finding friends in a crowd easier. For example, agree to meet friends at a specific spot so that you can find them more efficiently.

SHOWING INTEREST

Objective: Students will discover that everyone has unique interests that are both interesting and different.

Skills Addressed

- listening
- conversation

(Continued)

(((‹ SIDEBAR 5.4 *(Continued)*

Introduction: As a group, discuss what makes people want to interact with one another, their interests, likes, and dislikes. Explain that it is sometimes difficult to discover other people's interests. In the following activities, students will have a chance to think about the things that make them interesting and different. They will have a chance to share their uniqueness as well as discover the interests of their peers.

Materials: blindfolds (optional)

Activity

1. Divide students into groups of three.

2. Each group discusses the following questions:

   a. What makes you different from your peers?

   b. What is one thing that you do or have done that makes you proud?

3. Explain that one person in each group will answer the question first. The other members in the group must listen and may ask probing questions. The focus must remain on the person answering. Each person has two minutes to answer.

4. After everyone has spoken, bring the whole group back together and have each person describe one unique thing about a member of their small group.

5. Ask the students to take time during the next week and ask a person who was not in their group about the thing that makes him or her unique.

Source: Condensed and adapted with permission from N. Crow & S. Herlich, *Getting to Know You: A Social Skills/Ability Awareness Curriculum for Students with Visual Impairments and Their Sighted Peers.* (Louisville, KY: American Printing House for the Blind, forthcoming).

RECREATIONAL LISTENING

A large part of our ability to socialize comes from participating in extracurricular activities. When people socialize they often talk about what they enjoy doing, such as hobbies, sports, travel, and leisure-time activities. One leisure-time activity that students with visual impairments often enjoy is recreational listening. Recreational listening can take many forms, including listening to music, radio, television, computer games, audiobooks, sports, live performances, and sounds of nature. Exposing students to the variety of recreational listening available to them can help to provide another social outlet for individuals with visual impairments. Some students may not even realize the enjoyment that can come from the types of activities listed above. In addition to the recreational listening activities mentioned in Chapter 4, older students may enjoy the following:

▶ Once students have completed their work, or if students have reached an important milestone, allow them to choose some form of recreational listening, such as listening to music or a book or even a watching a movie with descriptive video (as described in Chapter 4).

▶ Encourage students to invite a friend to take part in a listening activity once a week or once a month, such as watching a descriptive video or playing an accessible computer game (see Resources section for sources of such games).

▶ Have students keep a log of their recreational listening. Review the log periodically and make suggestions for exploring other types of listening activities.

▶ Encourage parents to organize family listening opportunities such as attending a performance or a sports event. Another fun activity is for the family to go on a nature "listening walk" or hike. During a listening walk everyone is silent and listens to the sounds around them. After a set period of time each person shares what he or she heard, for example, birds, airplanes, lawn mowers, dogs, people, wind in the trees, and so on.

▶ There are many fun, commercial games available that rely on listening skills.

CONCLUSION

Students in middle school and high school need to "*learn to listen* so they can *learn by listening*." This process includes refining their ability to listen to classroom instruction actively and critically and engaging in collaborative discussions with their teachers and classmates. They also need to use fine-tuned listening skills as they utilize accessible technology for many curricular tasks. Middle and high school students thrive socially if they have learned how to fully interact with their peers because they have learned to listen. Learning to listen skillfully helps open the gateway to adulthood.

REFERENCES

Bancroft, N. R., & Bendinelli, L. (1982). Listening comprehension of compressed, accelerated, and normal speech by the visually handicapped. *Journal of Visual Impairment & Blindness*, *76*(6), 235–237.

Best, A. B. (1991). *Teaching children with visual impairments*. Philadelphia: Open University Press, Milton Keynes.

Boyle, E. A., Rosenberg, M. S., Connelly, V. J., Washburn, S. G., Brinckerhoff, L. C., & Banerjee, M. (2003). Effects of audio texts on the acquisition of secondary-level content by students with mild disabilities. *Learning Disability Quarterly, 26*, 203–213.

Common Core State Standards Initiative. (2010). Common core state standards for English language arts and literacy in history/social studies, science, and technical subjects. Retrieved from www.corestandards.org/the-standards.

Crow, N., & Herlich, S. (Forthcoming). *Getting to know you: A social skills/ability awareness curriculum for students with visual impairments and their sighted Peers.* Louisville, KY: American Printing House for the Blind.

Evans, C. (Ed.). (1997). Changing channels—audioassisted reading: Access to curriculum for students with print disabilities. Proceedings from National Conference of the Council for Exceptional Children, Division on Visual Impairments. Salt Lake City, UT.

Expanded core curriculum for blind and VI children and youths. (2007). Retrieved June 28, 2007, from www.afb.org/Section.asp?SectionID=44&TopicID=189&SubTopicID=4&DocumentID=2117.

Feeney, R., & Trief, E. (2005). *College bound: A guide for students with visual impairments.* New York: American Foundation for the Blind.

Ferrington, G. (1994). Keep your ear-lids open. *Journal of Visual Literacy, 14*(2). Retrieved July 18, 2011, from http://wfae.proscenia.net/library/articles/ferrington_earlids.pdf.

Goddard, K. M., Isaak, M. I., & Slawinski, E. B. (1998). Are the congenitally blind better at attending to auditory information? *Acoustical Society of America ICA/ASA '98 Lay Language Papers.* Retrieved June 4, 2007, from www.acoustics.org/press/135th/goddard.htm.

Harley, R. K., Truan, M. B., & Sanford, L. D. (1997). *Communication skills for visually impaired learners: Braille, print, and listening skills for students who are visually impaired* (2nd ed.). Springfield, IL: Charles C Thomas.

Hatlen, P. (1996). The core curriculum for blind and visually impaired students, including those with additional disabilities. *RE:view, 28*(1), 25–32.

Hatlen, P. (2004). Is social isolation a predictable outcome of inclusive education? *Journal of Visual Impairment & Blindness, 98*(11), 676–677.

Hatlen, P. H., & Curry, S. A. (1987). In support of specialized programs for blind and visually impaired children: The impact of vision loss on learning. *Journal of Visual Impairment & Blindness, 81*(1), 7–13.

Hoben, M., & Linstrom, V. (1980). Evidence of isolation in the mainstream. *Journal of Visual Impairment & Blindness, 74*(8), 289–292.

Huebner, K. M., Merk-Adam, B., Stryker, D., & Wolffe, K. (2004). *The national agenda for the education of children and youths with visual impairments, including those with multiple disabilities* (rev. ed.). New York: AFB Press.

International Society for Technology in Education. (2007). *NETS: National curriculum/ content area standards.* Retrieved May 30, 2007, from www.iste.org/standards.aspx.

Jones, R. (2007). Strategies for reading comprehension: Summarizing. Retrieved June 27, 2007, from www.readingquest.org/strat/summarize.html.

Kapperman, G., & Sticken, J. (2000). Assistive technology. In A. J. Koenig & M. C. Holbrook (Eds.), *Foundations of education* (2nd ed.). Vol. 2, *Instructional strategies for teaching children and youths with visual impairments* (pp. 500–516). New York: American Foundation for the Blind.

Kuns, J., & Amandi, A. (Eds.). (March 2007). Electronic book access. *In Proceedings from 48th annual conference of the California transcribers and educators of the visually handicapped.* Santa Clara, CA. Available on CSB website at www.csb-cde.ca.gov/ technology.htm. San Francisco, California School for the Blind.

Lee, D., & Hatesohl, D. (1993). Listening: Our most used communication skill. University of Missouri Extension. Retrieved July 17, 2011, from http://extension.missouri.edu/p/CM150.

MacCuspie, P. A. (1990). The social acceptance and interaction of integrated visually impaired children. (Unpublished doctoral dissertation). Dalhousie University, Halifax, Nova Scotia, Canada.

Mangold, S. S. (1982). *A teachers' guide to the special educational needs of blind and visually handicapped children.* New York: American Foundation for the Blind.

Manhattan Beach Unified School District. (2003). *Educational technology use plan.* Manhattan Beach, CA: Manhattan Beach Unified School District.

Presley, I., & D'Andrea, F. M. (2009). *Assistive technology for students who are visually impaired: A guide to assessment.* New York: AFB Press.

RFB&D. (2007). *RFB&D's learning through listening: Program at a glance.* Princeton, NJ: Recording for the Blind & Dyslexic.

Rosenblum, L. P. (2006). Developing friendships and positive social relationships. In S. Z. Sacks & K. E. Wolffe (Eds.), *Teaching social skills to students with visual impairments: From theory to practice* (pp. 163–194). New York: American Foundation for the Blind.

Tellefson, M. (1999). Compare these reading rates: What do you think? *WAER Newsletter.*

Thum, Carl P. (2001). Taking lecture notes. Hanover, NH: Dartmouth College Academic Skills Center. Retrieved May 24, 2011, from www.dartmouth.edu/~acskills/docs/ taking_notes.doc.

Tuncer, A. T., & Altunay, B. (2006). The effect of a summarization-based cumulative retelling strategy on listening comprehension of college students with visual impairments. *Journal of Visual Impairment & Blindness, 100*(6), 353–365.

Wolffe, K. E. (2006). Theoretical perspectives on the development of social skills in adolescence. In S. Z. Sacks & K. E. Wolffe (Eds.), *Teaching social skills to students with visual impairments: From theory to practice* (pp. 81–116). New York: American Foundation for the Blind.

Chapter 6

Listening Skills for Orientation and Mobility: Hearing the Whole Picture

Maya Delgado Greenberg and Wendy Scheffers

Most people take their hearing for granted. I can't. My eyes are my handi-cap, but my ears are my opportunity. My ears show me what my eyes can't. My ears tell me 99 percent of what I need to know about my world.

—Ray Charles, testimony before congressional subcommittees for Labor, Health and Human Services, and Education, 1987, quoted in *Ability Magazine*, 1995

CHAPTER PREVIEW

- ► Listening Skills and Independent Travel
- ► Listening in the Early Years: Attaching Meaning to Sound
- ► Listening to Acquire Information: Everyday O&M in Preschool and Elementary School
- ► Listening and Community Travel in Middle School and High School

Carol, a 15-year-old high school student, shifts her heavy school bag as she tucks her long white cane under her arm and locks the front door. She flips her long black hair out of her face, angles her chin up, then grins. Carol has no light perception due to retinal blastoma, a form of eye cancer, but she can tell from the heat on her face that it is going to be a beautiful sunny day.

Carol strides down the street toward her bus stop, her cane lightly tapping back and forth in front of her. She pauses when she hears a garage door opening ahead and on the right, waits for the car to back out and pull away, and then continues walking to the intersection. Traffic is heavy that day, so it is easy for her to hear that traffic is flowing in front of her on the perpendicular street. Carol waits for the next green light, listening carefully for the traffic pattern to shift. The cars in front of her stop, and the cars next to her on the parallel street surge forward. Carol steps out confidently. After crossing the street she steps up onto the sidewalk and slows as she hears a group of people chatting—they are probably waiting at her bus stop. Her cane taps the bus pole with a familiar clink and she stops and faces the street. Carol pushes the button on her talking watch to hear the time; then she hears the deep rumble of a bus approaching. The doors whoosh open; she confirms the bus number with the driver and steps up into the bus.

The ability to travel independently is a cherished freedom for all people, as it is for Carol, and it starts to develop early in a child's life. Many developmental milestones are measured by the ability to move purposefully. Children's movements are celebrated as they grow, from the first time they reach toward their parent's voice to the moment they take their first steps to the day they cross the street independently.

LISTENING SKILLS AND INDEPENDENT TRAVEL

Children with visual impairments need adaptive skills to travel safely and independently. The body of knowledge and specialized techniques for safe and independent travel used by individuals who are visually impaired is known as *orientation and mobility* (O&M). *Orientation* is the understanding of how the world is laid out and the ability to use the senses to gather information, recognize the current location, plan a route, and problem solve. *Mobility* is the ability to move safely and efficiently. Orientation and mobility skills, which begin to develop in infancy and continue to grow throughout life, are interdependent, and both are necessary for travel. Because the ability to interpret sensory input and move accordingly is the basis of later O&M skills, development of these skills needs to be supported through careful attention by a collaborative team of parents, educators, and an O&M specialist.

O&M specialists are highly trained professionals who teach people of all ages, from infants to senior citizens, who are blind or have low vision. O&M skills are taught by an O&M specialist through carefully sequenced instruction. Children with visual impairments, some of whom have additional disabilities, typically receive O&M

instruction through the school system. They are taught to use all available sensory systems to gather information about the world around them and to travel safely at home, at school, and in their community. To assist them in safe travel, they often learn to use tools and technology, such as long white canes, an accessible Global Positioning System (GPS), and low vision devices such as small monocular telescopes which are used to view objects at a distance. O&M instruction is individualized to meet each child's needs.

For a person with a visual impairment, hearing assumes a predominant role in allowing the individual to move through the surrounding environment successfully and safely. Vision and hearing are the two primary senses used to gather orientation information from a distance (Guth, Rieser, & Ashmead, 2010). For children with visual impairments, hearing becomes a primary sensory system for gathering environmental information beyond arm's reach. Children who are visually impaired do not have better hearing than sighted children, but out of necessity they often develop more effective and finely tuned listening skills.

Because listening skills are so essential for children of all ages to help them make sense of the environment and move independently, this chapter is devoted to the topic of listening and O&M. It begins with an overview of how the sense of hearing can be utilized for travel. The chapter then discusses the development of listening skills related to O&M in infants and toddlers, and continues with a description of O&M listening skills for school-age children that can be developed through experiences with O&M specialists, parents, teachers, family, and friends. The final section addresses sophisticated listening skills for preteens and teenagers that typically require instruction from a certified O&M specialist. The chapter highlights listening strategies that can assist in the development of O&M skills for children who are visually impaired or blind. Unless otherwise indicated, the content in this chapter applies to both children with low vision and children who are blind.

Becoming an Active Listener

While hearing can be passive, listening is an active process. For all children, it takes considerable practice to learn how to effectively interpret sounds and words. Children also need to learn how to integrate auditory information with other sensory information through touch, smell, and any remaining vision. Listening skills are important for children with low vision as well as for children who are blind. Listening can provide effective orientation information from a distance and can be less fatiguing and more efficient than relying solely on low vision.

Information gathered through listening can greatly compensate for reduced vision or blindness. Children can learn to identify a sound source, determine its location, and move toward it. They can learn to associate locations with sets of environmental sounds. Sounds provide information about the size and layout of a space, the presence of objects, and the location of landmarks. Auditory information can help a traveler analyze traffic patterns, create mental maps of an area, and plan a route.

While academically successful students may be able to understand and recall verbal directions in the correct sequence, they may not have mastered the listening skills needed for effective O&M. Listening skills for travel are complex and involve interpreting subtle properties of sound. In addition to remembering verbal travel directions, other skills necessary for safe travel are the ability to identify sounds, interpret properties of sound, and plan movement in relation to sound.

To become proficient travelers, children with visual impairments need to become active learners and listeners. Sighted children's lives are filled with incidental visual learning opportunities, as they see the layout of space and learn about the relationship of objects to one another. Using vision, it is simple to glance at a destination, size up the travel path, plan a route, and start moving. Children with visual impairments benefit from direct instruction in how to use their other senses to learn the spatial and environmental concepts that sighted children learn easily through vision.

It is impossible to make generalizations about the development of listening skills that apply to every child. While all children go through general developmental stages, the way that each child grows and changes is highly individualized (Brazelton, 1983; Ferrell, 2011). Additionally, infants and children with visual impairments frequently have other disabling conditions that can affect their development and learning (Lueck, Chen, Kekelis, & Hartmann, 2008; Warren, 1994). Another factor that can hinder the progression of skills is that some well-meaning people believe that blind children are incapable of doing things on their own and that it is unsafe for them to move around independently. Discouraging children who are visually impaired from exploring can impede their development of listening, orientation, and mobility skills.

Listening and O&M

O&M listening skills are used in routine activities throughout the day. Upon hearing a familiar deep voice, a baby uses spatial awareness and motor skills to reach out and touch his father's face. A young child uses listening skills when she gets out of bed in the morning, hears her brother talking in the kitchen, and then walks to the table for breakfast. During physical education class, a third-grade student uses sound localization and tracking to kick an approaching audible ball. A teenage student listens carefully to the traffic pattern before he crosses the street to go shopping at the mall.

For every person who is visually impaired, well-developed O&M skills are essential to live and work independently and successfully. These skills involve the finely tuned, advanced ability to apply the sense of hearing to understand and navigate the surrounding environment. Adults need to nurture these listening skills beginning when the child is an infant. With continued structured learning experiences, the child will build on and fine-tune these skills as he or she grows older.

A traveler with well-developed O&M listening skills:

▶ is aware of and compares sounds

▶ associates objects and their sounds

▶ identifies sounds

▶ localizes sounds—detects the direction and distance of a sound source (and orients and moves in relation to that sound)

▶ identifies environments or activities based on sets of associated sounds

▶ attends to sounds and verbal information—auditory attention span

▶ attends to one sound from a sea of background sound—auditory figure-ground discrimination

▶ uses sounds as landmarks and reference points to establish orientation in a familiar area

▶ uses environmental sounds to locate silent objects and detect properties of objects and space (and to orient and move in relation to that information)—auditory space perception

▶ orients and moves in relation to a moving sound source—sound tracking

▶ remembers multiple-step instructions or information in the correct order—auditory memory and sequencing

▶ listens to verbal information and asks clarifying questions

▶ uses sounds to create and update a mental map of the environment while traveling

▶ recognizes "danger sounds" and responds quickly

▶ uses technology, such as computers with speech output, to access auditory travel information

Note that as this chapter focuses on O&M, this list is different from the Listening Skills Continuum in Appendix A at the back of the book.

Parents, families, and teachers are all crucial members of the O&M team in teaching concepts and reinforcing safe travel. Parents are the most important teachers in a child's life, for while the child might have one or two lessons with an O&M specialist each week, children and parents are together every day. When a child is encouraged to apply O&M skills both at home and at school, these skills develop much more rapidly, and typically become fluid and automatic.

Hearing Impairments and O&M

Since listening skills play such a pivotal role in the development of environmental awareness and safe travel skills as well as the ability to participate in learning and literacy activities, it is important for parents, teachers, and other adults to be alert to the possibility that a child's hearing may be impaired. Sidebar 6.1 provides questions to consider to help determine whether a child's hearing needs to be assessed by a physician or specialist. (See Chapter 7 for more information on assessing students with multiple impairments, Chapter 8 regarding students who have a hearing impairment in addition to a visual impairment, and Chapter 9 regarding students with auditory processing and related issues.)

A child who does not respond to sounds or cannot accurately localize sound may have a hearing loss. All young children, especially children with visual impairments, need to have their ears checked regularly. Even children who do not seem uncomfortable

---

(⟡ Sidebar 6.1

Does the Child's Hearing Need to Be Assessed?

O&M tasks require complex use of listening skills, and teaching these skills may bring to light possible hearing issues. Considering the following questions will help a parent or teacher determine whether a child needs to be assessed by a physician or specialist. The first step is usually to have the child's ears checked by a physician to see if he or she has a ear infection. If there is no infection to treat, there are a number of specialists who can help evaluate and treat issues related to hearing, auditory processing, and other related skills. These include audiologists, school psychologists, resource specialists, speech and language pathologists, and sensorimotor specialists. Audiologists are health care professionals who evaluate and treat hearing loss disorders. School psychologists can assess auditory processing. Resource specialists can also assess certain elements of auditory processing. Speech and language pathologists evaluate, diagnose, and treat speech and language disorders. Sensorimotor specialists are occupational or physical therapists who have received additional training in how individuals access, integrate, and respond to input from their sensory systems.

1. Does the child detect sounds (such as voices or cars) when others do? Does the child need to be closer than others in order to hear the sounds clearly? Does the child detect only loud sounds? Does the child attend primarily to low- or high-frequency sounds? If the child misses sounds that others hear and a physician has ruled out an ear infection, arrange for an evaluation by an audiologist.

(Continued)

((SIDEBAR 6.1 *(Continued)*

2. Can the child accurately listen to a sound and figure out where the sound source is in space (localize sounds)? If the child cannot accurately localize sound and a physician has ruled out an ear infection, arrange for an evaluation by an audiologist.

3. Does the child consistently miss some steps in following instructions or scramble the order of instructions? This could be an indication of an auditory processing issue. If the child seems confused by verbal directions, make sure the terms used are clearly defined and question the child for comprehension. Instead of a general question such as "Do you understand?" ask specific questions such as "What are you going to do first?" "What is next?" or "Tell me what you are going to do." If the child still struggles with remembering and sequencing auditory information, refer the child to specialists in the school system such as a school psychologist, resource specialist, or speech and language pathologist for further assessment.

4. Does the child have difficulty focusing on a specific sound source in a noisy environment or become easily distracted by environmental sounds? This could be an indication of an auditory figure-ground discrimination problem. If a physician has ruled out an ear infection, consider referring the child to a speech and language pathologist, resource specialist, or sensorimotor specialist for further assessment.

5. Does the child find normal-volume sounds to be loud or painful? With relatively loud sounds present, does the child become frightened or lose the ability to attend to other sensory input? Does the child try to avoid certain sound activities? If so, have the child's ears checked by a physician to see if he or she has a ear infection. If no infection is found, consider referring the child to a sensorimotor specialist for an assessment.

may have a low-grade infection that can affect their hearing. The early years, during which infants and toddlers are prone to frequent ear infections, are a critical time for developing auditory skills. Even a temporary hearing loss can impede the development of communication, balance, and orientation (Anthony, Bleier, Fazzi, Kish, & Pogrund, 2002), but medical treatment for ear infections can be very effective.

For children who are visually impaired who have a permanent hearing loss, it is best to begin intervention at an early age. Many children who are visually impaired with hearing loss in one ear can learn to localize sound to some extent. If a hearing aid is prescribed, it is essential to select one that allows the child access to both speech and environmental sounds. The ability to localize sounds should also be considered (Lawson & Wiener, 2010a). (For more information on listening skills and children with both visual and hearing impairments, see Chapter 8.)

LISTENING IN THE EARLY YEARS: ATTACHING MEANING TO SOUND

As infants and young children learn about the sounds they hear around them, they begin to attach meaning to sound, the most basic development of listening skills. There are many emerging listening skills that develop at this age. A young child with good listening skills:

▶ notices sound

▶ listens to a specific sound

▶ localizes the position of the sound source

▶ compares how sounds are the same as, similar to, or different from other sounds

▶ notices if a sound is loud or soft

▶ notices if a sound is high or low

▶ notices if a sound is long or short

▶ identifies common sounds

▶ associates sounds with objects

▶ reaches toward a sound

▶ moves toward and away from a sound

▶ determines if a sound is near or far

▶ determines if a space is small or large from reflected and reverberated sound

▶ identifies a familiar location by listening to environmental sounds

Children typically acquire to some extent the early listening skills that contribute to attaching meaning to sound through play and incidental learning experiences (Lawson & Wiener, 2010b). Given how important listening skills are to children who are visually impaired for developing their orientation and mobility, however, basic listening skills should also be explicitly addressed through structured learning experiences by each child's family and early intervention teachers.

The ability to hear develops in the womb (Kisilevsky, Pang, & Hains, 2000). After birth, the infant is surrounded by a rich sensory environment of sound, taste, touch, movement, and smell (and for babies with low vision, sight). Over time, sounds become associated with other sensations. For most infants, the soothing sound of a parent's voice quickly becomes associated with warmth, gentle touch, and food. As the association of

Strategies for Teaching the Meaning of Sounds to Infants and Young Children

Throughout each day there are many opportunities for teaching the meaning of sounds to infants and very young children. Listed here are some examples of ways to help infants and young children learn that sounds are associated with objects, people, and places:

- Create a quiet environment. The sounds in a typical home may be overwhelming to an infant who is not accustomed to filtering out the sounds of TV, radio, dishwasher, fans, and other household noises. A quiet indoor environment allows the child to focus on isolated sounds of people and objects.

- Establish routines, allowing for natural repetition and consistency of experiences. For a sound to have meaning, a child needs multiple experiences with the sound source. For example, for each mealtime, encourage the child to participate in the routine by touching the silverware drawer as it is opened to get the baby spoon, touching the door of the humming refrigerator as the adult opens and closes it, and "helping" to wash the dishes.

- Set up daily playtimes in predictable spaces with items that make interesting sounds to encourage exploration and purposeful reaching.

- Whenever possible, link listening to touch, movement, and any remaining vision when explaining a sound to the child. A multisensory learning experience coupled with a verbal description helps the child link the sound to an object. For example, when the child hears nails clicking on the hardwood floor, a collar jingling, and a bark nearby, call the family dog over so that the child can touch, smell, and explore the dog so the sounds have meaning. Describe what the child is touching with statements such as, "Oh, here is the collar. Listen to it jingle when you shake it."

- Allow the child time to notice and listen to sounds without interrupting. After the child has listened for a reasonable time, provide a simple and timely description of the sound and what made it. (For specific examples, see Sidebar 2.6, "Enhancing Listening Comprehension during Everyday Experiences.")

- Encourage children to ask about sounds and to search for the sound source. When infants notice a sound, describe what it is and whenever possible let them touch it. Model how to ask about sounds by saying, for example, "I wonder what is making that sound? Let's go find out."

- When identifying sound-making objects, incorporate the use of simple spatial concepts (for example, "The noisy airplane is *up in* the sky," or "The bells are *in* the box").

- Comment on environmental sounds and identify the setting, such as the humming of the refrigerator in the kitchen, sounds of traffic on the street, or the beeping of the cash register at the store.

- When going places with a child, tell him or her where you are going before beginning to travel, and ask questions to help him or her anticipate what to expect. For example, "We are going to the park. Do you think that there will be lots of other children on the swings today? Do you think we will hear the geese honking by the lake?"

sounds with people and objects emerges, so does the beginning of purposeful listening and movement. Attaching meaning to sounds is the most basic level of early listening skills. (See Sidebar 6.2 for strategies for teaching the meaning of sounds to infants and young children.)

Localization

Infants with visual impairments demonstrate sound localization skills, that is, the ability to detect the direction and distance of a sound source, in various ways as they grow. The ability to localize sounds develops quickly in the first six months of life, and then improves gradually until age 7 (Anthony & Lowry, 2005). Very young infants often become quiet and stop moving as they attend to a sound and instinctively try to localize its position. As their neck muscles strengthen, infants may react to a sound by turning toward it. At 1 month, babies can identify their parents' voices (Bayley, 2005). By 3 to 4 months, they can localize a familiar sound in a horizontal plane at ear level (Johnson-Martin, Jens, Attermeier, & Hacker, 1991; Kukla & Thomas, 1978). As the developmental chart in Table 6.1 indicates, sound localization skills begin horizontally at ear level, eventually expanding to below and above ear level, and in front of, behind, and above the child. While many people are likely to place a sound-making object in front of an infant, a child's ability to localize sounds coming from in front of the child does not fully develop until 21 to 24 months (Kukla & Thomas, 1978).

As babies randomly move their arms and legs, they contact objects and people. The resulting tactile sensations and sounds reinforce attempts to move, touch, and explore the world. Over time these initially random movements are shaped into purposeful reaching and exploration. By around 11 months of age, many babies with visual impairments can combine sound identification and localization skills to consistently reach toward sounds (Fraiberg, 1977). Sound localization and intentional reaching for an object or person are the beginning of mobility! (For more information on listening skills for infants and toddlers, see Chapter 2.)

Table 6.1 presents some developmental milestones related to localization, other basic listening skills, and movement skills in infants and young children. Although typical age ranges for the development of these skills are presented, it is important to remember that each child develops at his or her own pace. The table provides a sequence of skill development to help parents and teachers determine the child's current skill level and understand what is next in the developmental sequence.

TABLE 6.1

The Development of Listening and Movement

For people of all ages, listening skills are used to identify objects, people, activities, and locations. This information provides the motivation for an infant or young child who is visually impaired to lift his or her head, point or reach, crawl, and walk; the development of listening skills and movement are intrinsically connected.

Although there are typical age ranges associated with the emergence of movement and listening skills, each child develops at his or her own pace. Consequently, the information presented here represents general guidelines for the progression of skills, not a specific guide to the rate of skill acquisition.

Skills	Age	Sources
Pre-ambulatory Movement		
Repeats limb movements to create sound	Birth to 1 year	Oregon Project
Turns head to sound	4 months	Bayley Scales 3
Turns head to localize sound while in sitting position	Birth to 1 year	Oregon Project
Turns head toward sound on the side at ear level	4 to 7 months	Assessment of Auditory Functioning
Turns head toward sound on the side below ear level	7 to 13 months	Assessment of Auditory Functioning
Reaches to sound	9 to 16 months	Fazzi et al., 2002
	11 months	Fraiberg, 1977
Turns head toward sound on the side above ear level	13 to 21 months	Assessment of Auditory Functioning
Turns head toward sound in front, then behind, and directly above	21 to 36 months	Assessment of Auditory Functioning
Whole-Body Movement		
With auditory cue, scoots or crawls to a familiar toy	Birth to 1 year	Oregon Project
Crawls on hands and knees	10 to 24 months	Fraiberg, 1977
	10 to 25 months	Fazzi et al., 2002
Walks without support	9 to 13 months	Bayley Scales 3
	1 to 2 years	Oregon Project
	12 to 20 months	Fraiberg, 1977
	13 to 32 months	Fazzi et al., 2002
Uses sound for orientation	13 to 30 months	Fazzi et al., 2002
Use of Reflected Sound*		
Reaches toward a wall or stops before contacting it	Preschool	Preschool O&M Screening
Walks next to wall without contacting it	Preschool	Preschool O&M Screening
Detects openings on a wall	Preschool	Preschool O&M Screening
Detects a two-foot-wide object while stationary from six feet away	4 years	Myers & Jones, 1958
Detects small objects (12 to 20 inches wide) from two feet away	4 to 12 years	Ashmead, Hill, & Taylor, 1989

The following sources include assessment tools for children with and without visual impairments as well as research studies:

Assessment Tools

Assessment of Auditory Functioning of Deaf-Blind/Multihandicapped Children is an assessment tool that measures how a child uses residual hearing in the classroom. It also contains descriptions of typical development in hearing and sound localization skills in infants. D. Kukla & T. T. Thomas, *Assessment of Auditory Functioning of Deaf-Blind/Multihandicapped Children* (Dallas, TX: South Central Regional Center for Services to Deaf-Blind Children, 1978).

Bayley Scales of Infant Development, 3rd ed., were created to evaluate the developmental status of young children from age 1 month to age 42 months. They consist of three scales: Mental, Motor, and Behavioral Rating Scale. N. Bayley, *Bayley Scales of Infant Development,* 3rd ed. (San Antonio, TX: Psychological Corporation, 2005).

Preschool Orientation and Mobility Screening is an assessment screening tool designed for use by O&M specialists to determine a child's current level of O&M functioning, help identify areas of need, and identify the need for O&M services. It includes a section on auditory skills. B. Dodson-Burk & E. W. Hill, *Preschool Orientation and Mobility Screening* (Alexandria: VA: Association for the Education and Rehabilitation of the Blind and Visually Impaired, Division IX, 1989).

Oregon Project for Preschool Children Who Are Blind or Visually Impaired, 6th ed., includes the Oregon Project Skills Inventory, which consists of 800 developmental skills organized in eight developmental areas: Cognitive, Language, Social, Vision, Compensatory, Self-Help, Fine-Motor, and Gross Motor. Each of these eight areas contains developmentally sequenced skills arranged in the following age categories: birth to 1 year, 1 to 2 years, 2 to 3 years, 3 to 4 years, 4 to 5 years, and 5 to 6 years. The Skills Inventory is a criterion-referenced assessment that enables educators to measure the performance level of a child who is visually impaired or blind and determine skills to be taught. S. Anderson, S. Boigon, K. Davis, & C. deWaard, *The Oregon Project for Preschool Children Who Are Blind or Visually Impaired: Skills Inventory,* 6th ed. (Medford: Southern Oregon Education Service District, 2007).

Other Sources

D. H. Ashmead, E. W. Hill, & C. R. Taylor, "Obstacle Perception by Congenitally Blind Children," *Perception and Psychophysics,* 46 (1989), pp. 425–433.

E. Fazzi, J. Lanners, O. Ferrari-Ginevra, C. Achille, A. Luparia, S. Signorini, & G. Lanzi, "Gross Motor Development and Reach on Sound as Critical Tools for the Development of the Blind Child," *Brain and Development,* 24 (2002), pp. 269–275.

S. Fraiberg, *Insights from the Blind: Comparative Studies of Blind and Sighted Infants* (New York: Meridian Books, 1977).

S. O. Myers & C. G. E. F. Jones, "Obstacle Experiments: Second Report," *Teacher of the Blind,* 46 (1958), pp. 47–62, cited in W. R. Wiener, R. L. Welsh, & B. B. Blasch (Eds.), *Foundations of Orientation and Mobility,* 3rd ed., Vol. 1, *History and Theory,* p. 132 (New York: AFB Press, 2010).

*Reflected sound has not been extensively researched in young children, and there are no existing developmental charts or assessment tools for young children regarding use of reflected sound at the time of this publication. The age references for use of reflected sound are primarily from research studies.

Predictable Spaces

Frankie, a 10-month-old baby, is learning how to move and play. He has no light perception due to retinopathy of prematurity, a retinal condition associated with his premature birth. Every day his mother puts him on a blanket between the wall and the side of the couch in the living room, creating a predictable space to help define the boundaries of his environment. She places a play gym over him with suspended household objects hanging above his torso. He wiggles and waves his arms, and his hand brushes metal measuring spoons. He startles as the spoons rattle, becomes still as he listens to the sound, and then intentionally reaches out to grab the spoons. He giggles and coos as he shakes them. His mother waits until Frankie is done with his initial exploration before describing what he is doing, "Oh, you found the spoons! They were over your head."

Frankie associates the clanking sound with the spoons, localizes the sound, and then reaches out to them. His repeated experiences in this predictable space have helped him develop localization and reaching skills. Understanding where objects and people are in space encourages him to turn his head and reach. Soon this awareness will provide the impetus to crawl and walk.

Predictable spaces—also called play spaces or defined spaces (Lowry, 2004)—are defined areas with tactile boundaries and distinct objects placed within to encourage movement and foster early listening skills. Some predictable spaces have walls within reach on three sides and objects or a "roof" above. With the world brought within arm's reach, the infant is encouraged to reach out in all directions. Predictable spaces can teach object permanence, the concept that a silent object out of sight and contact still exists. Developing object permanence and an understanding of the position of self in relation to objects can create the motivation to reach for, crawl toward, or walk toward objects. Exploration in a predictable space stimulates motor growth and develops spatial orientation (Nielsen, 1992), both essential and critical elements in the development of effective O&M skills.

Predictable spaces can be constructed out of household objects, furniture, playpens, or crib gyms. Elements that can be incorporated into a predictable space include textured blankets and household objects. A resonance board, a low platform made of birch, can be used as a floor to amplify sound and stimulate movement (Nielsen, 1992). Pegboard is a good material for construction of the walls and ceiling, as household objects can be easily attached with short elastic cord. It is crucial that the cord be short and well-secured so that it cannot be looped around the child's neck or become a choking hazard. If preferred, predictable spaces can be purchased. For example, Dr. Lillie Nielsen, a specialist on children who are visually impaired who have multiple disabilities, has created a commercially available space called a "little room" (Nielsen, 1992). (For additional ideas on selecting and introducing toys and play environments, see Chapter 2.)

An environment with consistently placed objects allows the child to explore the space, locate and compare objects, and return to preferred objects. This develops not

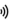

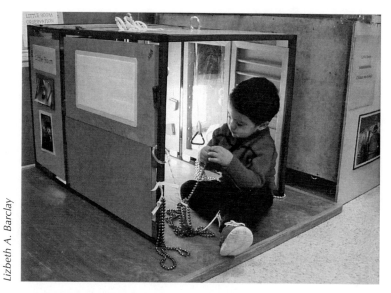

Predictable spaces encourage reaching, movement, and spatial awareness in infants and young children.

Lizbeth A. Barclay

only self-to-object awareness, but also an understanding of the relationship of objects to other objects, which is a critical element in developing spatial orientation. (For additional information about predictable spaces, see Chapter 7.)

Listening Behavior

As described in Chapter 2, infants with visual impairments may exhibit different listening behavior than sighted children. Sighted children often turn to and look at a sound source. When children who are visually impaired attend to sound, they may become quiet or cock their heads to the side. Turning the head from side to side to listen with both ears from different angles can help the child who is visually impaired localize the sound. Some people may misinterpret this behavior to mean that the child is looking away and not paying attention. As children who are visually impaired often "look" at something with their ears, turning the head may indicate that they are being very attentive and are merely trying to localize a sound.

Reflected Sound

Sounds reflected off walls and objects can provide young children with environmental information. "The native ability of human beings to sense space by listening . . . does not require special skills—all human beings do it: a rudimentary spatial ability is a hardwired part of our genetic inheritance" (Blesser & Salter, 2007, p. 1). Sounds can seem more intense in a small enclosed space and more "echo-y" in a large room. Many people can hear how sounds seem different when standing in front of a solid wall in comparison to an open door. Sounds can also be muffled by an object between the listener and the sound source. As young children begin to explore, they can use such differences in sound to help map out their world.

Adults can teach children the usefulness of reflected sound by making sounds and helping the child reach out to large objects, walls, or open spaces that cause differences in sound reflection. For example, an adult could tell the baby, "Listen to how the sound changes," and then hold the baby and walk slowly down a quiet enclosed hallway, encouraging him or her to touch the wall. As the adult makes intermittent tongue-clicking sounds at the child's ear level, the baby can hear how the sound subtly changes at the open door frame. The adult can point out when the sound changes and have the child reach out to confirm that there is open space at the doorway. Similar activities include listening near open and closed windows, gaps in furniture, or an open car window. (The use of reflected sound for traveling is discussed in more detail later in this chapter under "Auditory Space Perception.")

Experiential Learning

As discussed in earlier chapters, hands-on experiences with common sound-making objects help the child make sense of everyday sounds. Sighted children see people making sounds every day as their sibling flushes the toilet, their father puts away the pots and pans, and their mother rustles the newspaper. In order to learn what these sounds are, children with visual impairments need to push the lever on the toilet, play with pots and pans in the kitchen, and crumple the pages of a newspaper. Adults need to facilitate hands-on contact with sound-making objects for their children who are visually impaired as much as possible throughout the day. These direct experiences help children who are visually impaired identify sounds and associate them with objects, people, locations, and activities. Later, children learn naturally that a combination of sounds tells a story about what is happening in the world around them. For example, the garage door opening, the dog barking, footsteps nearing, and then the door creaking open means that someone is coming home.

Purposeful Movement toward Sound

Listening skills and motor development are intrinsically intertwined. Sounds provide the motivation to move and thus help promote motor development. In order to interact with sound-making objects, the infant needs to develop motor skills. Motor skills allow the child to explore the world and learn about properties of sound and space. Development in one domain fuels development in another, enhancing the child's overall growth and learning.

Scooting or crawling to a sound source emerges after infants understand that a desired object or person is nearby, but too far away to reach. Maintaining attention to a sound source while struggling to use undeveloped muscles to crawl is difficult, as most of the child's attention is on movement. Although each child's development is highly individualized, crawling skills usually develop at around 11 months (Ferrell, 1998). This purposeful movement of the whole body is a huge developmental landmark that most parents joyfully celebrate. The child can now access the world beyond arm's reach. Once crawling or walking skills develop, children can move through space and discover for themselves if they are near or far from a sound source. (For information on strategies to help children develop motor strength and mobility, see Sidebar 6.3.)

As motor skills improve, young children devote less energy and attention to movement and more to the world around them. Now they can practice more complex sound localization skills, such as traveling to an intermittent sound source. They can also begin to develop sound-tracking skills, traveling in relation to a moving sound source. Playing a simple game of "I'm going to get you," where the child and the adult take turns chasing each other, can be a fun way to practice tracking and moving toward and away from sounds. Movement and listening games help children not only to practice sound localization, but also to learn that sound provides information about depth and distance. As Ferrington (1994) noted, "Although sound is three dimensional it is the sound generated by moving objects, or the movement of the listener in relationship to the sound, that strengthens the perception of three dimensionality" (p. 59).

The ability to move independently gives the child more control over the world. Children can move toward a sound in order to get a desired object or attention from a person. They can also escape from a noisy environment or uncomfortable sound by moving away. Children can learn that a particular sound represents a specific place in their house or yard. Adults can help facilitate this use of sound for orientation by intentionally placing permanent sound-making objects throughout the home and yard, such as a ticking clock in the kitchen or wind chimes at the back door (Lueck, Chen, Kekelis, & Hartmann, 2008).

Community Destinations

Rasheedah is a 3-year-old who is thrilled to go shopping with her father today. She has 20/600 acuity in her left eye and no light perception in her

Strategies for Developing Motor Strength and Mobility in Infants and Young Children

Understanding what sounds represent can provide the motivation for infants and young children to move and touch the sound source. Conversely, the ability to move allows children to explore a sound source and develop a more complete understanding of their world. The following suggestions can facilitate the development of these skills and abilities:

- Vary the position of the infant while he or she is being carried, sitting, and lying down to stimulate muscles, develop balance, and encourage exploration.

- Infants need to spend time on their stomachs to develop the neck, back, arm, and hand muscle strength needed for crawling. Give infants many opportunities across the day to spend time on their tummies on the floor or on an adult's chest for as long as they will tolerate.

- When teaching an infant to locate and reach to sound, keep in mind that infants first learn to listen to a sound and figure out where it is in space (localize) near ear level. Whenever it is practical, present sounds initially next to the child at ear level. Over time, vary the position of sounds by moving them below, above, in front of, and behind the child.

- To encourage localizing and reaching, make intermittent sounds from a close-by stationary position. This helps the child attend to the location of the sound, not just the duration of the sound (Nielsen, 2005). As infants are more likely to reach out to a sound-making object that is within arm's reach, the sound should be presented close to the child (Litovsky & Clifton, 1992). For example, intermittently shake a favorite rattle within arm's reach of the child and encourage him or her to reach for the toy. Repeat the game, varying the position of the rattle.

- Create predictable play spaces with interesting household objects in consistent locations to foster exploration and develop object permanence. For example, at the baby's changing table, hang a sound-making mobile in a fixed position. Encourage the child to explore and play with it; over time, the child will learn the location of the mobile and will reach for it without prompting. When children get older, provide a predictable play location on a mat next to a kitchen drawer filled with safe kitchen items to enjoy.

- If a child shows interest in a sound, move him or her close to the sound source and encourage touching and exploring.

- As the child begins to scoot, crawl, or walk toward sounds, keep distances short and motivating sound-making objects stationary. Many people are tempted to coach the child to move greater distances by stepping back or pulling the sound source farther away, but keeping the sound source stationary helps the child learn not only how to localize sounds, but also how to estimate distances.

- Create an organized home environment that will allow the child to successfully and safely locate desired objects or destinations. Maintain a consistent furniture arrangement with limited clutter on the floor. Make sure that all objects are stored in a predictable location in drawers, cabinets, or shelves.

right eye resulting from a toxoplasmosis infection. She wears nonprescription glasses to protect her left eye from any injury that could reduce her remaining vision. Rasheedah walks hand in hand with her dad to the grocery store, her long white cane sliding on the hard concrete in front of her. The automatic door opens with a whoosh and they suddenly hear the clattering of the grocery carts and the beeping cash registers. They pause and her father says, "The door opened! Do you hear the carts in the grocery store? Let's go inside." Rasheedah's cane clinks against the metal shopping cart inside the door. She helps pull the cart into the aisle. When her father says, "Time to go up in the cart," he puts her cane in the basket and then lifts her into the seat. As they move down the aisles, they pause to touch the food, look at the items closely, and drop them into the cart. The cans make a loud noise when they drop. Dad asks Rasheedah to reach "way up" to get the big bag of pretzels. It has a crackly-sounding wrapper and needs to be handled gently. At the checkout stand, Rasheedah helps place the food on the conveyer belt. Her father puts his hand under hers and guides her to feel the belt and food as they move forward. The next time she hears the belt move she tells her father, "The pretzels are moving!" Her dad gives Rasheedah her own paper bag for the pretzels. They put the pretzels in the bag and place it in the cart. She can't wait to get home to show her grandpa.

For children of all ages, it is stimulating to visit destinations in the community. The unique sets of sounds and sensations of the world outside the home create a rich variety of learning opportunities. The more exposure children have to different environments, such as parks, grocery stores, and other homes, the more prepared they will be for independent travel in these places later in life.

Fun family trips like the one Rasheedah experienced with her father increase a child's understanding of the world, developing vocabulary, spatial concepts, listening skills, and positive memories. Similar experiences can happen just about anywhere: at the playground, the doctor's office, or the mall. Connecting words, touch, and sounds helped Rasheedah link the sound of the conveyor belt with the movement of the food on the counter. To help children who use long white canes to interpret what their canes are contacting, they need to use both their canes and their hands to explore the world around them. A cane moving over grass sounds different from a cane moving on cement, plastic, or wood, and initially taking the time to explore a new walking surface with hands will help the child to later identify the sounds the cane makes during travel.

While in different community environments, it is important for the young child to have hands-on experiences as much as possible. Short, simple verbal descriptions

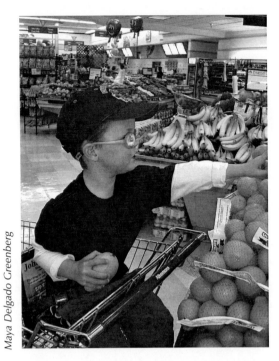

Maya Delgado Greenberg

Hands-on experiences develop children's understanding of the world.

of objects and sounds add to community learning opportunities. If possible, an adult needs to preview with the child what to expect. For example, at the grocery store you can say, "Soon you will hear the automatic door open." If there is an unanticipated sound, pause to give the child time to listen; then you can describe it by saying something like, "Oh, that was the rattling of a metal grocery cart." It is crucial to keep the descriptions concise and to the point. A running commentary can interrupt the child's learning experience, distracting the child from listening carefully and connecting his or her hands-on experiences with what he or she is hearing. The adult's voice can also mask environmental sounds and the child may miss opportunities to learn from the rich combination of sounds in the community.

After hands-on experiences, sounds alone will come to have meaning. Children who are blind need to have hands-on experiences with a sound-making object. Children with some vision may be able to see a sound source, like a conveyor belt, but may not be able to see it clearly enough to understand what is happening unless they also touch it, have it described to them, and listen to its sound. This experiential process helps children with low vision connect what they feel and hear with what they see. Once this connection is established, children with low vision can use vision to verify what is heard and hearing to verify what is seen.

A recording of familiar sounds gives children the ability to hear the sound over and over again. Just as sighted children usually love photographs, children who are visually impaired often enjoy sound recordings. Children can record the sounds of their vacation—the crashing of the waves on the beach or the squeals of joy of passengers on amusement park rides. To give the sound recording a context, they can also record a short description of the location and what the sounds mean, with parents helping as needed. Bringing home a sound image from a vacation, park, or shopping trip allows the child to recall and share experiences with others.

Children learn to identify activities and places by their sounds between the ages of 3 and 4 (Anderson, Boigon, Davis, & deWaard, 2007). They come to associate a set of sounds with a particular environment. For example, after many trips, they come to associate the sounds of automatic doors, grocery carts, beeping cash registers, and conveyor belts with a grocery store. The learned association that connects sounds, places, and activities is the product of years of experiences, learning, and development as children learn to fine-tune their ability to interpret and attach meaning to sound. This skill readies them for one of the most significant community destinations: school.

LISTENING TO ACQUIRE INFORMATION: EVERYDAY O&M IN PRESCHOOL AND ELEMENTARY SCHOOL

As children get older and prepare for preschool and kindergarten, they enter a new era with regard to listening skills. The school environment fosters purposeful listening to gather information, a more complex skill than learning to attach meaning to sound. There are many emerging skills for a young school-age child who is listening to acquire orientation information. The school-age child with well-developed listening skills:

- ▸ stays focused on auditory information for several minutes, increasing the number of minutes over time
- ▸ localizes sound while moving
- ▸ travels to or away from an intermittent source of sound
- ▸ hears if a space is big or small
- ▸ hears the presence of silent objects
- ▸ uses hearing to detect features of silent objects, such as size, shape, and density
- ▸ identifies people, objects, and activities auditorily
- ▸ identifies familiar and unfamiliar locations by listening to environmental sounds
- ▸ uses sound sources for orientation and to create a mental map
- ▸ listens to a specific sound within a noisy environment
- ▸ understands spoken information
- ▸ remembers verbal directions in the correct order
- ▸ listens for car sounds before crossing the street (with adult supervision)

Attending school is an exciting and challenging experience for young children. The school environment naturally encourages children to develop complex listening skills. Once students with visual impairments begin school, they, like all students, are formally engaged in learning activities, and their listening abilities are used to gather information. In the realm of O&M, they are similarly moving to a new level of acquiring orientation information to negotiate more complex community environments that are characterized by sudden dynamic shifts in many different environmental factors, such as crowds, hallways and stairs, and loud and distracting noise levels. For this reason, they need to refine their abilities in such areas as sound localization, auditory figure-ground discrimination, auditory space perception, and auditory memory and sequencing. As their vocabularies grow, children learn to follow multiple-step directions. They begin to apply their listening skills in new ways now that their attention spans have increased. They practice picking out specific sounds in a noisy environment. They improve their ability to track moving sounds and to move in relation to sound. Children with visual impairments often learn to tune in to subtle properties of sound in order to detect silent objects and understand the space around them. These new skills allow them to gain information about their expanding world of school and community.

Direct instruction by an O&M specialist becomes increasingly important as children develop the foundational listening skills for travel that they will use for the rest of their lives. Because children learn best when family members, caregivers, teachers, and specialists work as educational partners, the O&M specialist's key role as a team member involves identifying O&M listening skills to be taught by parents, teachers, and other service providers in addition to directly teaching adaptive strategies and use of mobility tools. These skills need to be reinforced by a variety of people throughout the day. Consistent support and instruction from the whole team make for a smooth learning process as the child learns how to apply listening skills in order to travel in more complex environments and process verbal information effectively.

Sound Localization and Tracking

When the recess bell rings, the first-grade class eagerly lines up at the door. As the class starts to exit, Carlos, a 6-year-old boy with albinism, turns back to get his hat. He knows that his eyes won't hurt if he wears his hat on the sunny playground. He shoves his black and orange Giants baseball cap onto his head and walks quickly to catch up with his class. The other students are too far away for him to see them, but he can hear their footsteps and excited voices down the hall. As he passes the open door to a classroom being remodeled, the banging of a hammer and the whine of an electric saw suddenly dominate, masking all other sound. Carlos fixes his eyes on the light of the open door at the end of the hallway until he gets past the sound and can hear his classmates again. As he exits the building, he pauses. Carlos can hear the space open up—it sounds different than the enclosed hallway. It is hard for him to see with the glare outside, so he cocks his head to listen for the voice of his best friend, Dave. Carlos turns his head to the right as he focuses on the sound of his classmates' feet stomping on the plastic steps of the playground structure. He hears a familiar shout, turns his body toward the sound, and runs to join Dave by the tire swing.

In the course of a typical school day, children have many opportunities to use complex applications of sound localization skills. Moving throughout the school and within the classroom requires children with visual impairments to move in relation to stationary sound sources, such as a pencil sharpener, as well as auditorily track multiple moving sources, the other children and teachers. Activities that require moving quickly in relation to the sounds of moving objects and people, such as those performed in physical education class, particularly stimulate a child's ability to distinguish between a stationary and a moving sound source, judge its distance, and assess which direction it is moving. By elementary school, motor skills have usually developed to a point where children can move in relation to sounds in a variety of ways: toward, away, or alongside. Sound localization "emerges as a perceptual skill of paramount importance going beyond the usual listening skills of a sighted person. It allows the visually impaired traveler to locate objects within the environment and travel safely through that environment" (Lawson & Wiener, 2010a, p. 111). (For strategies to help students develop effective sound localization and tracking skills, see Sidebar 6.4.)

Sounds that are associated with a distinct fixed position, such as the ticking clock on the kitchen wall, can serve as *landmark sounds*. Landmark sounds establish orientation

---

((⟨ Sɪᴅᴇʙᴀʀ 6.4
Sound Localization and Tracking Activities

The following sound localization activities can also be used to teach and reinforce concepts of position, direction, and distance. Begin teaching with a stationary sound source while the child is still, and then increase the difficulty by first moving the sound source and then asking the child to move in relation to the sound (Brothers & Huff, 2008).

- **Child stationary with a stationary sound source.** Have the child sit in a quiet indoor location with a stationary constant sound source, such as a radio or a ticking timer. Encourage the child to point to and label the sound location using specific terms, such as "the sound is in front of me," or "the sound is up over my head." Repeat the exercise, changing the position of the sound source by moving it in different positions in relationship to the child, above or below, in front of or behind, and next to the child.

(Continued)

- **Child stationary with a moving sound source.** Have the child point toward a constant sound source and then track it as it is moved in a variety of ways (for example, up and down, left and right, and around). Help the child label the way the sound is moving.

- **Child moving in relation to a stationary sound source.** Have the child turn in relation to a stationary sound source to place the sound in front, behind, and on the right and left sides. Ask the child to move toward and away from the sound source. With younger students, this activity can be turned into a game of "Simon says." Vary the game by "hiding" an interesting sound source, such as a boom box, for the child to find. Whenever possible, use an interactive sound source that the child would enjoy playing with once the object is located.

- **Variation: Free walking** (Guérette & Zabihaylo, 2011). In a large area without obstacles, stand 15 to 20 feet in front of the child. Talk to the child and have him or her point to your location. Continue to talk while the child walks toward you without a cane or guide, stopping when she thinks she has arrived close to you. Repeat the activity, but after the child points in your direction, stop talking and have the child walk toward you. This activity helps the child localize the sound source and judge how far it is from her current location. It also helps the child learn to maintain a straight line of travel without constant tactile or auditory cues. Finally, it allows her to enjoy the freedom of movement without holding a cane or a guide's arm.

- **Child moving in relation to a moving sound source.** Have the child track a slowly moving sound by walking parallel to it without contacting it. Guide the child if needed; then have the child try it independently. This is a prerequisite skill for efficient community travel and safe street crossings. This skill can be easily practiced anytime when walking next to a street with sounds of moving vehicles present.

- **Make it fun!** Play games with sounds in different environments. Go on a sound scavenger hunt to find a list of different sounds, play "I hear with my ear" (a variation of the children's game "I Spy"), or make up your own game. Encourage the child to point toward sounds, guess their source, and name their position and location. Whenever possible, have the child travel to a sound source and experience it hands-on. Children typically enjoy recording sounds. Go for walks to record sounds in a certain position (in other words, on one day record sounds on the right, on the next day the left, then in front, behind, above, or below).

- **Mix it up!** The activities listed here can be modified in the following ways:
  - ‣ change the pitch or volume of the sound source
  - ‣ change the location of the sound source (in other words, up or down, left or right, in front or in back)
  - ‣ alternate between a constant and an intermittent sound source

- Seek out naturally occurring opportunities for the child to localize sound. Point out how the hum of the refrigerator is to the left of the kitchen door and how the sound of the car moves as it passes by. Keep in mind that high-pitched sounds can be more difficult to localize than low-pitched ones. Children with low vision may benefit from closing their eyes (or if comfortable with it, using a blindfold) during these activities to help them focus on auditory information.

within a familiar space. Children who have a good mental map of an area can localize the landmark sound and use it as a reference point to locate other silent objects within that space, such as the sink, table, and stove.

Auditory Figure-Ground Discrimination

Children with well developed auditory figure-ground discrimination skills can pick a particular sound—the figure—out of a sea of background sound—the ground—such as when Carlos listened for his best friend's voice on the playground. This is also known as selective listening, the ability to attend to a specific sound, and then shift attention from one sound to another as needed. The relevant and background sounds together make up *soundscapes*, "acoustic environments that include both natural and human-made sound" (Ferrington, 2003, p. 43).

Even for children with excellent figure-ground discrimination skills, background sounds within a soundscape can be loud enough to mask other significant sounds. These background sounds may be a specific identifiable sound or residual sound (the background noise of a community when no specific identifiable sounds can be heard). When such a masking sound is present, the child needs to either wait for the masking sound to stop, use tactile or visual information to travel, or get assistance from others. When Carlos's ability to hear his classmates was blocked by loud construction sounds, he had to project a line of travel toward where he had last heard his classmates and rely on visual information in order to move in the right direction.

For infants, the environment needs to be calm and quiet in order for them to attend to sounds. As children get older, they need to develop figure-ground discrimination skills by listening in incrementally noisier and more complex soundscapes. Sounds can stand out naturally due to their volume, pitch, or proximity. It takes practice, however, to selectively listen to a specific sound, such as someone's voice, that might be soft, far away, or partially masked by other sounds. While some children can do this relatively easily, others need direct instruction in how to attend to or ignore specific sounds. Adults can help by acknowledging distracting sounds and redirecting the child's attention back to the relevant sounds. For example, if the child turns his or her head toward the open window as a loud truck passes, the adult can note, "There goes a truck. Now it's time to pay attention to what I am saying." If the child's auditory figure-ground discrimination skills do not improve with direct instruction, consultation with a specialist, such as a speech and language pathologist, is advised. (For strategies to help students develop the ability to differentiate between figure and background sound, see Sidebar 6.5. For more information on auditory processing concerns, see Chapter 9 on language and learning disabilities.)

It is vital for children to learn how to "keep an ear out" for sounds that could indicate danger while traveling in the community. Children need to learn how to take

((⸱ SIDEBAR 6.5
Activities to Develop Auditory Figure-Ground Discrimination Skills

The following activities can help children practice distinguishing important sounds from background noise in the environment:

- Go on sound hunts. Listen for categories of sounds, such as motor sounds, nature sounds, beautiful sounds, or soft sounds. Use of an audio recorder can motivate and focus the child's listening.
- When in a complex soundscape, such as a mall or party, ask the child to listen to different sounds. Practice shifting attention from one sound to another, including the background sounds, nearby sounds, soft sounds, and loud sounds.
- When listening to music, ask the child to name the different instruments and number of vocalists.
- At intersections, point out when loud engines mask quiet car sounds. Also, ask the child to point to the sound of a specific vehicle and track it as it moves by. These auditory figure-ground, sound localization, and sound-tracking skills help prepare the child for street crossings later in life.
- Note rhythmic sounds in the community, such as footsteps, raindrops, and traffic patterns at intersections.

((⸱ SIDEBAR 6.6
Teaching Tips for Developing Active Listening

It takes considerable practice to learn how to effectively interpret sounds and words. The following suggestions can help a child become an active listener:

- Use hands-on activities to incorporate other senses when teaching listening skills.
- Ask the child to identify sounds and guess what activity is creating them to foster curiosity and awareness.
- When traveling together with a child, take periodic breaks from conversation to walk quietly together. This allows the child to listen to sounds and assess where he or she is in space.
- Understand that children become distracted by interesting sounds. Patiently acknowledge the other sounds, and then redirect attention back to the task at hand.
- When masking sounds block the ability to listen, use the "teachable moment" to model one of the following problem-solving strategies:
  1. Wait for the masking sound to end.
  2. Move away from the masking sound.
  3. Use tactile or visual methods to travel safely (for example, trail the wall with a hand or use a long white cane).
  4. Get assistance from others.

- After the experience, talk with the child about which strategy you used and why.
- Introduce new information when the child is stationary. Keep in mind that when children are in motion they have to attend to safety, balance, orientation, and mobility.
- Notice what information is available through listening alone, without visual cues. Help children understand that others may see things that they cannot hear, and they might hear things that others do not notice. When correcting a mistaken conclusion that a child has made based on auditory input, first acknowledge his or her accurate listening before correcting the misperception based on visual information.

⟮ SIDEBAR 6.7
Safety Awareness Activity

Before children who are visually impaired can travel independently, they need to be street-smart—they need to be alert to the possibility of danger and know how to respond to it. One way to help children develop such an awareness is to brainstorm with them a list of sounds that could mean danger, as well as possible safe responses. Here are some examples:

Possible danger sound: Person talking in an angry tone or with slurred speech.
Possible responses: Move away by changing the route or crossing to the other side of street. If the person tries to talk to you, do not respond. Instead, turn your head away and walk away with a confident gait and quick pace.

Possible danger sound: Barking dog.
Possible responses: Call out to see if the dog's owner is present. Find out if the dog is friendly and on a leash. Cross to the other side of the street or change the route.

Possible danger sound: Footsteps behind or car slowly following in an isolated area that could mean that someone is following you in order to rob or hurt you.
Possible responses: Move purposefully to a more populated area, go to the nearest store or home for help, or call 911 on a cell phone. Ideally, do not travel in isolated areas, especially alone.

Possible danger sound: Speeding car running a red light or stop sign.
Possible responses: Stay on the sidewalk. If in the street, use your judgment to decide if you need to pause, maintain your pace, or speed up.

---

responsibility for their own safety. Adults can help children learn active listening by pointing out sounds such as screeching tires, people shouting, or barking dogs and talking about what they mean and how to react. Modeling active listening and responding helps prepare children to be attentive and responsive when they later encounter similar situations as independent travelers. (See Sidebar 6.6 for teaching tips to develop active listening skills and Sidebar 6.7 for activities to develop safety awareness.)

It is unsafe for children with visual impairments to use headphones to listen to music or text while walking. Headphones create a self-imposed hearing loss and mask not only danger sounds, but also other important sound cues.

Sensitivity to Sound

Every child has unique sensitivities to sound. Some children struggle with loud sounds, experiencing them as too loud, even painful. Reactions to uncomfortable sounds can vary widely, from acting irritated to covering one's ears to dropping to the ground in fear. These reactions block the ability to attend and can be a serious safety concern.

Adults can help desensitize children who are alarmed by sounds. When possible, the adult needs to show the child the source of the sound and allow for hands-on exploration of the object with the sound off. Then have the child experience the sound from a distance. It is best to forewarn the child before activating the sound and to keep the duration brief. When the child seems comfortable with the sound from a distance, slowly decrease the distance and increase the duration of the sound. For example, for a child who is alarmed by the sound of the leaf blower used by the school gardener, allow the child to touch and explore the leaf blower while it is off. Talk with the child about how it works and what the whooshing sound it makes means. Next, try having the leaf blower turned on at a distance from the child so the sound appears soft and not threatening. Praise the child for remaining calm. Once the child has learned to tolerate the sound from a distance, slowly move it closer in stages, stopping as soon as the child shows signs of discomfort and backing off to a place where the child remains calm. Over time, the child may learn to tolerate the sound of the leaf blower. However, the desensitization process can take days, weeks, or even longer, depending on the child.

If a child's reaction to sound interferes with learning, it is important to determine the reason. Children who react strongly to everyday sounds need to be checked by their pediatrician for ear infections or neurological concerns. It is increasingly common for children who are very sensitive to sound to be assessed to see if they have "auditory defensiveness" as a symptom of sensory integration dysfunction, a neurological condition in which the brain is not able to effectively process the sensory information it receives. There is anecdotal evidence that sensory integration therapy by a specially trained occupational or physical therapist can help some auditorily sensitive children moderate their reactions to sound. Sensory integration therapy generally consists of exercises to either stimulate or calm parts of the nervous system. While this therapy has not yet been thoroughly researched (Green, 2001, p. 23), there is a growing body of professionals, parents, and clients who firmly believe that it has positive outcomes where other therapies have failed (Ayers, 2005).

Auditory Space Perception

Most people are unaware that listening skills can be used to locate silent objects and to detect properties of silent objects and space. "When our ability to decode spatial attributes is sufficiently developed using a wide range of acoustic cues, we can readily visualize objects and spatial geometry: we can 'see' with our ears" (Blesser & Salter, 2007, p. 2). People can learn to use hearing to detect the location, size, shape, density, and distance of silent objects (Kish, 2009; Stoffregen & Pittenger, 1995). They can also learn to determine the characteristics of a space, including size, layout, and types of objects within the space. These elements combine to create an "aural architecture" (Blesser & Salter, 2007, p. 2). It is possible to hear where a wall begins, hear an open door in a hallway, detect the presence of a silent object nearby, or detect a change in acoustics when entering a room.

This kind of spatial listening is called *auditory space perception* (Ashmead et al., 1998). Research shows that there are many kinds of auditory space perception. One type involves *echolocation*: listening to sound, usually produced by the traveler, as it reflects and reverberates off objects to detect the presence, shape, size, and density of objects and the layout of space (Kellogg, 1962; Rice, Feinstein, & Schusterman, 1965; Stoffregen & Pittinger, 1995). *Sound reflections* are sound waves that bounce off objects, and *sound reverberations* are the prolongation of a sound after the original source has stopped producing sound waves (Lawson & Wiener, 2010b, p. 91). Another type of auditory space perception involves *sound shadows*, where sound is blocked by objects similar to the way that light is blocked by objects. A third kind of auditory space perception is a subtle auditory perception of low-frequency ambient sound waves that build up along nearby surfaces (Ashmead et al., 1998). (Sidebar 6.8 provides more information on auditory space perception.) Advanced travelers may be able to use echolocation, sound shadows, and the buildup of low-frequency ambient sound waves simultaneously. Auditory space perception is still not fully understood, and there may be even more elements of sound used in spatial listening that have not yet been explored.

Although most children with visual impairments spontaneously develop spatial listening skills from an early age, O&M specialists should help them to further develop these skills (Ashmead et al., 1989; Lawson & Wiener, 2010a), while some children do not develop auditory space perception on their own and need direct instruction and practice (Worchel & Mauney, 1950). A recent study by Teng and Whitney (2011) indicates that it takes relatively little practice to gain the basic echolocation skills necessary to locate and discriminate the size of small objects when seated in a quiet environment. In this study the researchers proposed a new way to quantitatively measure echolocation acuity, the vernier technique, which may prove to be a useful tool for people who want to objectively measure echolocation proficiency at near tasks

How Auditory Space Perception Works

ECHOLOCATION

Reflected sound can be used to detect silent objects. Sound reflections occur when an object reflects mid- to high-frequency sounds from a sound source back toward the listener. In this case, the listener perceives "extra" sound coming from the direction of the object (Ashmead et al., 1998, p. 630). The sound is usually generated by the traveler. Research shows that the most effective sound for echolocation is a tongue click produced by the tip of the tongue pulling down off the roof of the mouth near the front teeth (Martinez Rojas, Alpuente Hermosilla, Sanchez Montero, & Lopez Espi, 2009, p. 328). Sound reflections can also be used to determine the size of a space; a small space immediately reflects high-frequency sound back at the listener from all directions, whereas a larger space has a longer lag-time in the sound reflections.

Travelers can also interpret the size of a space by tuning in to the duration of sound reverberations—the prolongation of the sound after the original sound source has stopped producing sound (Lawson & Wiener, 2010a, p. 91). "A listener gets useful information because the reverberation time depends on the size and surface properties of a bounded space, such as a room" (Ashmead et al., 1998, p. 630). A large space has a long reverberation time; a small space has a short reverberation time. Additionally, a space filled with hard surfaces has a longer reverberation time than a space with soft, sound-absorbing materials.

Reverberated and reflected sound can be used to interpret the relative size and shape of a space. It can be used to detect objects and determine the size, shape, location, distance, and density of objects (Anthony et al., 2002). With practice, some people have learned to use spatial listening to differentiate between trees and awnings, estimate the size of silent parked cars nearby, and locate objects as narrow as street-sign poles. Following are some examples of the use of echolocation:

- A child walks down the middle of the hall at her school, her cane tapping on the linoleum. The sounds of her feet and cane reflect off the walls on either side, helping her maintain a straight line of travel. She pauses when she reaches the intersecting hallway because it sounds different when the space opens up. She is detecting the absence of the reflected and reverberated sound.

- Walking down a quiet street with his cane, a child makes periodic clicks with his tongue. He clicks, then abruptly stops, ducks, and reflexively puts his hand up to protect his head from contacting a tree branch. He is responding to the clicking sound reflecting off of the branch.

- A child sits in his car seat next to the open car window on the right side of the car. He turns his head toward the rush of sound each time the moving car passes parked vehicles, poles, and trees. He is hearing the sound of the car engine reflecting off of the objects nearby.

SOUND SHADOWS

Visual shadows are created when an object blocks light waves. Sound shadows are created in a similar way, when an object between the sound source and the listener blocks sound waves. This allows the traveler to detect the silent object that is blocking the sound. The sound seems muffled to the listener because there is missing sound, especially in the high-pitched upper-frequency range. In order to easily detect a sound shadow, the listener needs a clear and steady source of sound. Following are some examples of how sound shadows can be used during travel:

- A child walks down the hall toward the office, listening for the intersecting hall to his classroom. He hears softly muffled voices in the classroom hall as he approaches; then suddenly the talking becomes clear and louder. The walls of the office hall created a sound shadow until he reached the intersection of the two halls.

- A child walks down the sidewalk listening to the roar of traffic on her left. Midblock, the sounds of the traffic become muffled. She reaches to the left and her cane lightly taps the tire of a parked car. The car created a sound shadow between the girl and the sound of the traffic.

LOW-FREQUENCY AMBIENT SOUND WAVES

A 1998 study (Ashmead et al.) demonstrated how travelers use a "buildup" of low-frequency sound waves to detect the presence of walls. Ambient ("background") sound creates an accumulation of sound pressure near walls, floors, and ceilings that can be detected as far away as three to six feet. This type of buildup is present even in seemingly silent environments when the traveler is quietly moving. Although travelers may not be aware that they can hear the sound, they can detect the presence of a wall and use that information to travel smoothly next to it without contacting it. For example:

- In a seemingly silent carpeted hallway, a child quietly walks a few feet away from the wall. Although the hall is silent, she is aware of the wall and is able to maintain a straight line of travel due to the buildup of low-frequency ambient sound waves along the wall surface. She pauses when the hallway ends at the quiet living room. She is detecting that the buildup of sound waves is no longer at her side.

for assessment purposes. Sidebar 6.9 provides strategies for teaching auditory space perception.

Parents and teachers can augment O&M instruction by pointing out when the child is using auditory space perception. For example, if children reach for a silent object, change their line of travel to step around a silent object, pause at the end of a hallway, or ask about a silent object that was not contacted, the adult can acknowledge the use of spatial listening. This helps children learn that listening can be used to detect silent objects and determine properties of space. This can be a difficult concept for children younger than 6 or 7 to understand (Kish & Bleier, n.d.). Many travelers use spatial listening skills but are unaware that they are applying them (Kish, 2009). People often experience spatial listening as either an intuitive feeling that they are about to contact something or as a sensation of pressure on the face.

((• SIDEBAR 6.9
Strategies for Teaching Auditory Space Perception

Because the environment plays such an important role in auditory space perception, choosing the appropriate environment is a key factor in teaching students to utilize these skills. Following are some strategies and activities that help in developing auditory space perception skills:

SELECTING THE APPROPRIATE ENVIRONMENT

- Start in a controlled indoor area such as a hallway with open doors. While spatial listening can be used outdoors, other sensations or conditions such as wind and shade can interfere with the learning process (Wiener, 1980).

- Begin teaching object detection using large objects or hard wall surfaces in clear, uncluttered space. It is easiest for a beginner to detect single large objects at head height. Over time, introduce more and smaller objects at different heights in more complex soundscapes. Be aware that loud environments may mask sound reflections, sound shadows, and buildup of sound waves.

- Introduce detection of objects close by, and then slowly increase the distance.

- When teaching how to detect reflected sound, select a space such as a tiled hall that is acoustically "live," filled with hard surfaces to reflect sound. Bathrooms, kitchens, and most public building hallways and stairwells are typically "live" spaces.

- When teaching how to detect the buildup of low-frequency ambient sound waves, select quiet places and avoid making sounds. For example, walk barefoot or with soft soled shoes and avoid talking during travel. Walking near a wall in a quiet carpeted location with fabric curtains is ideal.

- When teaching how to detect sound shadows, start with a loud consistent sound source and large objects, for example, the roar of traffic on a busy street blocked by a large parked truck. Over time, use softer sounds and smaller objects, such as the sound of a fountain blocked by a bush, or the sound of one moving car blocked by a streetlight pole.

TEACHING CONSIDERATIONS

- Because the child will be listening to subtle changes in sound, the adult needs to first guide the child instead of asking the child to listen while walking (the child holds the arm of the adult and walks next to and slightly behind the adult). This allows the child to place all his or her attention on listening.

- Once the child is able to use auditory space perception when guided, the child is then ready to work on the use of spatial listening during independent travel.

- The adult needs to not interrupt while the child is listening for auditory space perception cues. Before beginning travel, ask the child to listen for changes or differences in the sound (Brauner, 2009). Ask the child to raise a hand or say "now" if a change in the sound is detected. At that point, stop and discuss what the child is hearing.

- Some children generate sound reflections by clapping, clicking their tongues, hooting, whistling, stomping, snapping fingers, or banging the cane. The crisp and distinct sound of a tongue click produced by the tip of the tongue pulling down off the roof of the mouth near the front teeth gives good reflective feedback (Martinez Rojas et al., 2009) and is superior because it emanates from a source close to the ears (Kish & Bleier, n.d.).

- Natural environmental sounds, such as footsteps, voices, or the light tapping of the long white cane, also generate sound reflections.

- Students need to be aware that creating self-generated sounds may draw attention or be considered socially inappropriate. It is a personal choice about whether and where to use self-generated sound or naturally occurring sound.

- Children with low vision can close their eyes (or if comfortable with it, use a blindfold) to help them focus attention on auditory input.

- Auditory space perception should always be used in conjunction with a mobility system, such as a long white cane. It is not safe to use it as the only means for independent travel.

ACTIVITIES FOR PRACTICING AUDITORY SPACE PERCEPTION

- Encourage the child to climb in and out of a large box while talking or making silly sounds. Have the child note the presence or absence of reflected sound, and how outside sounds seem muffled from inside the box.

- Hold a large, smooth, flat surface (such as Plexiglas or a large serving tray) in different positions near the child's head. Ask the child to talk or make sounds and determine the location of the flat surface by listening to the reflected sound. Have the child reach out to touch the surface to confirm the location.

- Any of the examples in Sidebar 6.8 can be turned into teaching activities. For example, following is an activity for detecting sound shadows: Locate a relatively quiet hallway that has an open doorway or intersecting hall containing a sound source, such as people talking or a radio playing. Ask the child to walk with you down the hallway and to listen carefully for when the sound becomes loud and clear. Start far away from the opening and walk toward it together, guiding the child. Point out how the sound is muffled by the walls until reaching the opening, and explain that this is called a sound shadow. Repeat the activity and ask the child to point or say "now" when the opening is detected.

Kish (2009), an O&M specialist who is blind, has noted that children who lose their vision later in life or who have low vision usually require direct instruction to develop auditory space perception because visual information is still so primary for them that it distracts them from focusing on subtle auditory cues. However, research shows that when given structured opportunities to practice, sighted people can quickly learn to use echolocation to discriminate size and location of small objects (Teng & Whitney, 2011). Children with low vision can learn to use spatial listening to some degree to supplement visual information. They may initially benefit from closing their eyes (or if comfortable with it, using a blindfold) when learning to use auditory space perception to help them focus on auditory input. Additionally, hearing fluctuations from chronic ear infections, allergies, or colds can prevent a child from developing auditory space perception. Because there are so many elements of sound involved in spatial listening, however, children with a hearing loss may still be able to learn to use some types of auditory space perception (Carlson-Smith & Wiener, 1996). (See Chapter 8 for more information about children with visual impairments and hearing loss.)

It is vitally important that children with visual impairments fully develop their auditory space perception skills. Being able to auditorily detect the presence of silent objects and walls greatly assists orientation and allows for more fluid and efficient travel in a variety of settings. Auditory space perception can decrease the need to rely on tactile travel techniques, such as trailing a wall with a hand or contacting objects with the long white cane.

Auditory space perception should not be used as the sole means for independent travel, however. Spatial listening is an orientation skill, not a mobility system. It can be used to detect objects, but it cannot detect curbs or other drop-offs or low-lying obstacles. Sound shadows, reflected and reverberated sound, and the buildup of sound waves can also be masked by other environmental sounds or weather conditions. The ability to use already developed auditory space perception can be reduced by temporary hearing loss caused by colds or allergies. Auditory space perception is a valuable orientation tool that supplements the information from a primary mobility system, such as a long white cane, dog guide, or human guide.

Auditory Memory and Sequencing

Sound is a fleeting event: Once created, it ceases to exist. The "temporal nature of sound requires extensive use of short term memory" (Ferrington, 1994, p. 55). Accordingly, auditory memory and sequencing play a crucial role when interpreting and remembering verbal information for O&M. The ability to remember the correct order of sounds on a route or route instructions is as important as being able to identify and interpret properties of sound. Processing verbal information involves complex memory skills, for the precise meaning of a sentence cannot be known until the speaker completes it (Ferrington, 1994). Children need good auditory memory and sequencing skills in order to learn concepts and comprehend instructions and conversations. While some information can be immediately used and then forgotten, most O&M information, such as directions to the store or emergency phone numbers, needs to be remembered over long periods of time.

Researchers have found that at least 50 percent of an elementary student's typical school day is spent listening (Ferrington, 1994). The ability to remember directions in the correct order helps children participate in group activities and travel. To be successful, children need to attend to instructions, ask clarifying questions, and take notes if needed. Countless daily activities require auditory memory and sequencing skills, from packing a backpack before leaving for school, participating in physical education activities, and making correct turns in a route to correctly dialing a telephone number.

It is easiest to follow a one-step direction, such as "stop," but the ability to follow multiple-step directions usually develops at an early age. Typical preschool children can follow up to three-step instructions (California Department of Education, 2010; Johnson, Attermeier, & Hacker, 1990). An example of a three-step direction is: "Stand up, push in your chair, and line up by the door." In order to remember complex multiple-step instructions (for instance, the sequence of turns in a route or the digits in a telephone number), children need strategies to help them recall the information in the correct sequence. It is good practice to model how to ask questions and restate content. The adult can also ask the child questions such as "Can you repeat what I said?" and model an answer if needed, by repeating, "First stand up, next push in the chair, then line up." Encourage the child to ask questions and repeat directions. If the child seems confused, prompt, "Did you need to ask for help? Do you know what I mean when I say, 'line up'?" When explaining complex directions to a child, keep in mind that it is generally difficult to attend to instructions, orientation, and safety simultaneously. It is easier for the child to listen to and restate instructions while stationary. Observe children who are following instructions and let them know right away if they have made a mistake or if they are on the right track. Sidebar 6.10 provides activities and strategies to help students develop auditory memory and sequencing skills. (For additional information on auditory memory and sequencing, see the Listening Skills Continuum in Appendix A at the back of the book.)

Children have different learning styles for processing verbal information. Some prefer to get a verbal preview of all the steps in a task, others learn best if someone talks them through each step as they do it, still others prefer to write down the steps and read them as they complete the task. To help children remember information, give them opportunities to practice the task or use the information. For example, if a student needs to remember how to pack her backpack, provide opportunities across the day to pack and unpack it and to help other children to pack their backpacks, as needed. After completing an activity, help the student place the information into long-term memory by asking her to describe what she just did. You can make the description process fun by asking the student to dictate a story, reenact the activity with props, draw a picture, teach another child how to do it, or write a journal entry.

Auditory Memory and Sequencing Activities

The following strategies can be used to help children remember or retrieve information. Try a variety of techniques and see what works best for each child.

REPETITION AND RHYTHM
- Use mnemonics, a pattern of letters, to assist recall of a sequence of words. An example of mnemonics is learning a catchy phrase such as "**n**ever **e**at **s**limy **w**orms" to help remember the cardinal directions, **n**orth, **e**ast, **s**outh, and **w**est.
- Use alliteration, a series of words that start with the same consonant sound or letter (for instance, "turn **l**eft at the **l**ibrary").
- Create a song or chant about the information.
- Use repetition when giving instructions or information. Introduce the topic clearly, then give the detailed information, and conclude by summarizing the main points.
- Ask the child to repeat the information in his or her own words.
- Have the child teach the instructions to another person.
- Have the child give route directions to a guide or driver during travel.

STORIES
- Make up a short story starring the child doing an activity and remembering important information. When possible, use props or act it out together to make it fun and engaging. For example, create a story about the child getting ready for school: first getting dressed, then eating breakfast, brushing his or her teeth, packing his or her backpack, and leaving on time.
- Have the child dictate a short story involving the information to be remembered. Record it in print, braille, or audio format. For example, have the child dictate her morning routine, and then review it together.

NOTE TAKING
- Use a device such as an audio recorder, or voice output device to record the information. The child can listen to it later as needed.
- Write or braille the information using an accessible computer or personal digital assistant (PDA). This allows the child to review the information independently at his or her own pace. If the child cannot use a computer independently, use single switch devices or adapted keyboards, or have the child dictate the desired information to be written and then reviewed.
- Have the child write or braille the instructions and then read them aloud.
- Create a tactile schedule using whole or partial real objects to represent tasks or activities. For example, a fork could indicate that it is time for lunch, and a piece of a sponge could indicate that it is time to wash the dishes. Verbally review the schedule together.

TEACHING TIPS
- Get the child's attention by standing within arm's reach and using his or her name.
- When presenting a new set of directions, note how many steps the child is able to remember. You may need to decrease the number of steps in order to ensure success.
- If the child needs to learn a task with multiple steps, such as tying shoes or learning a route, start by teaching the first step. Once the child has mastered one step, then add a second step. Over time, add the other steps until the child has learned the whole sequence. Another option is to begin with the last step, then gradually add the previous steps.
- See the teacher/adult strategies described in Chapter 8 for more teaching tips.

Weather Factors

It is necessary to practice listening skills in a variety of weather conditions, as weather can dramatically change sounds. Wind can mask or shift the sounds; for example, it can make a sound in front seem like it is coming from the side or even behind the traveler. Wind can make it difficult for the traveler to hear and localize or track sounds accurately. Fog or snow deadens sound. In addition, because people usually reduce their car speed in reaction to adverse driving conditions, the sounds of car engines and tires can be quieter, making detection of vehicles more difficult. Rain intensifies some sounds, such as car tires, while masking other sounds, such as car engines.

Clothing can also affect access to sounds. Plastic rain hats, waterproof jacket hoods, or umbrellas magnify the sound of rain and act as a sound barrier to important environmental sounds. Waterproof cloth rain hats are superior to umbrellas and plastic rain hats in allowing the traveler to listen to environmental sounds with less distortion. It is best to select hats with a wide brim that keep the head dry but that do not cover the ears, especially for street crossings. Insulating hats should not cover the ears unless absolutely necessary in cold conditions. In very cold conditions, the traveler may choose to wear a hat or hood that covers the ears but needs to uncover the ears for all street crossings or other situations where cars could be encountered, such as driveways or parking lots.

LISTENING AND COMMUNITY TRAVEL IN MIDDLE SCHOOL AND HIGH SCHOOL

As children enter adolescence, they often become more independent travelers, both at school and in the greater community. The O&M-related listening skills that the individual developed as a child are the foundation as preteen and teenage travelers begin to build the more complex skills they will need in adult life to travel to college, to work, and for recreation. There are many emerging listening skills for preteens and teenagers who are applying auditory information to community travel. A preteen or teenager with well-developed listening skills:

▶ uses auditory space perception while traveling in complex environments

▶ determines the relative speed of moving sound-making objects (in other words, slow or fast)

▶ aligns body and line of travel parallel or perpendicular in relation to the sound of moving vehicles

▶ updates mental map of current location by listening to sounds

▶ selectively listens to one sound within complex soundscapes

▶ listens to verbal information and asks clarifying questions

▶ recalls multiple-step directions in the correct sequence

▶ recognizes "danger sounds" and responds quickly

▶ locates correct position to cross the street

▶ determines if an intersection is a safe place to cross based on sound

▶ selects a safe time to cross the street based on sound

▶ monitors traffic sounds during street crossings in order to adjust pace as needed to safely complete the crossing

▶ uses technology to access auditory travel information

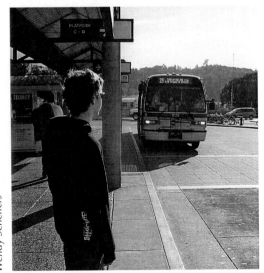

Wendy Scheffers

A teenager with low vision listens and looks for his bus.

Middle and high school students use their listening skills to travel in increasingly complex environments as they move toward adulthood. They travel to community destinations using sound to identify location, locate landmarks, avoid protruding hazards, and select a line of travel. Travelers frequently need to solicit travel information from others by asking specific questions, repeating the information, and taking notes as needed. These advanced listening skills develop best with direct instruction from an O&M specialist and support from school staff and parents.

The O&M specialist often partners with an assistive technology specialist or a teacher of students who are visually impaired to co-teach use of accessible technology.

Technology

Li, a 17-year-old high school senior who is blind due to retinopathy of prematurity, is getting ready to go to his new bank to deposit a paycheck. His fingers fly over the keys on his personal digital assistant (PDA), which includes a GPS and both voice and braille output. He enters a search for his bank, listens to the address and phone number announcement, and then keys in the command to create a walking route to the bank. Li presses the PDA keys to preview the route. After listening carefully to the route instructions and street names, he imagines the shape and distance of the route. He then picks up the phone and dials the bank to determine the location of the automatic teller machine (ATM). The bank employee explains that the ATM is to the left of the front doors, and then proudly adds that there is a talking sign above the ATM. Li confirms that the headphone jack to the ATM is working. He hangs up, packs his headphones and talking sign receiver, slings the GPS system over his shoulder, and heads out the front door with his cane.

Technology has revolutionized the field of O&M. It can provide the traveler access to information that previously was available only through visual means, such as the name of the street on a street sign or the change to a walk signal for the pedestrian at an intersection controlled by traffic signals. Information for travel planning can be gathered through tools such as telephones, accessible computers or PDAs, and GPS systems. The field of accessible technology is constantly evolving to improve ease of access for the user and to integrate multiple functions into small portable devices such as cell phones and touch screen tablets.

Two types of technology specific to O&M are electronic orientation aids (EOAs) and electronic travel aids (ETAs). EOAs, which include accessible GPS with speech or braille output, provide real-time travel and location information. For example, talking signs, also known as remote infrared audible signage, utilize transmitters at certain locations to broadcast recorded messages, such as street names, ATM locations, room names, and bus stops, which travelers can access with a handheld receiver. Another EOA, the accessible pedestrian signal (APS), provides a sound, vibration, or verbal message when the "walk" sign is displayed at a traffic signal–controlled intersection (Barlow, Bentzen, & Franck, 2010). ETAs are devices that emit sounds or vibrations that can be used to obtain information about the travel environment, such as the location and size of objects (Penrod, Smith, Haneline, & Corbett, 2010). While most commonly used by adults to supplement information from another mobility system, such as a long white cane, there has also been some success reported in teaching visually impaired infants and young children to use ETAs to scan, listen, and then reach for objects (Ferrell, 1984; Hill, Dodson-Burk, Hill, & Fox, 1995).

Good auditory memory and sequencing skills are needed to remember the steps for using each form of technology, as well as when soliciting information for route directions, public transit, or appointments. It has become very common for stores and businesses to use automated telephone menu systems that require the user to listen carefully and respond to voice prompts.

Planning travel requires students to gather and synthesize information about addresses, landmarks, routes, and public transportation. Taking notes in braille, in print, or on a PDA with voice output is a common system for recalling and retrieving complex travel information or a description of the steps in infrequently traveled routes. Another option is to record the steps using an audio recorder. Environment or route information can be recorded as an "auditory map." Auditory map information includes sequenced route instructions or other travel information such as detailed descriptions of streets, intersections, stores, and landmarks.

Talking tactile maps, interactive talking tablets that plug into a computer and use a database of map information and tactile overlays, can provide accessible map information (Bentzen & Marston, 2010), enabling the user to efficiently get an overview of the layout of a large area and conceptualize multiple possible routes of travel. This valuable tool requires the user to have good spatial orientation and the ability to interpret tactile graphics. The traveler must also have the capacity to pay close attention to auditory cues and remember multiple pieces of information. Similarly, talking information kiosks (sometimes found at transit stations, college campuses, and parks) that provide maps with voice output as well as touch-sensitive screens or three-dimensional displays can be a wonderful aid to the traveler (Bentzen & Marston, 2010). Talking information kiosks not only require the user to attend to verbal prompts and remember multiple pieces of information, but also to filter out distracting sounds of a potentially loud and chaotic environment.

Listening to the Whole Picture

Li follows the verbal prompt from his GPS system to turn right on Main Street. He shifts his attention from the GPS to the sounds on the street. He listens to the building line along his right and the rush of parallel traffic on his left side to maintain a straight line of travel. Li hears something in front of him and detours around a tree. He shifts his focus back to the GPS as it announces the upcoming intersection, and then returns his attention to the change in sound as the building line ends. Knowing that he is close to the intersection, he turns down the volume of the GPS system, focuses on detection of the upcoming curb with his cane, and starts listening for the beep of the APS locator tone. The motor of a leaf blower roars to life, drowning out all other sounds. Li sighs in exasperation as he realizes he will not be able to cross the street independently. He hears a woman next to him talking on a cell phone. She says good-bye and Li seizes the opportunity to ask, "Excuse me, may I take your arm to cross Baker Street?"

A traveler needs to use good judgment to selectively listen to specific sounds within a soundscape and to know when to shift attention from one sound to another. The traveler who uses an EOA, such as a GPS, has additional auditory information to integrate. Sometimes EOA information can distract the traveler from hearing or attending to other significant sounds. When EOA announcements are masking important environmental sounds, the EOA needs to be turned down or off. Likewise, it is not safe to travel while using headphones, particularly for street crossings. The only headphones that do not block outside sounds are special bone-conducting headphones that do not cover the ears. This type of headphones can be used to listen to recorded travel instructions or GPS information as needed for orientation purposes. It is important to realize that listening to information on any type of headphone can be distracting and that it is a judgment call whether having access to the travel information is worth the potential risk of missing other environmental sounds.

The presence of masking sounds requires the traveler to wait until the masking sound stops, change the route, switch to tactile or visual orientation methods, or get assistance from a passerby. If there are masking sounds or the residual background sounds of the community are too loud, a traveler who is blind should not attempt a street crossing because there may be a dangerous moving vehicle present that he or she is unable to hear (Scheffers & Myers, 2010b).

Business districts and school campuses are challenging to navigate safely and efficiently. These areas have many obstacles, such as poles, sandwich boards, shopping carts, store displays, pedestrians, newspaper stands, and trees. Travelers can navigate these areas more efficiently if they use multiple levels of listening skills. Auditory space perception can be used to avoid obstacles, such as trees, or locate a landmark, such as an open courtyard space, as well as to locate a walkway or travel a straight line next to a wall. Sound tracking can also be used to maintain a good line of travel next to moving parallel traffic, or to detect a veer from the intended line of travel. In the vignette that opened this section, Li used all of these skills, in addition to good judgment about safe travel.

Travelers use sounds to identify their travel environment. They draw on past experiences to discriminate between the sounds typical of a residential area and those typical to a business district, as well as to determine the types of nearby businesses.

They also need to learn to independently identify sounds that could mean danger and respond accordingly, as discussed in Sidebar 6.7; this is an essential safety skill for young adults to develop fully.

Good travelers create a mental map of their route and update that map as they move. In a familiar environment, sounds can be used to locate landmarks and verify location. Landmark sounds associated with an exact location, such as a fountain or automatic door, can be used to update mental maps as the traveler moves through space. Other sounds such as car engines or voices provide cues about nearby objects but do not indicate an exact location. Sounds can also be used to locate travel paths, streets, businesses, or public assistance in an unfamiliar area. To locate hard-to-find destinations, the traveler can create auditory landmarks. For example, a traveler can install wind chimes, a wireless doorbell activated by remote control, or a radio with an automatic timer as an auditory landmark for home.

Travelers can become disoriented as a result of masking sounds, distractions, illness, weather, and obstacles along the route. It can be extremely frustrating and disorienting for a traveler when the environment and the traveler's internal mental map do not match. Recognizing that there is a problem is the first step in reestablishing orientation. The traveler needs to then attend to available sensory information to determine location. Landmark sounds, tactile information, auditory space perception, and sound localization can all be used to get back on track, as the next part of Li's trip illustrates, as can seeking assistance from a passerby.

Li thanks his guide, and then continues down the street independently. He hears more traffic, the rustling of shopping bags, and pedestrian footsteps and voices. He notes that he has moved from his residential neighborhood to the nearby business district. He hears a man muttering to himself, cursing and slurring his words. Li grips his GPS system closer to his body, lifts up his chin, and steers away from the voice with a quick, confident stride. Walking briskly down the block, he begins listening for the next intersection, Davis and Main. He hears an espresso machine and realizes that in his distraction he has lost track of where he is. He is not near Davis Street but is actually next to the coffee shop at Carl Street and Main, one block short of Davis Street.

Advanced listening skills work in tandem with a mobility system, such as a cane or dog guide, allowing for more efficient travel. As dog guide travelers do not have the tactile information provided by a cane, listening skills play an even more important role in their travel (Guérette & Zabihaylo, 2011). While most dog guide schools do not accept students under the age of 16, practicing listening and O&M skills at an early age prepares travelers who may choose to use a dog guide later in life.

Monitoring Safety for Travel

All travelers, sighted or visually impaired, need to evaluate their ability to travel independently at any given time. Environmental issues such as neighborhood safety, masking sounds, the level of residual sound in the community, weather conditions, construction, or unexpected large obstacles can affect the ability to travel safely. Illness, stress, and the effects of medication, drugs, and alcohol can also impact hearing, attention, and concentration, and therefore travel safety. As teenagers begin to experiment with boundaries and take risks, parents and teachers need to discuss candidly the way drugs and alcohol can negatively affect the ability to listen and travel safely. When it comes to O&M, impaired judgment can be dangerous and even fatal. Whether it is internal or environmental factors affecting safety, travelers need to know when to set out on their own and when to get assistance from a passerby, friend, or family member.

Street Crossings

Li hears the roar of perpendicular traffic as he approaches the intersection of Main and Carl. He turns down the volume on his GPS system and focuses on the traffic sounds. Li steps forward to the edge of the curb, and then adjusts his position to line up with the traffic sounds. He shifts his attention between the parallel and perpendicular traffic sounds and makes final adjustments of his position on the street corner so that he will make a straight street crossing in the crosswalk zone. He listens for any sound shadows caused by large parked vehicles. Li is relieved that there are no obstacles to block his hearing and conceal him from drivers. He focuses on the traffic patterns and hears a long green light phase for vehicles on Main and a shorter one for Carl. Li positions his cane and gets ready to step forward as he anticipates the green light to cross Carl. As the vehicles on Main surge forward in the lane nearest to him, Li turns his head to listen for right-turning traffic and any car that might be running the red light, then steps off the curb. While he crosses the street, he shifts his attention to listen for traffic in each lane and adjusts his pace accordingly. Li steps up onto the sidewalk, pauses to confirm his location using traffic sounds, and then turns toward his bank on the corner.

Street crossings require an incredibly complex application of multiple listening skills. Travelers with visual impairments may use spatial listening (auditory space perception) to check for obstacles and visibility problems at the intersection. Many key features of an intersection can be discovered using auditory figure-ground discrimination and sound localization. Travelers need to verify their position and alignment on the

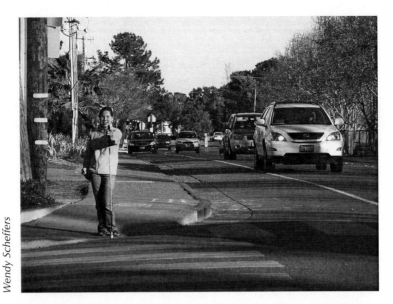

Wendy Scheffers

When preparing to cross the street at a stop sign–controlled intersection, a traveler listens for approaching cars in the near parallel lane.

corner by tracking the sounds of moving traffic and localizing the sounds of idling traffic (Barlow et al., 2010; Pogrund et al., 1993; Rosen, in press; Scheffers & Myers, 2010a). The traffic control at the intersection can be determined by listening to traffic patterns on the two streets. Travelers also need to use their listening skills to analyze the intersection shape, volume and speed of traffic, width of the street to be crossed, and direction of traffic flow (Rosen, 2011; Scheffers & Myers, 2010a).

After analyzing the intersection, travelers use their judgment to decide if they are at a safe place to cross the street. If they are not, they need to solicit assistance from another pedestrian or change their route to cross at a safer intersection. If they are at a safe place, travelers need to then select a safe time to cross. Depending on the traffic control, the safe street crossing timing varies from crossing the street with an "all clear" (no motor sounds at the intersection) to crossing with the surge of near parallel vehicles (Rosen, in press; Scheffers & Myers, 2010b). Some intersections have an APS that emits sound and vibration when the "walk" sign is displayed. Some APS devices have locator tones to help pedestrians locate the pedestrian pushbutton. The sounds from these signals should always be used in conjunction with other strategies to confirm a safe time to cross the street.

As the traveler prepares to cross a street, traffic should be monitored through use of an auditory scanning plan (and for travelers with low vision, an auditory and visual scanning plan) before and during the crossing (Barlow et al., 2010; Scheffers, 2010). A straight line of travel can be maintained by walking near the idling engines on the perpendicular street and parallel to the moving traffic. Travelers also need to listen for potential danger sounds such as sirens, the roaring engine of a fast-approaching car, or screeching tires. While this may seem overwhelming, juggling the sounds of traffic can become second nature to many people with visual impairments, in the same way sighted people master the complex motor, visual, and auditory tasks required to drive a car.

Research indicates that sighted children do not develop the necessary attention and judgment needed to cross streets independently until at least 10 years of age (Percer, 2009). For a student who is visually impaired who is learning to cross a street using only auditory cues, it may be even later before the student has the patience, practice, experience, and good judgment to independently cross a street safely. Although listening to traffic sounds should be introduced in the preschool years, children typically do not cross streets independently until they are much older. Through instruction with an O&M specialist, travelers learn to analyze intersection sounds and determine if there is a safe place and time to cross the street. Given the safety issues involved, travelers need to carefully listen to all the relevant sounds at every intersection. Once a student who is visually impaired demonstrates consistently safe intersection analyses and street crossings during O&M lessons, parents then need to weigh the safety of their community and the maturity of their child to make the final decision about independent street crossings.

CONCLUSION

Whether moving within the home, listening to instructions in physical education, or crossing the street, children with visual impairments need to rely on listening skills to move safely and efficiently. Listening can be used to identify sounds, label environments, plan a route, determine a line of travel, locate objects, and analyze complex travel environments. O&M listening skills develop best with organized instruction by a collaborative team of the O&M specialist, family, teachers, and other educational or medical specialists. From birth to adulthood, children's understanding of the world expands as they learn to listen, opening new worlds of discovery and preparing them for independent adult life.

REFERENCES

Ability Magazine (Interviewer) and Charles, R. (Interviewee). (1995). *Ability Magazine.* Retrieved August 23, 2006, from http://abilitymagazine.com/charles_interview.html.

Anderson, S., Boigon, S., Davis, K., & deWaard, C. (2007). *The Oregon project for preschool children who are blind or visually impaired: Skills inventory* (6th ed.). Medford: Southern Oregon Education Service District.

Anthony, T. L., Bleier, H., Fazzi, D. L., Kish, D., & Pogrund, R. L. (2002). Mobility focus: Developing early skills for orientation and mobility. In R. L. Pogrund & D. L. Fazzi (Eds.),

Early focus: Working with young children who are blind or visually impaired and their families (2nd ed.) (pp. 326–404). New York: AFB Press.

Anthony, T. L., & Lowry, S. S. (2005). Sensory development, session 2. In *Developmentally appropriate orientation and mobility*, Module 3 of the Distance Education Training: Blind, Low-Vision Program for the Infant Hearing Program, Early Intervention Training Center for Infants and Toddlers with Visual Impairments, Mount Sinai Hospital, Toronto, Ontario, Canada. Retrieved on July 30, 2010, from www.mountsinai.on.ca/care/infant -hearing-program/blind-low-vision/module-3/attachments/OM2_Session%20Notes.pdf.

Ashmead, D. H., Hill, E. W., & Taylor, C. R. (1989). Obstacle perception by congenitally blind children. *Perception and Psychophysics, 46*, 425–433.

Ashmead, D. H., Wall, R. S., Eaton, S. B., Ebinger, K. A., Snook-Hill, M., Guth, D. A., & Yang, X. (1998). Echolocation reconsidered: Using spatial variations in the ambient sound field to guide locomotion. *Journal of Visual Impairment & Blindness, 92*, 615–632.

Ayers, J. A. (2005). *Sensory integration and the child: 25th anniversary edition.* Los Angeles: Western Psychological Services.

Barlow, J., Bentzen, B. L., & Franck, L. (2010). Environmental accessibility for students with vision loss. In W. R. Wiener, R. L. Welsh, & B. B. Blasch (Eds.), *Foundations of orientation and mobility* (3rd ed.) Vol. 1 (pp. 324–385). New York: AFB Press.

Barlow, J., Bentzen, B. L., Franck, L., & Sauerburger, D. (2010). Teaching travel at complex intersections. In W. R. Wiener, R. L. Welsh, & B. B. Blasch (Eds.), *Foundations of orientation and mobility* (3rd ed.) Vol. 2 (pp. 352–419). New York: AFB Press.

Bayley, N. (2005). *Bayley scales of infant development* (3rd ed.). San Antonio, TX: Psychological Corporation.

Bentzen, B. L., & Marston, J. R. (2010). Teaching the use of orientation aids for orientation and mobility. In W. R. Wiener, R. L. Welsh, & B. B. Blasch (Eds.), *Foundations of orientation and mobility* (3rd ed.) Vol. 2 (pp. 296–323). New York: AFB Press.

Blesser, B., & Salter, L. R. (2007). *Spaces speak, are you listening? Experiencing aural architecture.* London: MIT Press.

Brauner, D. (2009). I hear with my little ear—Teaching auditory object perception (AOP) to young students. *AER Report, 26*(3), 1, 10–12.

Brazelton, T. B. (1983). *Infants and mothers: Differences in development.* New York: Dell.

Brothers, R. J., & Huff, R. A. (2008). *The sound localization guidebook* (4th ed.). Louisville, KY: American Printing House for the Blind.

California Department of Education, Child Development Division. (2010). *Desired results developmental profile—Preschool, DRDP-PS (2010), Sacramento, CA.* Retrieved July 27, 2010, from www.cde.ca.gov/sp/cd/ci/drdpforms.asp.

Carlson-Smith, C., & Wiener, W. R. (1996). The auditory skills necessary for echolocation: A new explanation. *Journal of Visual Impairment & Blindness, 90*, 21–35.

Dodson-Burk, B., & Hill, E. W. (1989). *Preschool orientation and mobility screening.* Alexandria, VA: Division IX of the Association for the Education and Rehabilitation of the Blind and Visually Impaired.

Fazzi, E., Lanners, J., Ferrari-Ginevra, O., Achille, C., Luparia, A., Signorini, S., & Lanzi, G. (2002). Gross motor development and reach on sound as critical tools for the development of the blind child. *Brain and Development, 24*, 269–275.

Ferrell, K. A. (1984). A second look at sensory aids in early childhood. *Education of the Visually Handicapped, 16*, 83–101.

Ferrell, K. A. (2011). *Reach out and teach: Helping your child who is visually impaired learn and grow.* New York: AFB Press.

Ferrell, K. A., with Shaw, A. R., & Deitz, S. J. (1998). *Project PRISM: A longitudinal study of developmental patterns of children who are blind or visually impaired. Final report.* Greeley: University of Northern Colorado. Available at www.unco.edu/ncssd/research /PRISM/default.html.

Ferrington, G. (1994). Keep your ear-lids open. *Journal of Visual Literacy, 14,* 51–61. Retrieved from http://jcp.proscenia.net/publications/articles_mlr/ferrington/earlids.html.

Ferrington, G. (2003). Soundscape studies: Listening with attentive ears. *Journal of Media Literacy, 49–50*(1), 42–45. Available at http://journalofmedialiteracy.org/index.php/past -issues/17-media-literacy-a-the-arts/233-soundscape-studies-listening-with-attentive-ears.

Fraiberg, S. (1977). *Insights from the blind: Comparative studies of blind and sighted infants.* New York: Meridian Books.

Green, G. (2001). Evaluating claims about treatments for autism. In C. Maurice (Ed.) & G. Green & S. Luce (Co-Eds.). *Behavioral intervention for young children with autism: A manual for parents and professionals* (pp. 15–28). Austin, TX: Pro-Ed.

Guérette, H., & Zabihaylo, C. (2011). *Mastering the environment through audition, kinesthesia, and cognition: An O&M approach for guide dog travel* [DVD]. New York: AFB Press.

Guth, D., Rieser, J., & Ashmead, D. (2010). Perceiving to move and moving to perceive: Control of locomotion by students with vision loss. In W. R. Wiener, R. L. Welsh, & B. B. Blasch (Eds.), *Foundations of orientation and mobility* (3rd ed.) Vol. 1 (pp. 3–44). New York: AFB Press.

Hill, M. M., Dodson-Burk, B., Hill, E. W., & Fox, J. (1995). An infant sonicguide intervention program for a child with a visual disability. *Journal of Visual Impairment & Blindness, 89*, 329–336.

Johnson, N. M., Attermeier, S. M., & Hacker, B. J. (1990). *The Carolina curriculum for preschoolers with special needs.* Baltimore, MD: Paul H. Brookes.

Johnson-Martin, N. M., Jens, K. G., Attermeier, S. M., & Hacker, B. J. (1991). *The Carolina curriculum for infants and toddlers with special needs* (2nd ed.). Baltimore, MD: Paul H. Brookes.

Kellogg, W. N. (1962). Sonar system of the blind. *Science, 137*, 399–404.

Kish, D. (2009). Flash sonar program: Helping blind people learn to see. Retrieved July 26, 2010, from www.worldaccessfortheblind.org/node/131.

Kish, D., & Bleier, H. (n.d.). Echolocation: What it is, and how it can be taught and learned. Retrieved August 3, 2011, from www.prcvi.org/files/workshops/echolocation.pdf.

Kisilevsky, B. S, Pang, L. H., & Hains, S. M. J. (2000). Maturation of human fetal responses to airborne sound in low- and high-risk fetuses. *Early Human Development, 58,* 179–195.

Kukla, D., & Thomas, T. T. (1978). *Assessment of auditory functioning of deaf-blind/ multihandicapped children.* Dallas, TX: South Central Regional Center for Services to Deaf-Blind Children.

Lawson, G. D., & Wiener, W. R. (2010a). Audition for students with vision loss. In W. R. Wiener, R. L. Welsh, & B. B. Blasch (Eds.), *Foundations of orientation and mobility* (3rd ed.) Vol. 1 (pp. 84–137). New York: AFB Press.

Lawson, G. D., & Wiener, W. R. (2010b). Improving the use of hearing for O&M. In W. R. Wiener, R. L. Welsh, & B. B. Blasch (Eds.), *Foundations of orientation and mobility* (3rd ed.) Vol. 2 (pp. 91–117). New York: AFB Press.

Litovsky, R. Y., & Clifton, R. K. (1992). Use of sound-pressure level in auditory distance discrimination by 6-month-old infants and adults. *Journal of the Acoustical Society of America, 92,* 794–802.

Lowry, S. S. (2004). *Defined spaces.* Chapel Hill: Early Intervention Training Center for Infants and Toddlers with Visual Impairments, FPG Child Development Institute, University of North Carolina at Chapel Hill. Retrieved August 15, 2006, from www.fpg .unc.edu/~edin/Resources/modules/OM4.cfm.

Lueck, A., Chen, D., Kekelis, L., & Hartmann, E. (2008). *Developmental guidelines for infants with visual impairments: A guidebook for early intervention* (2nd ed.). Louisville, KY: American Printing House for the Blind.

Martinez Rojas, J. A., Alpuente Hermosilla, J., Sanchez Montero, R., & Lopez Espi, P. L. (2009). Physical analysis of several organic signals for human echolocation: Oral vacuum pulses. *Acta Acustica United with Acustica, 95,* 325–330.

Myers, S. O., & Jones, C. G. E. F. (1958). Obstacle experiments: Second report. *Teacher of the Blind, 46,* 47–62. In B. B. Blasch, W. R. Wiener, & R. L. Welsh (Eds.), *Foundations of orientation and mobility* (2nd ed.). New York: AFB Press, 1997.

Nielsen, L. (1992). *Space and self.* Copenhagen: Sikon Press.

Nielsen, L. (2005). The listening ability of a child who is blind. Vision Australia. Retrieved August 3, 2006, from www.visionaustralia.org.au/info.aspx?page=1484.

Penrod, W. M., Smith, D. L., Haneline, R., & Corbett, M. P. (2010). Teaching the use of electronic travel aids and electronic orientation aids. In W. R. Wiener, R. L. Welsh, & B. B. Blasch (Eds.), *Foundations of orientation and mobility* (3rd ed.) Vol. 2 (pp. 462–485). New York: AFB Press.

Percer, J. (2009). *Child pedestrian safety education: Applying learning and developmental theories to develop safe street-crossing behaviors.* Report No. DOT HS 811 190. Retrieved July 20, 2010, from the U.S. Department of Transportation, National Highway Traffic Safety Administration Reports Online: www.nhtsa.gov/DOT/NHTSA/Traffic%20Injury %20Control/Articles/Associated%20Files/811190.pdf.

Pogrund, R., Healy, G., Jones, K., Levack, N., Martin-Curry, S., Martinez, C., Marz, J., Roberson-Smith, B., & Vrba, A. (1993). *TAPS—Teaching age-appropriate purposeful skills:*

An orientation and mobility curriculum for students with visual impairments (2nd ed.). Austin: Texas School for the Blind and Visually Impaired.

Rice, C. E., Feinstein, S. H., & Schusterman, R. J. (1965). Echo detection ability of the blind: Size and distance factors. *Journal of Experimental Psychology, 70*, 246–251.

Rosen, S. (2011). *Step-by-step: An interactive guide to mobility techniques.* Study guide: Street crossing techniques. Louisville, KY: American Printing House for the Blind.

Scheffers, W. (2010). Basic and lane by lane scanning techniques. Section L of San Francisco State University SPED 792 Course Reader. Unpublished.

Scheffers, W., & Myers, L. (2010a). Intersection analysis. Section L of San Francisco State University SPED 792 Course Reader. Unpublished.

Scheffers, W., & Myers, L. (2010b). Street crossing timings. Section L of San Francisco State University SPED 792 Course Reader. Unpublished.

Stoffregen, T. A., & Pittenger, J. B. (1995). Human echolocation as a basic form of perception and action. *Ecological Psychology, 7*, 181–216.

Teng, S., & Whitney, D. (2011). The acuity of echolocation: Spatial resolution in sighted persons compared to the performance of an expert who is blind. *Journal of Visual Impairment & Blindness, 105*, 20–32.

Warren, D. H. (1994). *Blindness and children: An individual differences approach.* New York: Cambridge University Press.

Wiener, W. R. (1980). Audition. In R. L. Welsh & B. B. Blasch (Eds.), *Foundations of orientation and mobility* (1st ed.) (pp. 115–185). New York: American Foundation for the Blind.

Worchel, P., & Mauney, J. (1950). The effect of practice on the perception of obstacles by the blind. *Journal of Experimental Psychology, 41*, 170–176.

PART 2

UNIQUE NEEDS

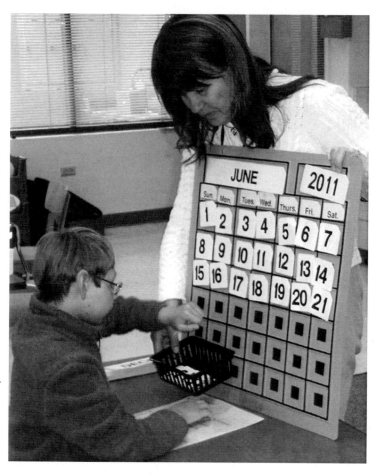

Chapter 7

Students with Additional Disabilities: Learning to Listen

Sandra Staples

Make the most of every sense; glory in all the facets of pleasure and beauty which the world reveals to you.

—Helen Keller

CHAPTER PREVIEW

- ▸ The Impact of Additional Disabilities
- ▸ Listening Skill Development and Instruction
- ▸ Promoting the Development of Listening Skills
- ▸ Strategies to Target Listening Skills
- ▸ Listening Skills for Recreation and Leisure
- ▸ Appendix 7A: Listening Skills Embedded into Alternative Functional Goals That Align with a Standards-Based Core Curriculum

Students who have visual impairments, including students who are blind, students who have low vision (those who have some usable vision), and students whose impairments include visual and additional disabilities, have in common difficulty perceiving and understanding visual information. They therefore need to be engaged in meaningful learning experiences that use other sensory modes (Downing & Chen, 2003). Students who have visual impairments, including those with additional disabilities, typically use touch and hearing to gain information, to respond to and interact with other people, to move within their environment, and to occupy their leisure time. The adults in the lives of these students—parents, caregivers, and educators—need to structure learning experiences for them that address the students' impairments in an individually appropriate way and provide opportunities both to learn through touch and to learn to listen. This chapter highlights the needs that may attend students with multiple disabilities as they learn and develop listening skills.

As stated in Chapter 1, research indicates that approximately 60 percent of the population of children with visual impairments is made up of children who have additional disabilities (Dote-Kwan, Chen, & Hughes, 2001; Ferrell, 1998; Hatton, 2001). Given that the incidence of multiple disabilities is notable, that the impact of additional disabilities on a student may be significant, and that the principles guiding effective instruction of listening skills pertain to all students who are visually impaired, including those with additional disabilities, this chapter incorporates many of the principles elaborated in Part 1 of this book.

Students who are visually impaired and who have another disability are a highly diverse group in which there is variability not only with respect to visual functioning but also with respect to the range of additional disabilities that may be present (Downing & Eichinger, 1996; Orelove & Sobsey, 1996; Sacks, 1998). Some students have visual and cognitive impairments, and perhaps also a neurological, health, or physical impairment, the combination of which is unique for each student, as are the ways in which this combination impacts and shapes the student's responsiveness and learning. Students with specific learning disabilites related to language and associated issues are the focus of Chapter 9; however, many other students with additional disabilties have significant learning challenges as well as significant support needs. It is this group that lies at the heart of this chapter.

This chapter discusses the listening needs of these students, offers strategies for creating environments and experiences that support learning to listen, and describes teaching strategies that target listening skill development. (In addition, Chapter 8 focuses on students with hearing impairments, with specific environmental and instructional considerations for working on listening skills with students who have a combination of vision and hearing loss.) Because of the complex ways in which learning can be affected when students have a visual impairment and additional disabilities, the chapter begins with vignettes of students to illustrate the variability of this group and their range of strengths and needed supports. Meaningful communication and functional relevance need to be the foundation of instruction in listening skills for all students with visual impairments but may be especially critical for students with additional disabilities. Thus, listening skills that support the development of a capacity for anticipation and readiness, movement and discovery, and language and understanding of auditory information are critical focuses for these students.

Embedded throughout this book is the acknowledgment that it is the effective partnership of parents, caregivers, educators, paraeducators, and other service providers that yields meaningful instruction in listening skills, reflecting respect for the whole student and the student's unique constellation of needs.

THE IMPACT OF ADDITIONAL DISABILITIES

When considering the listening needs of students who are visually impaired and have additional disabilities, educators and caregivers need to be mindful of the ways in which multiple disabilities can complicate learning. Their combined effect creates a unique set of learning characteristics with challenges of greater intensity than that suggested by considering each disability separately, and the disabilities need to be regarded as interactional rather than additive (Heller, Alberto, Forney & Schwartzman, 1996c). For example, for students with a visual impairment and additional disabilities that include a physical impairment, the educational implications are more complicated than "doesn't see well and uses a wheelchair." Students' positions in adapted equipment—their posture, balance, and range of motion—compromise not only their comfort and ability to attend to their environment but also how they are able to use their vision. In turn, and as described in Chapter 1, visual impairment affects how students experience and then understand the world as well as their awareness of people and objects in the environment. The interactive effects of combined disabilities affect how students gain access to materials, learning experiences, and the physical environment much differently than if only one of the impairments was present.

The interplay of a visual impairment and additional disabilities creates a constellation of effects that influences general functioning, responsiveness, attention, and learning and requires creative interventions and the collaborative efforts of parents, caregivers, educators, other service providers, and paraeducators. To ensure that the combined impact of a student's multiple impairments is reflected in the behavioral supports, accommodations, and instructional strategies that are implemented, it is important to be aware of the learning characteristics associated with the additional disabilities (Cushman, 1992; Downing & Eichinger, 1996; Sacks, 1998). The following sections provide descriptions of the learning characteristics and educational implications of specific additional disabilities in three broad areas that individually and collectively exemplify the ways in which multiple disabilities complicate learning:

> ‣ emotional disabilities, including challenging behaviors
> ‣ health impairment and cortical abnormalities
> ‣ physical impairment

Each of these sections is introduced by a vignette of a student. While each vignette has a primary focus, the interplay of multiple disabilities, as already noted, creates a cascade of effects—the unique characteristics of each student reflect challenges in more than one area. These descriptions of students with different disabilities set the stage for the second part of the chapter, which focuses on the development of listening skills and offers strategies for targeting listening skills for students with visual impairments and additional disabilities.

Emotional Disabilities and Challenging Behavior

Hana is sitting at her desk copying her spelling words from this week's lunch menu at school. She pushes down very hard on the keys of the braillewriter and voices each letter aloud as she writes: "M-i-l-k spells milk!" "T-a-c-o spells taco!" After she writes each word, she says "Good, Hana!" with enthusiasm.

Hana is 14 years old and in eighth grade at a middle school campus. She has a rare chromosomal abnormality, characteristics of which include microophthalmia and blindness, poor fine motor skills, poor proprioception, poor tactile perception, and cognitive challenges that can range from mild to severe. Hana likes jumping up and down, bouncing on large therapy-style balls, and drumming with her hands and fingers on any surface. Hana's development is patchy. She is learning to use a spoon but prefers eating with her fingers; she undresses herself but needs assistance dressing. She hums any melody played for her or sung to her. She recites the numbers 1 to 100 in English and Spanish and names the capital of every state when that state is named. Hana's peak skills and talents involve sound and memory for sound. They contrast dramatically with her eccentric verbal expression as well as significant challenges in aural comprehension.

Often, Hana's voice rises in pitch and she twists her fingers as she says "No, no." She swings her arm at, pinches, or grabs adults, school staff, or family members who move within arm's reach to calm her or try to determine the cause of her apparent agitation. Her parents are in the process of identifying whether part of Hana's cluster of disabilities includes autism spectrum disorder. Her educational team, which includes her parents, conducted a functional behavioral analysis to identify antecedents or circumstances that can trigger challenging behaviors from Hana and have put into place strategies that are effective in calming rather than escalating her behavior. They have identified preferred activities that provide motivation or redirection, as well as communication skills to teach or shape behavior, so Hana can either communicate her need or calm herself.

Hana reads and writes uncontracted, or alphabetic, braille and has an individualized literacy program that her teacher for students with visual impairments and her special education classroom teacher have developed in collaboration. She reads with eccentric hand mechanics, overlapping and twisting her two middle fingers, and presses down on the braille letters and words she is reading with a great deal of force. Most of Hana's educational program is provided in a specialized classroom. She joins her peers without disabilities each day for choir, lunch, and a guided reading activity in a language arts class.

The classroom teacher rings a bell and says to the class of students, "Spelling practice has ended. Put your spelling papers in the finished box. Then check your schedules." Hana continues to write and voice the letters she is writing. The teacher approaches her and says, as he puts his hand on her shoulder, "Hana, it's Mr. Conner. Spelling is over. It's time to check your schedule." She stills as Mr. Conner's hand touches her shoulder, and when Mr. Conner finishes speaking, Hana shouts, "Check your schedule! Check your schedule!" and flaps her hands near her shoulders. Mr. Conner removes his hand. Hana does not stand or move toward her personal schedule until the teacher approaches her as before, again placing his hand on Hana's shoulder, saying, "Hana, it's Mr. Conner. Stand up and check your schedule." Hana stands and continues to chant, "Check your schedule! Check your schedule" while bouncing in place. Her teacher touches Hana's forearm with the back of his free hand, in which he holds Hana's transition object, a Popsicle stick, and calmly says, "Hana, check your schedule." Hana traces Mr. Conner's arm to his hand, takes the Popsicle stick when she contacts it, and turns toward the shelves where her schedule is located.

Disruptions in routine can be difficult for Hana, and when there is a substitute in class or a rainy-day schedule for recess, she screams, bites her hand and arm, and sometimes pushes her desk over. Her team has introduced a special tactile symbol signifying "something different" when her regular routine is altered, such as when there is an assembly at school, to allow her to anticipate and learn to tolerate the change.

This is Hana's first year with a schedule written in braille. For the past three years she has had a schedule using objects. A Popsicle stick is still used as a concrete object to cue her to check her schedule for the next activity in which she is to participate. The educational team is continuing to pair the concrete cue with simple verbal information to help Hana learn to listen and attend to, interpret, and follow verbal directions.

Students with visual impairments and additional disabilities have conditions that can affect any of the body's major systems (visual, tactile, motor, neurological, hearing, digestive, endocrine, pulmonary, cardiac) to varying degrees, and multiple systems are often affected (Cushman, 1992; Silberman, Sacks, & Wolfe, 1998). Areas that can be adversely impacted can include comfort, stamina, tolerance for stimuli and processing of information, communication, and readiness for learning (Dunn, 1996). Often these effects are not fully appreciated as factors shaping a student's behavioral response to the environment or response to a personal state of being.

Some students who have visual impairments and additional disabilities exhibit behaviors ranging from ritualistic clapping or rocking to behavior that is self-injurious (such as head banging) or aggressive, either toward the environment (throwing things) or toward others in the environment (hitting, biting, pinching). Many of these eccentric behaviors are reactions to some facet of the environment, such as lack of control, surprise, proximity of others, type or intensity of sensory information, or need for sensory input. Sometimes such behaviors represent attempts to communicate personal need or personal discomfort, or frustrated attempts to gain attention (Gense & Gense, 2005b; Orelove & Sobsey, 1996). Careful observation and documentation of what may be very subtle behaviors can often yield information that the educational team can consider to determine the circumstances that trigger that behavior, the student's communicative intent, and strategies for adults to use in structuring the learning environment (Gense & Gense, 2005b; Mar & Cohen, 1998; Orelove & Malatchi, 1996). This process, while requiring an investment of time and energy, allows teams to structure the physical environment and develop effective communication strategies that lower stress levels for students and support regulating behavior.

To determine why a student is behaving in a certain way, educators and caregivers can consider the following questions:

▸ **Can specific triggers or factors that result in challenging behavior for a student be identified?** Common triggers might include changes in routine or transitions from one place to another or one activity to another. Physical aspects of the environment can serve to unsettle a student and result in challenging behavior as well. These might include noise; temperature; scents from food, cleaning materials, or perfume; lighting (too much, too little, or the effects of glare); and crowding or the student's perception that his or her personal space has been invaded. The student's physiological state and effects of hunger, thirst, illness, pain, and even discomfort from being positioned or seated in a certain way or for a period of time can affect levels of arousal and agitation. Medications and their side effects, as well as when they are or have been administered, are also considerations when attempting to identify factors that trigger a student's challenging behavior.

▸ **What function does the behavior serve?** Behavior often serves one of two functions: to get a need met, such as obtaining a desired object, gaining attention, or satisfying a physical need such as thirst or hunger; or to escape or protest a particular situation, including avoiding something the student perceives as unpleasant or painful, a task he or she feels unable to do, or a situation he or she does not understand.

▸ **What can be controlled in the environment that can change the student's behavior?** Communication is often one of the points of breakdown—not only the form of communication but also the way in which the physical environment is structured to communicate activities and expected behavior. Forgiving lighting (that is, lighting adequate for the individual needs of the student that does not produce glare) and reduced visual or auditory clutter can offer sensory comfort and manage stress levels for students, modulating agitation that can result in challenging behavior. Implementing consistent and predictable routines can be effective in organizing the student's world and easing transitions.

▸ **What is missing in the student's repertoire of skills that needs to be taught?** Again, the missing skills often relate to communication, whether it is a more conventional means of communicating need or a signal for attention. Other related behaviors that might require instruction include acquiring a means of self-calming, making choices, waiting, and taking turns with others, each of which draws upon listening skills.

Students who are visually impaired and have additional disabilities often exhibit behaviors that are similar to those considered characteristic of autism spectrum disorders. These might include rocking, flapping hands, or resistance to change (Gense & Gense, 2005a; McHugh & Lieberman, 2003). Their use of language can be eccentric: it can be very literal or concrete; there can be confusion regarding usage of pronouns; or it can show ranges of echolalia, in which students repeat sentences, questions, or phrases said to them (Gense & Gense, 2005a; Jamieson, 2004; Perfect, 2001). While some of the behavioral characteristics can be similar to those of autism spectrum disorders, this similarity does not necessarily mean the behaviors result from the same cause or diagnosis. Cass's (1998) summary of literature related to visual impairment and visual impairment with autism spectrum disorders suggests that stereotypic behaviors in blind children can be adaptive responses at a particular time in development and might be distinguished from those related to autism spectrum disorders on the basis of whether the individual responds to redirection and whether the behaviors continue throughout life (pp. 126–129). Gense and Gense (2005a) wrote that despite the appearance of similar behaviors in children who are congenitally blind and children with autism spectrum disorder, it is important for "the coexistence of these complex conditions to be explored and addressed" (p. 23). They emphasized the importance of developing educational programs that reflect consideration of the combined impact of visual impairment and the behavioral characteristics reflecting autism spectrum disorders.

Effective educational programs for students who have visual impairments and additional disabilities with challenging behavior and those for students whose additional disabilities include autism spectrum disorder do have in common strategies for addressing behavior that include use of predictable routines; preparing students for transitions; and environmental considerations that provide structure, consistency, and orientation (Chen, 1995; Dote-Kwan, 1995; Gense & Gense, 2005c; Jamieson, 2004; Smith & Levak, 1996b). Each of these strategies, several of which are described in Sidebar 7.1, serves to smooth the environment and lower stress levels for the student, minimizing behaviors that can interfere with development and learning, including the development of listening skills.

((Sidebar 7.1

Strategies for Working with Students Who Have Challenging Behavior: Structuring the Environment, Activities, and Communication

Many challenging behaviors have a communicative function and reflect the student's difficulty with transitions or a breakdown in communication. Structuring the environment and the student's day can often enhance meaningful communication between adults and the student, reducing challenges for the student and the subsequent challenging behaviors. Specifically, the physical environment, activities that take place in it, and communication with the student can be structured so that the student is able to answer the following questions in concrete and meaningful ways: Who are you? Where am I? What am I to do here? When is it over? What do I do next? Suggested strategies include the following:

- Gain a student's attention prior to communicating a direction, with judicious use of touch and understanding of the extent to which words or sound are meaningful to the student. For example, if an adult is gaining the attention of a student who does not understand words but who does alert to voices or change in the background sound, she might speak the student's name while simultaneously touching the student's shoulder, pairing sound and touch. When gaining the attention of a student who understands words, the adult might call the student's name and pause, waiting for the student to respond before touching the student on the shoulder.

- Consider a student's tolerance of touch, the quality of touch, and what that touch is communicating (Miles, 1999). For those students who tolerate tactile input, touch may need to be sustained so the student has an opportunity to process the tactile information and react to it. If the touch is too feathery or too slight, it may be irritating, potentially triggering a flight response. Pressure that is too deep can be uncomfortable or can communicate anger. The contact or touch should be provided at a location on the body that is not invading personal space (Chen, Downing, Minor, & Rodriguez-Gil, 2005; Downing and Chen, 2003). For example, touch near a student's face might be threatening; touch on the shoulder or forearm is often less personal. Consider the qualities of touch that Mr. Conner used to gain Hana's attention in the earlier vignette by placing his hand on her shoulder as he spoke directly to her.

- Structure the environment so that it communicates to the student the nature of the expected activity and, therefore, the behavior expected during the activity. For example, use of shelving can provide boundaries for a work space, further defined by the desk within the space, and the materials or work organized on the shelves can indicate the activity to be performed there. A throw rug can define the border of a leisure area, whose purpose is further defined by the materials in that space, such as a CD player and headphones, magazines or books for free reading, pillows, and a comfortable chair. In each instance, the physical environment and the materials in it communicate what students are going to do in that space and address the question not only of where they are but also of what they might be doing there and how they are expected to behave.

- Set up specific activities with routines to clearly communicate beginning, participating, and ending. Some activities may lend themselves to a left-to-right organization, with materials or manipulatives on the left, a defined work area (a mat or tray) in the middle, and a "finished" bin or basket on the right. This physical structure can communicate the task, how to participate in the task, and when the task will end. Like other routines, it must be judiciously supported and systematically taught within the context of meaningful tasks over time, so students can respond to, learn, and then internalize the sequence. For example, Hana has a tray on the left side of her desk, her braillewriter in the middle, and a shallow rectangular basket the size of a piece of braille paper on the right. The tray to the left has two papers in it: her spelling list containing four words and a page with her full name and address. Hana's job is to copy the spelling list. When she is finished, she places that paper in the basket to the right, the finished basket. When she finishes copying her full name and address, that, too, is placed in the finished basket. There are no more papers in the tray to the left,

(Continued)

((SIDEBAR 7.1 *(Continued)*

communicating to Hana that she is finished with that activity, which, over time, will become a signal or prompt to check her schedule on her own.

- Ritualize endings. Effective strategies to communicate the end of an activity can vary depending on the student and the activity. Some students may have the motor and orientation skills to respond to a signal or the presentation of a transition object to put items away or carry them to their usual location in the classroom. Other students may need a "finished" basket or bin brought to them. Communicating endings can be accomplished within the routine of the task, as described with Hana. Ritualizing endings can organize the learning environment for students and allow them to internalize when activities will end and to attend to the task at hand.

- The use of written or object calendar systems can convey what is going to happen, indicate where the student may be going, and answer the question, "What is going to happen next?" (Blaha, 2001; Blaha & Moss, 1997).

- A student's personal calendar or schedule can also be organized to accommodate a need for breaks or to alternate preferred and less-preferred tasks. Hana's schedule, for example, had bouncing on the therapy ball in the leisure area of the classroom, something she enjoys, after spelling. Schedules may also require adjustment if behavior problems for a student occur more frequently at a certain time of day, perhaps triggered by a specific activity or by the student's biobehavorial state.

Health Impairments and Cortical Abnormalities

Ten-year-old Micah and Ms. Terry, a paraeducator who works with his classroom teacher, are walking back to the classroom after taking the attendance folder to the office. As they pass the cafeteria, Micah stops walking and begins to fuss as he points inside. As she holds out a photograph of the class, Ms. Terry says, "Classroom, Micah. We're walking to the classroom." He continues to fuss and point at the cafeteria. Ms. Terry repeats, "Classroom, Micah. We're walking to the classroom," and touches his free hand with the photograph. Micah drops to the ground and begins to cry, one of his behavioral signals that his blood sugar level might be low. Ms. Terry says, "Juice, Micah? I think you need some juice," and again touches his hand with the photograph. He turns his head and looks down at what is touching his hand. He grasps the photograph, brings it to his face for closer inspection, and after a few seconds says, "Juice, classroom," and stands up.

Micah is part of a class of upper elementary school students that provides specialized instruction for students who have multiple disabilities. His medical diagnosis is optic nerve hypoplasia, and an MRI indicates hypoplasia, or underdevelopment, of the optic nerve, the optic chiasm, and the pituitary stalk, as well as partial absence of the corpus callosum, the band of neural fibers that connect the two hemispheres of the brain. He is administered a variety of replacement hormones due to the impact of his condition on his endocrine function. Micah does not like to be touched, particularly when he is agitated, and does not like wearing shirts with collars or tags at the neck, pulling at them or taking the shirts off. He gets overheated easily on hot days and gets lethargic and weak. Micah cannot yet control urination and sometimes floods his training pants.

Micah has a personal schedule that keeps activities varied and brief to accommodate a short attention span and tendency to get frustrated with long or complicated activities. He tends to handle and discard items after a few minutes of inspection and is often distracted by other movement in the classroom. Micah's responsiveness and participation vary from one day to the next and sometimes within a day. He is most actively involved in activities when he is given time to explore materials and when slow, deliberate gestures or modeling is used to guide participation. He follows verbal directions when they are paired with gestures and when the important information is offered up front, then restated in longer sentences to model appropriate language use.

Micah leans in to about 6 inches to visually inspect items before handling them. He has pronounced nystagmus, which affects the extent to which he can sustain fixation (that is, hold his gaze to visually learn about something or recognize it). He visually scans a tabletop or a row of his personal schedule with head movement and touches or picks up the object before verbally labeling it.

Micah probes surface changes (cement to grass, for example) with his foot and resists climbing the steps for the slide, suggesting difficulty with tasks involving depth perception. He has a wide-based stance and somewhat stiff-legged gait. Micah pauses to adjust his balance when walking and running and often staggers. The adults in his classroom are attentive to the quality of his movement and, on days when his balance fluctuates, adjust their proximity so they can steady him with a hand on his shoulder.

Micah walks from the speech room on campus to his classroom, occasionally needing redirection if he heads to the playground instead. At these times, his destination is either forgotten or not as attractive and fun as the playground. His team has introduced a transition object for him to carry to allow him an opportunity to check the destination and regulate his travel on his own. He needs reminders to continue to hold it and still tends to let it slip out of his hand, perhaps intentionally dropping it or perhaps forgetting to hold on to it.

Optic nerve hypoplasia (ONH) and cerebral/cortical visual impairment (CVI), two of the leading causes of visual impairment in children (Ferrell, 1998; Lueck, 2010; Roman-Lantzy, 2007b; Sacks, 1998), arise from conditions that are associated with either damage to the visual cortex or abnormalities of the optic nerve and midbrain. Each impacts neurological function and affects responsiveness, tolerance for stimuli, attention span, and learning.

Some students whose additional disabilities affect their health may have seizures, require procedures such as tube feeding or suctioning, or use devices such as a ventilator. Educators, caregivers, paraeducators, and other service providers need to be familiar with both daily and emergency health care plans. The behavioral clues that signal a physiological need for a student with additional disabilities are often subtle, whether it is the aura that foreshadows a seizure or a listlessness that suggests low blood sugar or illness. Adults need to be observant in interpreting these clues and ready to use meaningful communication methods to ready the student for what might happen next.

Optic Nerve Hypoplasia

Optic nerve hypoplasia (ONH) is characterized by an underdevelopment of the optic nerve as well as abnormalities of both the midbrain and structures of the endocrine system that lie at the base of the midbrain. The interplay of the medical complications resulting from compromised endocrine function and the neurological or processing disorders that stem from cortical abnormalities can have significant implications with regard to health, stamina, physiological state, attention, and learning. While some students have normal endocrine function, others have severe endocrine problems and have an array of medications and regular medical appointments to monitor hormone levels and growth. Some students are typical learners while others have significant learning challenges and require adapted teaching strategies to accommodate how they attend to and process information.

Cerebral or Cortical Visual Impairment

CVI is a neurological visual impairment resulting from damage to the brain rather than abnormality of the eye (Lueck, 2010; Roman-Lantzy, 2007a). CVI has been noted as the leading cause of severe vision loss in students who have visual impairments and other disabilities (Sacks, 1998, p. 26). It is the major cause of visual impairment in children in developed countries, and its incidence is increasing (Lueck, 2010, p. 589).

CVI results from damage to the posterior visual pathway or the visual cortex, resulting in a constellation of effects on visual behavior and visual processing, and can be one aspect of other neurological impairments. Asphyxia, a history of hydrocephalus, head injury, infections such as meningitis or encephalitis, or abnormalities of the brain can be causes of CVI. Cerebral palsy, epilepsy, cognitive impairment, and processing disorders are among the other neurological problems that result from injury to the brain that may also cause CVI (Liefert, 2003; Roman-Lantzy, 2007a; Smith & Levak, 1996b). Therefore, sensory, motor, and cognitive functioning each need to be considered when designing educational programming for students with CVI, since more than visual functioning is often affected (Jan, Groenveld, Sykanda, & Hoyt, 2006). This cluster of functional impacts highlights the need for students who have CVI to have the opportunity to develop listening skills as a compensatory skill for acquiring information for learning and for learning where to look and what to look for.

Physical Impairments

Four-year-old Yi is sitting in a corner seat at circle time in a blended preschool program. In this class, 16 children are developing typically and eight have Individualized Education Programs (IEPs) reflecting a variety of special needs, from speech and language to significant learning challenges. The co-teachers are early childhood educators, one whose background includes early childhood special education. Yi's medical diagnosis includes cerebral palsy, neurological or cerebral/cortical visual impairment, and developmental delay.

Yi's special corner seat offers upright support and is low to the ground, the same height as the other preschoolers sitting on small rugs. She has enough height so that her knees are bent and her feet rest flat on the floor. Yi directs her gaze toward the light coming through the open window in front of her, until one of the teachers, Ms. Mila, notices that she is not seated in her usual spot, next to the side of a bookcase and facing the teacher, with the window behind her. Ms. Mila approaches Yi slightly from the side and stands still as Yi visually alerts to the movement and turns her head. She says "Yi, it's Ms. Mila. Your seat is not in its correct place. I'm going to help you move." Ms. Mila crouches down slowly to let Yi follow visually. She places a hand on Yi's shoulder and waits for Yi to indicate in any manner that she is aware of the contact. When Yi blinks, Ms. Mila says, "Yi," and, still maintaining contact with Yi, moves her hand from her shoulder to under Yi's arm as a touch cue that she is going to pick her up. Ms. Mila again waits for Yi to respond to her voice and touch. When Yi moves her head, Ms. Mila places her other hand under Yi's thighs, says, "I am going to pick you up now," and slowly counts, "One, two . . ." Ms. Mila lifts her hands slightly with each number, and while keeping Yi's shoulders rolled slightly forward, picks her up as she says, "Three." Yi is carried while still in a sitting pose, so her body position won't have to be changed as she is lifted or reseated. This also keeps Yi's hips and knees bent and her body slightly folded, reducing the likelihood of a startle reflex or an extensor pattern, when her head and body hyperextend, making it difficult, and possibly harmful to Yi, when lifting her or assisting her in moving.

Yi's corner seat is moved and Ms. Mila uses the same communication strategies of pairing slight touch cues and counting to move Yi from being held to being seated. Once Yi is seated, Ms. Mila reaches toward the side of the bookcase and ruffles a silver metallic pom-pom attached there. Yi turns her head slightly to that side for a few seconds and then turns her head back to midline as she reaches for the pom-pom and pats it. "Yes, Yi. Circle time is next." Pom-poms are used in the opening singing activity during circle time and this pom-pom and this location are intended to communicate to Yi that it is circle time.

Some days Yi does not appear to visually respond to movement to the side or to the pom-pom. On those days, Ms. Mila pulls the pom-pom from the Velcro attachment on the bookcase and places it on Yi's lap. She then rests her hand on the side of the pom-pom and waits for Yi to reach for what is on her lap. When Yi reaches, her hand touches both the pom-pom and Ms. Mila's hand. If Yi pulls her hand away, Ms. Mila waits for her to reach forward again. Once Yi keeps her hand on the pom-pom or on Ms. Mila's hand, they reattach the pom-pom to the side of the bookcase. Hand-under-hand guidance—the adult's hand under Yi's—and slow movement are positive support strategies for Yi. She pulls away and clenches her fists if an adult tries to move her hands for her.

At this time, Yi's needs are anticipated and met by the adults in her environment, both at home and at school. When they initiate interaction, her educational team and parents respond to any movement from Yi, such as a blink, a head turn, or a vocalization, as intentional communication. Teachers and her family first try to gain her visual attention by making movement to the side, then talking to her as they use touch. Because Yi's responsiveness to visual cues varies from day to day or within a day, if she does not visually alert or respond, adults then pair touch and sound, using touch cues as they talk to her.

Yi communicates behaviorally, and adults have the challenge of interpreting her cries as distress, hunger, discomfort, fatigue, or frustration. During free-play time in the preschool classroom the noise level increases and both the activity level and movement in the room are unpredictable. Yi tends to cry and clench her arms and hands tightly at such times. She has a wheelchair for supported seating at tables or for travel. When she is positioned in it, if it is pushed forward or otherwise moved quickly, she startles reflexively and cries.

Many students who have visual impairments and additional disabilities have physical impairments that limit functional movement. Some physical impairments are classified as neurological or neuromotor impairments, affecting both nerves and muscles, including cerebral palsy, spina bifida, and traumatic brain injury (Heller, Alberto, Forney, & Schwartzman, 1996a; Rosen, 1998a). Other physical impairments have an orthopedic component, such as juvenile rheumatoid arthritis or missing limbs (Heller, Alberto, Forney, & Schwartzman, 1996a; Rosen, 1998b).

Physical impairments, particularly those with a neurological component, affect a student's ability to maintain balance or position or control movement. There are often a cascade of functional limitations that affect social interaction and communication, activities of daily living, stamina, and attention for learning.

Students who have physical impairments vary in the extent to which they have impaired learning. The range of learning characteristics for students may include those of typical learners, those of students with specific learning disabilities (as discussed in Chapter 9), and those with significant and complicated learning challenges. Physical impairments that have a neurological component have a higher incidence of cognitive or processing impairments as well as health conditions such as hydrocephalus or epilepsy (Heller, Alberto, Forney, & Schwartzman, 1996c; Rosen, 1998a).

Heller, Alberto, Forney, and Schwartzman (1996b) identified six variables that affect learning for students who have physical impairments (p. 37):

1. pain and discomfort
2. fatigue and endurance
3. functional physical and sensory limitations
4. adaptations, such as communication systems or positioning equipment and ambulatory devices
5. medication and treatment affects
6. absenteeism, often for medical appointments or procedures

Adaptations, the fourth of these variables, include placement of materials for the student's best access and use of assistive devices, such as communication systems, or positioning equipment and ambulatory devices, each of which is individualized based on the student's unique need and each of which draws on the expertise of teachers for students who are visually impaired, speech and language specialists, and physical therapists and occupational therapists. Students whose additional disabilities include physical impairment often have difficulty communicating, and just as often their attempts to communicate may not be understood by others (Heller, Alberto, Forney, &

Schwartzman, 1996c). The educational team needs to consider the form of communication, nonsymbolic or symbolic, for each student (Erin, 2000).

Nonsymbolic communication can begin as unintentional responses and might include any of the following (Erin, 2000):

> ▸ subtle changes in muscle tone
>
> ▸ eye gaze (which may be an eccentric gaze rather than a direct gaze for some students who have low vision)
>
> ▸ movement, ranging from slight movement such as a blink to a deliberate reach toward a person or object
>
> ▸ vocalization
>
> ▸ body language and gestures including facial expressions
>
> ▸ responding to real objects

For example, Yi communicates using a nonsymbolic form of communication. Adults interpret her subtle blinks as responsiveness. They follow through with spoken words and touch as a means of reinforcing her behavior and building intentionality.

Symbolic forms of communication might include the following (Erin, 2000):

> ▸ sign language
>
> ▸ picture communication systems or a communication board
>
> ▸ tactile symbols, ranging from parts of real objects to symbols
>
> ▸ print or braille
>
> ▸ speech

In symbolic communication, the symbol is not directly related to what is being communicated. For example, the transition object that cues Hana to check her schedule is a Popsicle stick, which has no real relevance to her schedule or the action of checking her schedule—it is simply a tactile symbol. Additionally, her personal daily schedule or calendar is written words; for her, the words are written in braille. Both types of communication for Hana, the student described in the first vignette, are symbolic forms.

Methods of communication are also classified as *unaided*, for example, hand or body movements or speech, or *aided*, involving the use of tools or equipment. Aided communication methods use either low technology, such as calendar systems and communication boards that use objects, tangible symbols, or icons, or high technology, such as electronic systems with digitized speech (Heller, Alberto, Forney, & Schwartzman, 1996c).

The emphasis in choosing the form or forms of communication a student will use needs to be on creating individualized systems that support the student's ability to make choices, convey a message, or make a request (Downing & Demchak, 1996). Many students have both aided and unaided communication systems available, depending on the activity, the environment, and whether they access the system by pointing, touching, or directing their gaze. Once the student's method or methods of communication have been identified by the educational team, including the caregivers, the skills to use alternative or augmentative communication systems—forms of communication other than speech—need to be taught and infused into ongoing and meaningful activities for the student, both at school and at home. Regardless of the form of the communication system, supporting the development of concepts and skills that enhance responsiveness and communication is interwoven with listening and the development of listening skills.

LISTENING SKILL DEVELOPMENT AND INSTRUCTION

As discussed in Chapter 1, vision and hearing are the primary senses that allow individuals to have access from a distance to other people, to things around them, and to the environment. Students who have visual impairments, including those who have additional disabilities, such as Hana, Micah, and Yi, need opportunities to become aware of, respond to, and understand information from the other distance learning channel: hearing. Hana and Yi are each learning to listen, to attend to sound, and to attach meaning to sound so they can anticipate and prepare for interaction. Hana and Micah are learning to listen as they acquire communication and language skills and build comprehension. They are learning to listen and to attach meaning to sound as they build on experiential knowledge and develop curiosity about and understand the world.

Auditory-Perceptual Development

Teaching effective listening within educational programs for students who have visual impairments, including those students who have additional disabilities, requires appreciation for the manner in which auditory-perceptual skills—skills that enable the individual to attach meaning to sound—develop as well as for the functions of hearing. As outlined in Chapter 1, hearing is a physiological process, one in which sensory information is passively received. Awareness of sound, indicated by a student's behavioral reaction to its presence or a behavioral reaction when it ceases, reflects processing of the sensory information taken in by the hearing system and the emergence of auditory perception.

Stages in the Development of Auditory Skills

The components of auditory-perceptual development described in Chapter 1 establish a foundation for instruction in listening skills (Harley, Truan, & Sanford, 1997)—part of the expanded core curriculum in the area of sensory efficiency for students who have visual impairments, including those with additional disabilities (Hatlen, 1996). Anthony and Lowry (2004) grouped the components of auditory perception into five stages of auditory development (presented in Chapter 2 in Table 2.1) and identified some of the behavioral responses a student might make that demonstrate individual skills. To review, the process of developing auditory perception proceeds through the following stages:

▶ Stage 1: The auditory-perceptual skills clustered in this stage of auditory development might include awareness of sound, followed by attending to and beginning to attach meaning to sound. Behavioral responses a student might exhibit that reflect those skills include reacting to loud and sudden sounds with a reflexive reaction or startle reflex and to soft, close sounds or a parent's voice with a change in expression.

▶ Stage 2: This cluster of auditory-perceptual skills includes beginning to localize sound, discriminate and recognize sound, and develop auditory memory. At this stage, infants or children respond to different voice tones, respond differently to different voices, and begin turning toward a familiar person speaking to them. Turning to voice alone indicates that the child has attached "permanence" to the person; the person exists beyond the student's physical contact and experience with the individual. As discussed in Chapter 1, this behavior reflects "distancing" (Bruce, 2005)—a gradual process of separating self from others and from objects—and indicates that the student holds the person or object in his or her memory. Localizing the position of that familiar person or object by sound alone requires not only auditory memory but auditory-discrimination skills, subtle attention to differences in sound intensity (loudness) and frequency (pitch), that facilitate perceiving space or localizing sound. This capability develops initially at ear level to either side.

▶ Stage 3: As infants or children gain experience and continue to acquire auditory skills, auditory discrimination and the recognition of changes in sound become refined. Infants/children begin to track or follow moving sound and manipulate objects intentionally to make sound. They begin to anticipate events based on what they hear, such as associating bath time with the sound of bathwater running or the ding of the microwave timer with food being ready. Children may also be upset by unfamiliar sounds. In addition to intentionally banging or shaking an object to make sound, they begin to cry out with purpose, to gain attention for a basic need, such as needing clothing changed or needing to be fed.

▶ Stage 4: Auditory comprehension skills become increasingly meaningful in regard to both sound and speech. Infants or children attach meaning to words and respond to their own name; they begin to sequence sounds and understand short, familiar phrases. Hearing speech over time, attaching meaning to sound and words, and experiencing the emergence of auditory-sequencing skills (see Chapter 1) inspire experimentation with sound and playing with inflexion. Children engage in vocal play with another person, and vocalizations begin to approximate words.

▶ Stage 5: The fifth stage of auditory skill development reflects the emergence of higher-order auditory-perceptual skills that support comprehension and the use of oral language. These skills include auditory-memory span, auditory sequencing, figure-ground discrimination, and auditory blending. Children follow simple directions without accompanying gestures and attend to someone speaking to them, not to background sounds. Their expressive vocabulary increases, as does their meaningful use of spoken language.

Functions of Hearing

Anthony and Lowry (2004, pp. 137–138) also described three functions of hearing:

▶ Primitive: the awareness of biological sounds (such as breathing and swallowing); awareness of background sounds, which might include startling to a loud sound or a door slamming, and include self-stimulatory play with one's own voice.

▶ Signal warning: monitoring of the environment, such as discriminating a change in background sound, attaching meaning to sound, and interpreting sounds to represent people or objects and identifying where they are located.

▶ Spoken communication: speech, which occurs with increasing comprehension of auditory information and understanding verbal language. Students respond to a name, understand familiar words, or follow directions, each of which reflects active listening and understanding. Speaking and using spoken language with intent and with purpose reflect not only hearing and understanding sound but also higher-order auditory-perceptual skills, such as blending sound.

Anthony and Lowry (2004) wrote that infants can develop "awareness of commonly occurring sounds in the immediate environment, leading to functional comprehension [understanding] and, later identification" (p. 144). By observing the response to sound of a child who is visually impaired, adults can be attentive to the child's auditory awareness and can support his or her understanding by pairing touch and sound. Lawson and Weiner (2010) noted that "a mother's or father's touch, when paired with her or his vocalizations, serves to stimulate the development of sound recognition and discrimination" (p. 114). Children respond differently to the voices of their mother and father, elevating the physiological process of hearing sound to a functional context. Awareness of sound at the body, and attaching meaning to that sound, allows students to shift from reacting reflexively to sound to attaching significance to, recognizing, and discriminating sound.

Examples of Effective Instruction

Creating effective instruction in listening skills for students with visual impairments, including students with additional disabilities, demands attention not only to the stages in the development of auditory skills but also to the functions of hearing to ensure that listening instruction is embedded within meaningful contexts and contains relevance for the student. It becomes the responsibility of adults to provide meaningful auditory cues that connect to a student's immediate experience by supporting listening skill development within naturally occurring routines and focusing on the function of hearing in that context, rather than on the specific auditory skill (Diaz-Rico & Weed, 1995a). As noted in Chapter 1, teaching auditory awareness by shaking sound-making objects near a student who has a visual impairment and additional disabilities is at best an experience unconnected to meaningful activity and at worst might be subjecting the student to something confusing or unpleasant from which he or she cannot escape. As illustrated in the vignettes presented earlier, adults need to provide carefully designed experiences that teach a student to alert to auditory signals and recognize the changes in the soundscape that cue someone's presence.

For example, in the earlier vignette presenting Yi, whose additional disabilities included physical impairment, listening instruction for Yi was embedded within social interactions with Ms. Mila getting ready for circle time. It was paced to offer Yi an opportunity to become aware of the sound of Ms. Mila speaking to her and to respond behaviorally, carefully nurturing the development of listening skills to support anticipation and readiness for change or for being handled. In this situation, the auditory skill—awareness of sound—is attached to a function of hearing—signal warning—which facilitates readiness.

Supporting the development of listening skills in this situation involves:

▶ pairing touch and sound (speaking)

▶ allowing time for the student to become responsive

▶ being attuned to subtle behaviors that communicate the student's readiness to respond

▶ acting on the student's response to positively reinforce the circular interaction between child and adult (Chen, 1999)

The listening experience was structured so that continuing the activity was contingent on Yi's response, ensuring her active participation—and allowing Yi to act rather than be acted upon.

Similarly, in the vignette describing Micah's health impairments and cortical abnormalities, the development of listening skills was embedded within a regularly occurring routine for Micah. Ms. Terry paced the interaction to help Micah learn to attend to, interpret, and act on verbal information—spoken communication. The interaction was also structured to reflect Micah's attention span, memory, and provide support in completing steps in a routine. The routine in this instance was taking the attendance to the office and walking back to class. In this instance, supporting the development of and teaching listening skills involves:

▶ pairing verbal information with a visual cue (the photograph of the classroom)

▶ allowing time for the student to become responsive

▶ increasing the level of prompting—that is, providing more assistance to the student to help produce the desired behavior—by offering the verbal message; then the verbal message paired with a visual cue—the photograph; and finally the verbal message, the visual cue, and a tactile cue, as Ms. Terry touched his hand with the photograph, paying careful attention to where Micah tolerates touch, and maintained the contact until Micah grasped the photograph on his own hand (prompting is described further in Sidebar 7.2)

▶ being attuned to subtle behaviors that suggest that the student's internal state is affecting the interaction

▸ offering vocabulary that can help the student listen to spoken communication and learn labels for what he or she is experiencing

The interaction was structured so that continuing the routine was dependent on Micah's response, with supports and judicious use of prompting to cue the desired behavior, allowing Micah to act, to regulate his own behavior, and to communicate his need.

((SIDEBAR 7.2
Levels of Prompting

A functional model for designing learning experiences for students with visual and additional disabilities—one that pays attention to the purposes of listening—uses meaningful contexts and routines and encourages students to respond to natural cues to execute a sequence of steps, complete a task, or participate in an activity. Many students, however, need to *learn* responsiveness to natural cues and require that the series of cues and prompts provided by adults to signal the next steps in a routine have relevance and intensity. Adults must consider the use of instructional prompts to support such students' active participation and also need to have a plan for systematically fading or discontinuing these prompts as the student integrates the steps in the routine, acquires skills, and requires prompting that is less intense or intrusive.

LEAST-TO-MOST INTRUSIVE PROMPTING HIERARCHY

The following prompts might be used to help a student perform the next step in a task, listed in order from the least to most intense or intrusive:

- natural cue or stimulus; the smell of food at mealtime; sitting at the table; or a mealtime tray on the student's wheelchair
- indirect verbal prompt; an adult says, "I am hungry."
- gesture; an adult points to the applesauce on the plate
- direct verbal prompt; an adult says, "Eat some applesauce."
- modeling; an adult holds his or her spoon and eats some applesauce from his or her plate
- partial physical assistance or tactile cues; giving the student a spoon; assisting the student in picking up the spoon with tactile cues at the wrist or forearm to reach forward so the student's hand contacts the spoon
- physical assistance; with co-active assistance (adult and student performing the task together), and positioned next to the student so physical movements are from the same direction and in tandem, student and adult grasp the spoon, scoop, and raise it to the student's mouth

With students who have visual impairments and additional disabilities, there are cautions in using certain prompts, particularly those involving physical assistance, related to these students' unique learning characteristics. Students who have visual impairments use their hands for learning, communicating, and connecting to the environment. Any physical assistance must respect both this aspect of their learning and their reaction to manipulation of their hands. Many students exhibit resistance to hand-over-hand instructional support, in which the adult physically moves a student's hands. This resistance is sometimes labeled defensiveness, but it may be an adaptive response to something students experience as physically intrusive. Students can also withdraw from the overuse of hand-over-hand prompting and assistance, having learned that they have little control over other people or over their environment. Learned helplessness, too, can be an adapted response. Avoiding either of these extremes requires prudent use of physical assistance. Co-active assistance, in which the adult and student move together as they perform a task, and hand-under-hand assistance, during which the adult's hands remain under those of the student as the adult does the activity, are more appropriate forms of physical prompting, should a student with visual impairments and additional disabilities require that level of support to participate in activities and routines.

GUIDELINES FOR INCORPORATING PROMPTS

Assessment and ongoing evaluation offer the educational team information regarding the type or combination of prompts that a student needs to actively participate in routines and activities incorporating the development of listening skills. Guidelines for incorporating prompts into the instructional sequence include the following:

- Begin with the prompt identified as the least intrusive that facilitates the student's participation in that particular activity.
- After providing the prompt, pause to allow the student time for processing and responding to the prompt.
- If the student does not respond, provide a prompt or a combination of prompts that increases the amount of support.
- Again pause to allow the student time to process the message and to respond.
- Because students sometimes attach significance to the prompt as a part of the routine and wait for it to be provided (verbal cues and prompts can be particularly difficult to fade), pair the prompt with other cues, such as an object or tactile cue, to provide meaning for the student, allow the verbal prompt to be faded, and support the student's meaningful participation and interaction in the routine—that is, meaningful listening.

Finally, in the vignette illustrating visual impairments and emotional disabilities or challenging behaviors, support for the development of listening skills was embedded within the transition routine for Hana. Her teacher, Mr. Conner, approached her and used spoken communication to identify himself and interact with Hana. He first offered an indirect verbal cue ("spelling is over") and a direct verbal prompt ("check your schedule"). When Hana simply repeated the last phrase and flapped her hands, he approached again, using a direct verbal prompt: "Hana, stand up. Check your schedule." Hana listened to, understood, and responded to the familiar direct verbal prompt to stand. However, when she continued to repeat the phrase "check you schedule, check your schedule" and bounce in place, Mr. Conner used touch to cue her to reach for a familiar transition object that signified that she was to check her schedule, pairing touch and her grasp of the transition object with the spoken communication "Hana, check your schedule."

Supporting the development of listening skills, the teaching of listening skills in this scenario involves the following methods:

▸ pairing spoken communication with touch

▸ pausing to allow Hana to organize a response

▸ being attentive to Hana's behavior, which communicated a mismatch between hearing and understanding

▸ increasing the level of communication support by adding a familiar communication object and reducing the communication to only the words that are paired with the object ("check your schedule")

This interaction reflected sensitivity to Hana's emerging understanding of spoken communication; she heard and repeated sound, in this case, words. She required the pairing of touch with spoken communication to direct her auditory attention to and then respond to Mr. Conner with purpose. She required pairing of a concrete communication object with spoken language to direct her auditory attention and demonstrate understanding—that is, active listening (discussed in Chapters 4 and 6).

In each of these scenarios, the interaction between adult and student was structured to reflect the interplay of visual and additional disabilities for the student and was paired with tactile or visual cues, or both, to ensure that meaningful communication had been provided. Each exchange was paced to allow time for the student to receive and process the message and to respond—that is, to be actively engaged and actively listening. Each interaction reflected the individual student's particular stage of hearing development and the perceptual skills for learning to listen. Teaching those skills and reinforcing those skills was embedded within naturally occurring routines and placed in a functional context, and each interaction was structured to ensure that continuing the activity and interaction was contingent on a response from the student, with cues and prompts provided with care to guide the student as necessary.

PROMOTING THE DEVELOPMENT OF LISTENING SKILLS

Whether students who have visual impairments and additional disabilities receive instruction in a typical classroom, a specialized class setting, or a community environment, the responsibility for delivering meaningful lessons, facilitating interactions, and smoothing the environment falls to the adults in their world—their parents, teachers, and other service providers. This process requires that educators understand the sensory functioning of students with visual impairments, including their additional disabilities, responsiveness to sound, and individual learning characteristics. In addition, educators need to consider the extent to which unnecessary noise interferes with learning and with learning to listen (Nelson, Soli, & Seltz, 2002), identify features of the environment that compromise hearing, and remedy circumstances that contribute unnecessary noise. Adults need to be mindful of their roles not only as communication and listening partners with students who have visual impairments, but also as models of listening behavior and active listening.

Individual Learning Characteristics and Sensory Responsiveness

Designing meaningful instruction in listening and creating opportunities to learn to listen requires knowledge of each student's general functioning and responsiveness, sensory functioning, and basic biobehavioral state. In addition to the clinical reports provided by medical professionals, the educators and specialists who make up the educational team need to conduct assessments in their respective areas and collaborate to develop recommendations regarding educational goals and the adaptations, accommodations, and behavioral supports the student requires for participation and learning. However, assessment is an ongoing process. "We must always be aware that the child is growing and changing. What is more, our knowledge of a child is always incomplete, because each child is an individual with myriad ways of interacting with the world and unique interests and needs" (Crook, Miles, & Riggio, 1999a, p. 96). Comprehensive instruction in listening skills involves evaluating the student's responsiveness to learning situations and interactions to shape instruction and plan appropriately for the next steps.

The assessment and ongoing evaluation process is more complicated when considering some students with visual impairments and additional disabilities. The variety of additional disabilities that might accompany a visual impairment, the extent to which sensory functioning varies, and the complex interplay of multiple impairments have unique impacts on the processing and organization of information, attending, comfort and alert state, movement, tolerance for stimuli, visual functioning, hearing, and attention to auditory information. Brown (2001) wrote, "Because of this broad and complex spectrum of difficulties, it is very likely that some of the sensory problems will go undiagnosed and unsuspected, and the significance and implications of the sensory problems, both individually and as a whole, will be overlooked" (p. 1). Ensuring that the possible multiple impacts of visual impairment and additional disabilities on sensory responsiveness is not minimized within instructional situations or during the ongoing assessment process requires careful planning and methodical observation. Strategies that can hone this process include the following:

> ▸ Collaborate with others: Draw upon the experience of those who know the student well and the unique perspective of other members of the student's educational team, which includes parents and paraeducators.

> ▸ Develop a sensory learning profile for a student to identify the intensity and combinations of sensory information that the student tolerates or requires for meaningful responsiveness, and the sensory information that provides motivation or inspires active learning. Developing such a profile involves gathering appropriate medical information and assessment reports (including medical reports regarding the visual and hearing systems), carefully observing the student in typical routines, activities, and environments to note both the qualities of the sensory information that the student responds to and the qualities and combinations of input the student prefers. This attention to sensory learning and learning modalities can be an appropriate part, and for some students with visual impairments, the primary component, of a learning media assessment (an assessment to help determine the student's optimal learning channels and subsequent learning media, such as use of objects, print, or braille, and modes of presenting auditory information). Anthony (2004) has created an "Individual Sensory Learning Profile" form that illustrates the type of information that would be useful in identifying a student's sensory learning characteristics and could be used to organize and record them.

> ▸ Consider the student's biobehavioral states as they affect level of arousal, such as sleep, drowsiness, awake and alert, crying, or agitated. Smith and Levak (1996a) describe the influences on level of arousal for a student as biological (hunger, tiredness, comfort, and health) and behavioral (emotions, interest, and environment). Health impairments, illness, medications, physiological factors such as hunger or fatigue, and a lack of

meaningful stimulation or sensory overload can all affect a student's level of arousal. Many students with visual impairments and additional disabilities have difficulty achieving and maintaining the level of arousal needed for attention and learning. Identifying a student's biobehavioral characteristics involves setting up an observation schedule and identifying environmental influences, including tolerance for sensory stimuli and medical and physiological factors. This assessment can identify and document the times of day during which a student is more alert, the environmental factors that enhance or maintain a desired level of arousal, and factors that adversely affect arousal, causing agitation or distress (Smith & Levak, 1996a; this resource contains an "Assessment of Biobehavioral State" form that can be used to document this type of assessment).

▶ Identify physical positions that minimize the student's difficulties with head and postural control and vestibular function (awareness of the body in space) and that facilitate his or her use of vision and hearing, allowing the student to attend to the interaction or activity rather than his or her own comfort or balance. For some students, appropriate positioning may be upright, supported seating; other students with poor vestibular function often prefer reclining (Brown, 2001) on a beanbag chair or in the corner of a couch. Some positions—for example, in side-lying equipment—can isolate a student and limit opportunities for social interaction unless adults in the environment ensure that those opportunities are deliberately provided (Palisano, 1992).

▶ Be attentive to subtle behavioral clues such as a blink, a slight movement, or a cessation of movement—a stilling or "quiet alert"—that communicate a student's awareness and responsiveness to sensory information or to interactions. Brown (2001) noted that some students may not turn or reach with intent but "will show they are aware of the stimulus by changing their breathing rate, or the tone of their muscles" (p. 3).

▶ Allow time. "Using vision and hearing is a very complex and sophisticated process and each stage in this process (being aware that there is something to see or hear, attending to it and locating it, recognizing and attaching meaning to it and responding to it in some planned way) may need a considerable amount of time" (Brown 2001, p. 3).

Supportive Listening Environments

Creating environments free of distracting or discomforting elements and supportive of learning activities is an important part of providing instruction to all students. However, as Cushman (1992) has pointed out, creating supportive listening and learning environments is especially important for students with disabilities: "Most [students] with multiple disabilities cannot organize their surroundings in a meaningful way and thus, are dependent on others to structure the environment for them. When setting up a space for these [students], consider factors such as acoustics and lighting, as well as physical layout" (p. 1.11).

Managing an environment that supports learning how to listen demands careful attention to acoustics, which refers to the ability of a space to transmit sound effectively, as well as ways to create spaces in which effective listening can take place. This attention to the qualities of a listening environment applies not only to the physical space but also to other variables affecting the extent to which an environment is acoustically friendly. Factors for educators to consider include the following:

▶ classroom acoustics, not only with how sound is produced but also with its effects

▶ the general level of arousal among students in the classroom

▶ the role of adults in the environment as models of listening behavior and as communication partners in listening experiences

Classroom Acoustics

A student's ability to hear or receive sound, the first component in auditory skill development, is often compromised by poor classroom acoustics. Making the classroom acoustically friendly can be a first step in creating effective listening environments. Nelson, Soli, and Seltz (2002) identified several justifications for "quiet learning spaces" (p. 2), including the following:

▶ Students through adolescence are developing language and require appropriate listening environments to understand spoken communication.

▶ Many students are learning in a language that is not spoken in their home. They are "listening in a non-native language and are susceptible to interference from background noise" (p. 3).

▶ Students with disabilities such as specific learning disabilities, auditory processing disorders, chronic illnesses, behavior challenges, and cognitive challenges have particular need for learning environments that allow "clear listening and communication" (p. 2).

▸ Students with hearing loss, even slight hearing loss, for whom sound appears both quieter and distorted due to an impaired hearing system, need learning environments that similarly offer clear listening and communication. There is often a misconception that hearing aids can remedy a hearing loss. Hearing aids, if recommended for a student, may amplify all sound, making it difficult to sort out background noise, and do not correct distortion. Students may be more aware of sound, but that sound may lack clarity. (See Chapter 8 for additional information on hearing aids and amplification systems.)

The unique educational needs of students who are blind or visually impaired, whose access to learning experiences is highly dependent on listening, need to be added to the list of justifications for considering the importance of acoustics in classroom environments.

Two variables that negatively affect classrooms as learning and listening environments are background noise and reverberation of sound (American Speech-Language Association, 2005). Excessive background noise and the extent to which sound reverberates both interfere with hearing and can create auditory distractions. For students who have visual impairments and additional disabilities, it is particularly important to minimize the effects of reverberation and the amount of background noise so students can learn not just awareness of sound but attention to relevant sound.

Reverberation results when sound waves are reflected off boundaries, such as a wall or other smooth, hard surface, after the source has stopped producing sound. One of its effects is what is known as a "smearing" of sound as the spaces between words become filled with reflected noise (United States Access Board, 2007). Reverberation adds noise, lowers the understanding of speech, and makes listening more difficult. Strategies for reducing the effects of reverberation involve increasing the absorption of sound by using acoustic tiles, placing rugs or carpeting on the floor, and using drapes or curtains at windows.

In addition to reverberation, some of the other sources of background noise that compromise effective listening environments include the following:

▸ fans, heating vents, and air conditioners
▸ computers, radios, and TVs
▸ chairs, as they are pulled in or pushed away from desks or tables

▶ fluorescent lights

▶ other students

▶ noise from hallways or adjacent classrooms

▶ noise from the playground

▶ street traffic

Addressing some of the sources of background noise requires changes in architecture and equipment, such as heating vents, air conditioners, and fluorescent lighting. However, their effects on the acoustic environment can be minimized for students with visual impairments and additional disabilities by considering the physical layout of the classroom and making sure that learning and work areas are not set up, for example, near the air-conditioning unit or heating vent. Some examples of low-technology modifications of the physical environment that can be implemented to reduce background noise and create quiet listening spaces are provided in Sidebar 7.3.

((SIDEBAR 7.3
Modifications for Creating a Quiet Classroom Environment

The following are some methods of creating a quiet environment in the classroom without substantial or expensive modifications:

- Put carpeting or rugs on the floor that can soften footfalls or sounds of chairs being moved as well as absorbing sound that might otherwise contribute to reverberation.
- Place tennis balls or felt on the bottom of chair legs and table legs that are on hard floors so they make less noise and slide easily.
- Wear soft-soled shoes.
- Keep doors and windows closed.
- Hang drapes or curtains, which can serve the twofold purpose of controlling classroom acoustics by absorbing some sound and reducing reverberation and by muffling outdoor sound that transmits through windows. For students who experience difficulty with glare, closed drapes also filter light and create an environment that is more visually friendly and accommodating.
- Attach a drop seal to the bottom of the classroom door to close the gap between the door and the floor to reduce hallway noise.
- Use partitions that have sound-absorbing qualities to create some of the boundaries that are used to define activity spaces; they can be adjusted in height to allow adults visual contact to that space and other areas of the classroom.
- Turn off computers when they are not being used.
- Eliminate competing noise from radios, television, musical recordings, or CDs that are playing in the background for ambience and not for instructional purposes.

Levels of Arousal

A dynamic learning environment has activity, movement, conversation, and students' vocalizations—in other words, noise. Some of the strategies that are effective in managing the physical environment as a listening space are equally effective in minimizing noise generated by regular classroom activity. However, when considering students who have visual impairments and additional disabilities, educators also need to balance active learning, encouraging language and responsiveness, and managing behavior while maintaining an effective listening environment for all learners. These require attention to the activity and arousal level of the class, prudent groupings or pairings of students, and thoughtful scheduling.

Assessment information, including evaluation of biobehavioral state, can yield useful information regarding factors that arouse individual students. Too much information or activity in the classroom can lead to sensory overload for some students, while with too little meaningful sensory input and activity, students may be underaroused or bored. Students with visual impairments and additional disabilities behaviorally communicate a mismatch between the overall arousal level of the classroom and their tolerance or need for stimulation, and may shut down, act out, or exhibit agitation, distress, or confusion. Maintaining a moderate level of arousal requires simplifying the environment and lowering the level of distraction, not only with regard to sound, but also with respect to visual clutter, the activity level, and the amount of movement.

Classroom Design

Classroom design that includes activity-specific areas or work areas that have specific functions can be an effective strategy for simplifying the classroom environment for students who have visual impairments with additional disabilities. The spatial environment can be organized to create defined and predictable spaces with consistent placement of materials. The areas, the activities, and the materials in them need to reflect students' interests and chronological ages. For example, while students of any age might have a leisure area for recreational reading or listening with a rug, comfortable seating, or pillows for reclining, bounded by shelving and a partition, the type of reading and listening material would differ for young learners versus high school–age students.

The arrangement of furniture and the materials in that space readily communicate to either age group of students where they are in the classroom (leisure area), the activities associated with that area (reading, looking at pictures, using headphones to listen to music or recorded stories), and what behavior or action might be expected (choice making, relaxation). Activity-specific work areas organize the physical space of the room and frame the type of activity that takes place in that space. They also help maintain a moderate level of arousal for students with visual impairments and additional disabilities by reducing the burden of problem solving with regard to where they are in the room and what they will be doing, as well as minimizing visual and acoustic distractions.

Classroom Management

The assessment and ongoing evaluation process also offers information regarding a student's responsiveness to the social environment. Students with visual impairments and additional disabilities, who may have limited connections to other people and to the environment, may find the experience of large-group activities confusing or fragmented. Their specific sensory impairments may limit access to the whole process of the activity, and they may not understand what is going on around them or what is expected of them. They may also miss antecedents to other students' pleasure or another student's distress and be confused by laughter or frightened by an outburst. Adults can build in structure and smooth the learning environment for the student by considering how space is used and how students are grouped within the space, as in the following example:

> *Yi, whose additional disabilities include physical impairment, became distressed and cried during the free-play time in the preschool classroom. The educational team considered ways to add meaningful participation for Yi as well as to reduce the activity and noise level. Rather than continue the existing schedule of the entire class first engaging in a general free-play time inside the classroom followed by outside play with sand and water tables, riding toys, and climbing, the staff organized three smaller groups of students and a rotation of the smaller groups through three activities: outside play; free play centered in a specific activity area of the classroom (for example, house area one week, block area another week); and finger painting and easel painting in an art area. The staff members were each assigned areas in which to facilitate interaction and support exploration with modeling and commenting. This reorganization resulted in the following benefits: a systematic use of physical space; a smaller number of students in the classroom during more open learning experiences; a contextual framework for free-play time that continued to support creative exploration in two outlets, art and play; and a more accessible and friendly social, learning, and listening environment for all of the students, including Yi.*

In this scenario, thoughtfully organizing students in small groups is a class management strategy that promotes listening behavior and smoothes the learning environment

(Jalongo, 1995). Inexperienced listeners have difficulty staying engaged during large-group activities in which they need to wait for a turn. Providing instruction in smaller groups more effectively promotes active learning and focused participation and allows more accessible and meaningful learning experiences for each student in the small group, particularly a student with visual impairment with additional disabilities. This also serves to lower the overall arousal level in the classroom, making it more student friendly and a more conducive listening and learning environment.

Managing Transitions

Similarly, managing transitions from one activity to the next through simple and predictable routines can support an effective listening environment and provide focus for students (Jalongo, 1995). Establishing a predictable schedule for daily activities offers consistency for students and creates a framework for transitions. Students understand in what order daily routines occur and can anticipate the activity and prepare for participation and for the transition from one activity to the next. In classrooms for younger students, a common routine to signal transition from free-choice or free-play time to the next activity is the teacher ringing a bell and beginning to sing a cleanup song, one in which the children join over time, and they learn that one activity has an ending before another begins. Students with visual impairments and additional disabilities may miss subtle cues that telegraph change, next events, or expected behavior. The use of strategies and supports such as personal schedules or calendar systems, routines, and ritualized endings offer meaningful communication regarding activities and transitions, as well as focusing the student's attention, encouraging readiness for learning and learning to listen.

Adults as Models of Listening Behavior and Communication Partners

Students with visual impairments, including those with additional disabilities, depend on the adults in their world to manage a classroom environment that is both relevant and acoustically friendly, and to structure learning experiences that are meaningful and accessible as they learn to listen. Students also depend on adults as models of appropriate listening behavior and as communication partners who invite interaction and are responsive to their communicative efforts. As Olsen, Miles, and Riggio (1999) have observed, "It becomes clear that the most important element of the environment is the people."

As models of listening behavior, adults need to establish a respectful environment that places value not only on the exchange between themselves and students but also on what students contribute to the interaction. This requires modifying "teacher talk" (Diaz-Rico & Weed, 1995a, p. 116) or "teacherese" (Miles, 1999, p. 71), which tends to be directive, controlling the flow in information from teacher to student, and takes the form of commands and questions to which the teacher already knows the answer.

One of the primary ways of modifying teacher talk is to embed communication and interaction into meaningful activities that invite conversation and listening. Not only do students with visual impairments, particularly students with additional disabilities, need to learn to receive a message, but they also need to experience the interaction in a positive way as they learn to attach meaning to sound and develop understanding. Appreciating the student's sensory functioning, responsiveness, and interests allows adults to select preferred activities, choose appropriate ways to create mutual attention on a topic, and use modes of communication that have relevance and engagement. Modeling listening behavior and embedding communication into meaningful routines can take many forms, depending on the student's learning characteristics and sensory losses. They require creativity and an unhurried and respectful focus on the student.

The following are some strategies for modeling listening behavior and acting as an effective communication partner with students who have visual impairments, including students with additional disabilities:

▶ Establish a learning climate that has respectful, attentive focus on students foremost, with minimal adult talk in which students are not also participants.

▶ Gain a student's attention prior to proceeding with an interaction. For some students with visual impairments, including those with additional disabilities, this requires only that the student's name be used prior to engaging in further interaction, allowing the student to alert, offer a response, and get ready to listen for more in the exchange. Gaining the attention of students who are less connected to people and to their environment involves judicious use of touch or pairing of touch and sound. For example, depending on a student's visual functioning, adults can use the following strategies:

● place their hand on the student's shoulder or rest their hand next to the student's hand

● voice a greeting or offer a gesture

● enter the student's visual field

▶ Each cue would be followed by a pause while the adult waits and listens for the student's response before continuing (Miles, 1999).

▶ Position oneself to maintain the appropriate tactile, auditory, or visual contact with a student to behaviorally communicate attention on the shared exchange and model active listening for the student (Miles, 1999). For example,

When Mr. Ortega prepares to greet Eli, a high school student with visual impairment and hearing loss, he enters Eli's study space but stands at arm's length so he does not fill Eli's visual field. Mr. Ortega places his hand next to Eli's and waits while Eli responds to the contact and visually traces Mr. Ortega's arm upward to his face, at which point Mr. Ortega says, "Good morning, Eli. I am Mr. Ortega." When he visually recognizes Mr. Ortega and hears his voice, Eli smiles and voices a greeting. In this scenario, Mr. Ortega positions himself to maintain visual, tactile, and auditory contact with Eli and to maintain that contact as Eli indicates responsiveness. By doing so, he models attention to Eli's attentive listening behavior.

▸ Respond to the signals and communication efforts of students with visual impairments, including those with additional disabilities, in modes that are meaningful to them (such as touch cues, speech, gesture, or co-active movement, or an adult moving together with the student), to convey that the communicative behavior was meaningful and that an adult was listening (Miles, 1999). For example, in the earlier vignette with Yi, Ms. Mila interprets Yi's turning of her head as intentional communication and replies using her name and touching Yi's shoulder.

▸ Initiate mutual attention on an object that can serve as a topic of conversation by pointing and holding the point so students who have low vision can visually direct attention to the shared referent and then actively reach for it on their own (Miles, 1999), as in the following example:

After gaining a student's attention, a teacher sitting across a small table from a student may slowly point to a bowl of popcorn at the side, holding the point as the student visually traces her arm to the bowl. The teacher maintains the point until the student reaches for the bowl, and says to the student, "A bowl of popcorn. Let's eat some popcorn for snack." Together they move the bowl between them.

▸ For students who require that touch be paired with looking and listening or with sound, initiate mutual attention on the object as the student is touching it, sliding one or two fingers under his or hers, inviting joint attention (see Chapter 2) and shared interaction through touch (Miles,

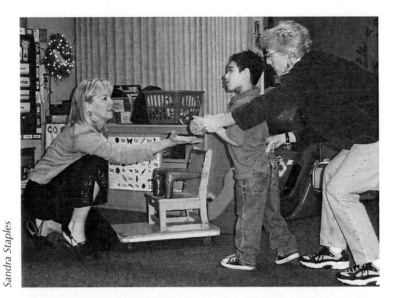

Sandra Staples

The teacher is inviting the student to move toward her with his transition object for circle time. The O&M specialist is a silent partner, offering physical prompts and support, but is not part of the communication exchange.

1999). In the previous example, the teacher may place the bowl of popcorn so it is touching the student's hand and wait for the student to move her hand to indicate awareness of the bowl. When she does, the teacher slides two of her fingers under the student's hand so they are both holding on to or touching the bowl. The teacher can continue their joint exploration by gently moving her hand toward the edge of the bowl, allowing the student to follow the movement of her hand so they can discover that popcorn fills the bowl.

▶ Engage in a resonance activity with a student, an activity that is structured to inspire or evoke a response from the student in order for it to continue. Consider an activity with movement or one in which both the adult and the student are handling and exploring an object that the student finds interesting and pleasurable. Then stop the movement or exploration and wait for the student to initiate repetition of the action, the beginning of turn taking (Miles, 1999).

▶ Work in partnership with a parent, a paraeducator, or another educator so one adult assumes the role of communication partner and the other the role of "silent" facilitator, providing appropriate levels of co-active prompting or co-active support to cue the student's response.

▶ Offer the important information first, particularly when interacting with students who have fluctuating attention or emerging listening skills, as Ms. Terry did when speaking to Micah: "Classroom, Micah." Ms. Terry then restated the important information in sentence form—"We're walking to the classroom"—to model conventional sentence structure and use of language.

▶ Modify language by slowing down the delivery and speaking clearly to allow students to separate words and to process and understand language (Diaz-Rico & Weed, 1995a).

▶ Express one function of communication at a time, with pauses for the student's response; use care to avoid expressing multiple functions, such as commenting, giving a directive, and asking a question at the same time, which "confuse[s] children with slower response and wait time" (Bruce, Godbold, & Naponelli-Gold, 2004, p. 87). For example, offer a greeting ("Eli, good morning"), pause for the student's awareness and response, indicating readiness for further interaction; then follow with a comment or question inviting further conversation ("What is on your schedule today?").

▶ Use intonation, gestures, and body language to maintain and extend a student's interest in an interaction or conversation, pausing often to invite the student's response or comment (Diaz-Rico & Weed, 1995a).

▶ Participate in an activity that has a central topic (often an object one student finds interesting) with a small group of students; model how to ask a question about the object and how to take turns (Aarnoutse, van den Bos, & Brand-Gruwel, 1998).

▶ Use reciprocal teaching in listening activities: Listen to a short passage aloud with a very small group of students, one of whom assumes the leadership role and reads a simple question that prompts, for example, predicting what might happen next; the adult participants model listening behavior as they listen to the short passage; then model listening to the question and offering a response that is on the topic; then model listening to others as they take turns answering (Aarnoutse, van den Bos, & Brand-Gruwel, 1998).

▶ Structure opportunities for students to eavesdrop on conversations so students can learn from other models of listening behavior. As Bruce, Godbold, and Naponelli-Gold (2004) wrote, a student can incidentally listen to a predetermined communication exchange involving "a request and an appropriate response to a request" (p. 87). These structured conversations can be expanded to include commenting on an object or activity and on how to listen to a communication partner's replies and enrich an exchange while keeping it on topic, as in the following example:

> *At snack time, a teacher sits at a table with a student and the paraeducator. One adult asks the other if she would like crackers or apple slices. The student has an opportunity to listen to the request ("Ms. Terry, would you like crackers or apple slices?") and then listen to a response ("I would like apple slices, please.") One of the adults can futher comment on the bright color of the apples, their crispness, or how juicy they are.*

STRATEGIES TO TARGET LISTENING SKILLS

Developing listening skills and integrating the components of auditory perception into the functions of hearing (primitive, signal warning, and spoken language) allow students to anticipate and become ready for interaction, develop curiosity about and understand the world apart from their own bodies, acquire language, and build on experiential knowledge. It falls to educators, caregivers, paraeducators, and other service providers to design and offer meaningful learning experiences for students with visual impairments and additional disabilities that foster the development of listening skills within contexts such as signals to change (for example, to change activity, change communication partner, or change position), inspiration for movement and discovery, and nourishment of spoken communication and understanding. As Miles and McLetchie (2008) stated, "Most importantly, we must take the responsibility of providing experiences that will maximize the [student's] opportunities to develop useful and meaningful concepts of the world" (p. 1).

Strategies for teaching listening skills have at their foundation the following principles:

▸ Active listening and active learning require that students with visual impairments and additional disabilities be involved, with the opportunity to act, not be acted upon.

▸ Sound is elusive and fleeting, and for students with visual impairments and additional disabilities who may have emerging connections with people and with the environment, sound may not have sufficient relevance to be meaningful on its own. Structuring activities to teach the awareness of sound requires judicious pairing of sound and touch, or sound and touch and visual cues.

▸ As noted in Chapter 1, understanding sound from a distance is tied to the development of object permanence. This is a gradual process that begins with the development of attachment to other people, then the understanding of objects. For students with visual impairments and additional disabilities, activities that emphasize meaningful engagement and interaction with other people, with the opportunity to develop those attachments, are central to the development of listening skills.

▸ Activities need to be individualized to accommodate and respect the unique interplay of visual impairment and additional disabilities for each student.

▸ Many students with visual impairments and additional disabilities have difficulty transferring skills from the isolated situations in which they are taught into other natural circumstances and environments. Listening skills cannot be separated into isolated instructional categories. They need to be embedded within natural routines to attain functionality and relevance for students, and they require the collaborative efforts of educators, paraeducators, caregivers, and specialists to do so.

Many of the strategies and charts of listening skills described in other chapters of this book that focus on specific age groups have relevance for students with visual impairments and additional disabilities in those same age ranges and grade levels. An additional table, Appendix 7A in this chapter, shows how listening skills and behaviors can be embedded into alternative functional goals for students with moderate and severe disabilities that align with a standards-based core curriculum in language arts that draw upon and enhance the development of listening skills. Like the charts in other chapters in this book, this listing of skills does not represent a prescribed scope or sequence of either listening skills or functional skills. Rather, the table is a tool for attaching functionality to listening skills and is intended to assist readers in the development of educational programming for students with visual impairments and additional disabilities. The lists of functional behaviors related to listening skills for each alternative standard is by no means exhaustive; these and any other functional behaviors considered need to be individualized for a particular student based on the student's learning characteristics and sensory functioning and further shaped by information gathered through assessment and ongoing evaluation.

The following sections focus on strategies that can be used with students who have visual impairments, including those with additional disabilities, to support them in their progress through the stages of listening skill development. These stages include building awareness of sound; sound, movement, and discovery; understanding auditory information; and auditory comprehension and spoken language.

Becoming Aware of Sound

Listening skills encompass a range of behaviors whose development needs to be encouraged and reinforced. As indicated in Chapter 1, auditory awareness is an early component of these skills. The following are emerging listening behaviors to encourage and reinforce in this area:

▶ quiets or stills when his or her name is called

▶ changes expression or stills when there is a change in sound

▶ repeats an action or movement that creates sound, in mutual-action (an experience that an adult and the student actively share) or joint attention with an adult

Listening begins with awareness of biological sound, such as one's own breathing or swallowing, then of background sound, and soon includes self-stimulatory vocal play (Anthony & Lowry, 2004). Infants who have visual impairments, including those with additional disabilities, frequently demonstrate this awareness in a unique manner—they tend to quiet when there is sound in the background and listen to their own voices when the background is quiet. As Rowland (1983) noted in her studies of language acquisition for blind children, listening is central to understanding the world beyond arm's reach; responding to sound by vocalizing would be "cluttering the auditory environment" (p. 127). Students exhibit a quiet alert in the presence of sound that signals their attention to that sound. Conversely, when it is quiet and nothing is competing for auditory attention, students may engage in self-stimulatory play with their voices, including a range of simple vocalizations, or recitation of familiar words, strings of words, or phrases.

Adults in the student's environment have critical roles to play as attentive communication partners in supporting and teaching emerging listening skills. As such, they acknowledge and reinforce behaviors that indicate awareness of sound and shape them to include environmental listening, awareness of differences in background sounds, and attaching meaning to sound. As an adult alerts a student to his or her presence by entering the student's visual field, providing touch and sound by speaking (the judicious pairing of visual, touch, and sound cues), and then pausing for the student's response, the adult and student are engaging in a dance of mutual action, turn taking, and resonance (van Dijk, 1991) that serves to establish the foundation for *contingent* listening experiences—listening activities that make the continuation of sensory experiences a consequence of the student's behavior or response (Chen, 1999). This back-and-forth dance—mutual interaction followed by a pause or break in the dance—evokes a response or reaction from the student. The adult in turn responds by continuing the action or activity, a natural reinforcement of the student's responsiveness and awareness.

The earlier case study of Yi and her interaction with Ms. Mila as her seat was repositioned for circle time exemplified a contingent listening experience that drew upon visual, sound, and touch cues. Once she was certain that Yi was aware of her presence, Ms. Mila crouched down slowly so Yi could visually follow her movement. She placed a hand on Yi's shoulder and waited for her to respond. When Yi blinked, Ms. Mila continued with their interaction by speaking Yi's name and helping her to move, acting on Yi's behavioral response. Proceeding with their activity was dependent or contingent on some action or indication of awareness from Yi.

Students who require that awareness of sound be a targeted skill area generally have limited awareness of their environment, including people and objects. The sensitive pairing of touch, sound, and (when appropriate) visual cues needs to be infused into interactions and activities. Naturally occurring activities invite opportunities to infuse awareness of sound into meaningful routines and to build responsiveness—readiness for interaction—much as the exchange between Yi and Ms. Mila did.

Other activities to support the development of listening skills and build awareness of sound for students that might otherwise be out of context for a student can be structured to include exploration and attention with a familiar adult. The activity then becomes one of participation and engagement with another person, instead of an isolating experience passively receiving sound. For example, activities using sound that produces vibrotactile feedback, or sound with enough bass or moderate volume to create vibration, can be used in structured activities that systematically support building awareness of sound (see Sidebar 7.4 for a description of such activities). Such listening activities are paced to allow the student's exploration, whether supported or independent, and structured so that continuing the activity is contingent on a response or reaction from the student to changes in the soundscape.

(((SIDEBAR 7.4

Activities That Target Developing Awareness of Sound

A sound source that creates vibrations can be used in activities that support a student's awareness of sound. Depending on the student's comfort and positioning considerations,* the adult and student can sit together, either side by side or across a small table, depending on the student's visual functioning, with both resting their hands on the speaker of a CD player or other sound source. If needed, the player can be on the student's lap or positioned on a table or wheelchair tray so the student's arm and hand touch its surface. If the student is more comfortable lying down on a mat, place the CD player or sound source next to and touching the student's body, close to ear level rather than at his or her knees, for example.

- Turn the sound on. If the sound has enough bass or is moderately loud, the speaker will vibrate under the hands of the teacher and student, as will the sides of the player. The adult and student can engage in mutual exploration and share joint attention on the vibration and the sound.

- Turn the sound off and closely observe the student for clues that he or she has noticed the change—that the vibrotactile feedback and sound have ceased.

- When the student makes any response, turn the sound source or player on again and continue mutual interaction and enjoyment.

- Over time, when the student's response to the sound is consistent, increase the distance from the sound source, reducing the amount of vibrotactile feedback. For example, the player can be within reach of the student but slightly to the student's side rather than directly in front of him or her, also offering experience with the sound's location.

- When the sound is turned on, and when the student offers a reaction that indicates that he or she is aware of the sound, allow the student a little time to orient, and then co-actively prompt the student to reach toward the now-familiar player, perhaps a distance as little as an inch or two. The co-active assistance can be as subtle as a light prompt at the student's elbow, or placing two or three fingers under the student's hand to invite the student to place her hand on the teacher's fingers and slowly reaching together. If the student pulls his or her hand away, the teacher can rest his or her hand next to the student's or at that same spot on the table. The student may return his or her hand to the teacher's and their shared reach for the sound can continue.

This process pairs the vibrotactile feedback—vibration the student can feel—with sound. As the tactile aspects of the experience are faded and become less salient, the student's attention is drawn to the sound. The activity can evolve into a listen-and-do activity, with the adult and student again sitting close to the sound source but with the sound off:

- When the sound is turned on, engage with the student in a preferred action: If the student enjoys clapping hands, clap hands together; if the student likes jumping up and down, jump up and down together; if the student likes rocking, rock back and forth or side to side together.

- Build in a wait time appropriate for the student: long enough to be attending to the lack of sound but short enough so the student doesn't get distracted or forget the game.
- Facilitate auditory and tactile associations by using hand-under-hand guidance to teach reaching to a sound source once the student has behaviorally indicated an awareness of the sound (Crook, Miles, & Riggio, 1999b). Again, this might be a reach of only inches.
- Handle other items that make sounds using co-active or mutual action. Keep in mind that objects should make sound only as long as they are handled and that students can habituate to constant sound. Make a pattern with the sound-making objects with intermittent pauses to add interest and build anticipation for more. Shake the item three or four times rhythmically; then pause; then repeat the sequence.

---

* The positions of the adult and student with a visual impairment will vary depending on several factors:
  - the need for proximity due to the student's sensory functioning
  - the positioning equipment the student may require for comfort and attention
  - the age of the student—when interacting with older students with additional disabilities, sitting side by side or across from each other but touching, arm to arm or hand under hand (adult's hand under the student's so the touch is not directive but inviting), may be more appropriate than body contact and the types of co-active movement that might be used with younger students with additional disabilities (Miles, 1999)

Sound, Movement, and Discovery

Emerging listening skills to encourage or reinforce in the area of movement and discovery related to sound include the following:

▸ repeats one's own movement or action that creates sound

▸ localizes the voice of a familiar person, for example, orients, reaches, or moves toward a communication partner

▸ localizes sounds of objects, for example, orients, reaches, or moves toward a familiar sound-making object

The typical sequence of hearing development—the development of listening skills and behaviors—begins with awareness of and attention to sound that is near if not at the body. With experience and with sensitive nurturing and reinforcement of students' responsiveness, students' auditory awareness and attention to sound extends to sources of sound farther away, and students have the opportunity to be drawn into spaces away from their bodies. The world that had been limited to what touched them becomes larger, filled with special people and interesting things to reach for, new places to discover, and novel things to touch and explore.

Nurturing these skills for students with visual impairments, including those with additional disabilities, draws upon the attentiveness of the adults in the student's world to features of the environment that affect sound and to their roles as effective communication partners to inspire attention to sound, orientation to sound, and reaching or moving to sound.

Using Predictable Spaces to Support Development of Listening Skills

For students with visual impairments who are just acquiring these skills, play spaces or defined spaces that are individualized for the particular student can be set up to facilitate building concepts of sound and experiences important for understanding that people and objects exist outside of the student's immediate experience. These spaces allow students to connect with the environment and learn that their actions can produce an effect, that the environment can be predictable, and that things can be rediscovered—and also that sound can have meaning and can be interpreted to represent things in the environment. Referred to elsewhere in the literature as "defined spaces" (Brown, Anthony, Lowry, & Hatton, 2004, p. 374), "a defined area" (Crook, Miles, & Riggio, 1999b, p. 155), or "a playbox" (SKI-HI Institute, 1989, p. 163), predictable physical spaces are based on the concepts described in the work of Lilli Nielsen (1992) regarding the "Little Room" (p. 54). These terms all refer to individually designed spaces in which objects that are meaningful or interesting to a student are kept in consistent locations. Predictable spaces, also discussed in Chapter 6, offer tactile access to a discrete environment and provide opportunities for students with visual impairments, including students with additional disabilities, to experience sound and associate sound with objects and space. They offer opportunities to learn to listen.

Nielsen's Little Room is a closed-in space with three walls and a Plexiglas ceiling that allows natural lighting for students with visual impairments and additional disabilities who use or are learning to use visual information while also letting adults observe the student's activity. It is sized so a student's roll or reach to either side brings him or her in contact with something interesting attached to or hanging from a wall or the ceiling. The locations of objects are consistent so that these accidental discoveries can be repeated and the objects handled again, building predictability and establishing a foundation for object permanence.

In a predictable space, students have opportunities for discovery, repeating actions, and comparing the experiences. They learn that:

▸ their movements create sound
▸ when they move in certain directions, they can touch, handle, and explore specific objects
▸ these objects make their own particular sounds

Active listening experiences in a predictable, defined space provide a frame of reference for understanding that sounds can represent objects. The environment of the space is consistent; an object can be relocated, reexamined, and handled repeatedly as it becomes something with permanence. With the attainment of the concept of object permanence, students become aware that sound emanating from an object as another person shakes it signifies that "there is something to reach for" (Nielsen, 1992, p. 61)— and their world expands beyond their bodies.

While effective learning opportunities for students with visual impairments, including those with additional disabilities, draw upon naturally occurring activities and the routines that are established within them, some specialized activities and unique learning experiences do not occur naturally or with adequate frequency. They need to be deliberately scheduled. Active learning opportunities in meaningful, predictable spaces are such activities. The predictable space needs to be located in an area of the room that is quiet and time in the space needs to be scheduled for students when the activity level in the room is minimized so the noise and vibration that students receive are from their movement and their contact with objects and materials in that space. This ensures that there is no confusion for students regarding what noise is relevant, what the source of a sound is, or where to direct their listening attention.

Nielsen (1992) identified several stages of spatial development that can provide a framework for observing students' activity while engaged in active learning in a defined, meaningful space:

1. Accidental movement resulting in the awareness that there are things and objects in that space.

2. Deliberately pushing or touching objects.

3. Grasping items and letting go followed by grasping and holding them.

4. Immediately and intentionally repeating a tactile activity or an auditory activity.

5. Handling objects in various ways.

6. Listening to the sound-making qualities of an object while handling it.

7. Reaching for objects in specific locations and comparing the tactile qualities of two objects, the sound-making qualities of two objects, or how to make different sounds with the same object. These behaviors also reflect spatial awareness and the emergence of mental mapping.

The activity within the defined space is student directed; a student needs to be left alone during his or her time in the space, without adults intruding or distracting the student with touch, movement, or talking. The time the student spends actively learning in a meaningful space may range from 15 to 30 minutes depending on the student's tolerance for sensory information. Initially limit the number of objects affixed to or hanging from the surfaces in the space to ensure that the environment is uncluttered and that the student has the opportunity to expect items in specific places as he or she develops deliberate exploration, object permanence, and mental mapping skills. Adults need to carefully observe the student's reactions and activity in the space and make notes of the exploratory behaviors that represent stages in listening and concept development, the qualities of the objects that the student finds interesting, and how the student responds to or repeats sound-making actions.

The student's activity in a meaningful space lends itself to joint attention and conversation with an adult afterward. The adult and student can mutually explore a basket of duplicates of items that the student handled and used to create sound in the defined space, re-creating the experience. The adult verbally labels the objects, building auditory memory and elements of communication. A paraeducator or other adult can serve as a silent partner, facilitating the student's reach and supporting attention on the primary communication partner and their mutual exploration of objects.

Complexity need not be a barrier to constructing spaces that offer consistency and encourage active learning and active listening. They can be constructed in many forms, from a simple, defined area on a rug using the side of the couch at home as one

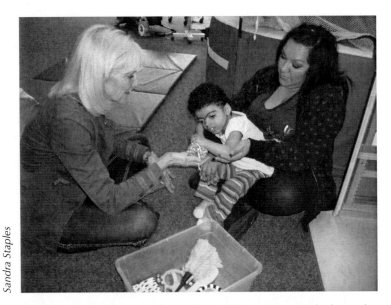

Sandra Staples

Teacher and student jointly explore objects that match those the student has handled in the predictable space. The paraeducator supports her reach and helps her attend to her teacher.

border and items of interest within arm's reach of the student, to Nielsen's commercially available Little Room. They can include a rug marking a defined space next to shelves in the classroom where preferred items are in consistent locations. Meaningful, predictable spaces can be three-sided frames constructed from PVC pipe, from which interesting objects can be hung; or they can be an area where heavy-duty Velcro is attached to a wall to hold preferred and interesting items a student can reach for, explore, grasp, and compare from his or her wheelchair or corner chair. For older students, predictable spaces may take the form of personal study spaces or "dens" (Smith, 2010), with walls or borders and materials that are of interest but reflect a student's chronological age. For example, the sound of a rattle may be a favorite one for an older student. However, a small rainmaker can make the same sound and have the same timbre, still matching the student's interests but affording the student and the learning situation an appropriate level of dignity.

Predictable spaces can be located on top of what is referred to as a resonance board, a hollow platform that vibrates when a student moves on it, pats it, or bangs it. These sources of sound and vibrotactile feedback serve to reinforce movement and inspire repetition of sound-making actions. When Yi, described in an earlier vignette, has time for self-discovery in a predictable space, she lies on a resonance board and sometimes bangs on it lightly with her hand or with her foot. As she feels the vibrations that result, she smiles and murmurs, which results in vibration of a kind different from the vibration she creates when she bangs her foot. The predictable space, whether made of PVC pipe or another creative option, creates a chamber that allows slight sound and vibration to reverberate and provide Yi with meaningful feedback from her actions. These active learning experiences are contingent listening experiences—the sensory feedback of sound and touch that Yi receives is in response to and dependent upon her own movement.

Environmental Listening and Sound Localization

The development of auditory awareness and attention to sound begins nearby: Students quiet to a familiar person who is both touching them and talking to them; students experiment with sound they can make, by vocalizing, patting something that touches their bodies, or shaking something their hands have contacted. With these experiences with sound that is close, the awareness of sound and listening skills extend to sound a little more distant. A student reaches for a familiar sound-making object or turns toward a familiar person talking to him or her, as in the following example:

Yi demonstrates a "quiet alert" when Ms. Mila touches her shoulder and calls her name. One day, after Ms. Mila calls her name but before she touches her shoulder, Yi turns and lifts her arm toward Ms. Mila's voice.

Yi's slight turn and reach toward her teacher's voice indicate that Yi not only is aware of sound but also is attentive to the location of the sound, the location of her familiar communication partner, Ms. Mila. Over time, within the familiar routines and interactions with Ms. Mila, Yi has been developing attachment; she begins perceiving Ms. Mila as someone who has permanence and attaches meaning to the sound of her voice alone. Yi's attentions to sound—her listening skills—now include people and objects beyond her body. Awareness of sound and attention to sound from a source not in direct contact with her body inspire turning for visual advantage and reaching toward that sound source, whether it is a familiar person or favorite object. Yi's world expands beyond what touches her and what she is touching.

Chapter 1 describes the process of "distancing" (Bruce, 2005) as students acquire an understanding of objects and people and hold them in memory. Students with visual impairments, including those with additional disabilities, need to know that objects and people continue to exist beyond their experience with them to develop memory of that person or object and attach meaning to sound alone. With that memory—the concept of permanence—students can attach meaning to the sound alone and be inspired to reach into space and to listen to and localize sound, building further concepts about and experiences with people, objects, and space in the environment, a process vital for students with visual impairments and students with additional disabilities as they develop purposeful movement and use listening to understand spaces and spatial relationships. Chapter 6 expands on this discussion of sound, movement, and discovery and applies it to orientation and mobility, one of the areas of the expanded core curriculum for students with visual impairments, including students with visual impairments and additional disabilities (Hatlen, 1996).

Supporting Environmental Listening and Sound Localization

A sound source on one side of the body or near to one ear is perceived differently than a sound near to the other ear, building sound localization skills or understanding of the direction of the sound source. Comparing qualities of sound includes not only the different sounds various objects make but also the subtle difference in sound a single object makes depending on where it is held. Auditory localization begins initially in the horizontal plane—that is, on either side of the body—and at ear level (Lawson & Wiener, 2010; Northern & Downs, 2002). It then develops to the side and below. Localizing sound that comes from a source behind or directly in front of a student is the last to develop.

As illustrated in the activities for targeting environmental listening and sound localization presented in Sidebar 7.5, supporting attention to sound that is from sources not in direct contact with a student's body requires adults to be attentive to the student's present awareness of sound. It requires understanding how auditory localization develops to support students as they become aware of space and sound in space. It

((SIDEBAR 7.5

Activities to Target Environmental Listening and Sound Localization

The following are suggestions for activities that can help students develop skills in environmental listening and sound localization:

- Be attentive to how auditory localization develops and to a student's current behavior regarding sound. Since localization develops first at ear level and to the side, approach the student slightly to one side while speaking to him or her. The adult can sit or crouch so his or her voice is at ear level and continue speaking. The adult can invite a reach toward his or her voice by using hand-under-hand assistance or prompting.

- For a student who has low vision, enhance some visual aspect of a sound-making object the student finds pleasurable as a means of reinforcing a head turn and building auditory localization skills. For example, add red stripes to a tambourine if a student likes its shaking sound. Once the student turns even slightly toward the sound of the tambourine, the additional visual aspects—the red stripes—may further capture and hold the student's attention, offering additional sensory reinforcement for turning to sound.

- If a student behaviorally communicates awareness of a sound in the environment, explore together what is making it so he or she can develop associations between sound and object and between sound and its location in the environment. Go to the source of the sound together with the student, acting as a guide or as the "motor" for a wheelchair, rather than bringing the source to the student, even if the source is small enough to do so. Helping the student to move to the sound source offers information related to space and location and to how sound changes with distance, and builds mental mapping of that space or room.

- As students who are becoming more skillful perceivers enter a room, stand with them in the doorway and ask them to listen for the voice of a familiar adult in the room, using communication modes and supports appropriate for that student (such as spoken language, photographs and labels, and gestures). For students with visual impairments and additional disabilities who have challenges with body awareness, asking them to point their noses at the sound can be an effective alternative to pointing with an arm or hand. Walk together to that person and engage in a pleasurable social exchange to reinforce the functionality of localizing sound. Begin this process when the familiar adult is within close proximity and is cued to the activity so that he or she speaks clearly and with adequate volume to gain the student's attention, gradually increasing the distance as the student demonstrates understanding and competence.

requires adults to continue as effective communication partners, initiating interaction that is meaningful for students and that inspires responsiveness while the adult remains slightly apart from the student. It requires controlling the environment so that students with visual impairments, including those with additional disabilities, are not confused about what noise or sound is relevant, what the source of a sound is, or where to direct their listening attention.

Understanding Auditory Information

Emerging skills to encourage or reinforce in the area of understanding auditory information, including auditory discrimination and auditory memory, include the following:

▸ recognizes and responds to familiar sounds: voices of familiar people, sounds of familiar objects

▸ responds to one's own name

▸ picks up or gives a named familiar communication object or icon

▸ anticipates regularly occurring events or activities based on environmental sound, such as the sound of water running cuing washing hands; a bell meaning change of class or checking the schedule

▸ anticipates an event based on a verbal cue or label, such as hearing the word *recess* and orienting or moving to the door

▸ follows a familiar one-step direction given in context

▸ shares information about an event with family members using communication supports, such as objects

As students with visual impairments and additional disabilities become more skillful perceivers of auditory information, they begin to discriminate differences in sound and differentiate people and objects based on their sounds alone. They attach meaning to sound and develop an inner receptive vocabulary that elevates listening skills and behaviors to a representational level. They begin to understand and attach meaning to words and associate those words with the activities or people that those words represent: the sound of water running in the bathtub represents a specific activity; the sound of a favorite person or parent's voice represents that specific person. Students with visual impairments and additional disabilities begin to understand and respond to their own names. They not only differentiate sounds and associate a particular sound with a specific object but also begin understanding labels. With the development of receptive vocabulary, students with visual impairments and additional disabilities have the opportunity to listen with intent and to make associations between sound and space and their location, between sound and an activity, and between sound and people in their environment. Their world not only has expanded beyond their bodies but also, with the emergence of meaningful receptive vocabulary tied to concrete experience, has become ordered.

The perceptual listening skills of discriminating differences in sound and differentiating people and objects suggest that students with visual impairments and additional disabilities are beginning to conceptualize. They tactilely or visually look for a specific item first based on its sound and then based on the label or word. The development of a receptive vocabulary and the emerging skills of attaching a label to an object or person allow students with visual impairments and additional disabilities to know what to look for and orient their attention appropriately and with intent.

Developing the ability to attach meaning to sound and differentiate objects and people based on sound is of particular significance for students with neurological visual impairments or CVI, who are able to use their vision more functionally when they are in familiar places and when they know what to look for. Some students with CVI require a verbal label or the sound of an object to visually orient to the object and reach for it or step over or around it. Developing these listening skills and behaviors allows them to direct their visual functioning and attach meaning to visual information. Many students who have neurological visual impairments or other cortical abnormalities that affect the processing of information have difficulty organizing stimulation from multiple modalities simultaneously and, for example, may close their eyes when localizing or attending to sound. Adults need to be astute observers of often subtle behaviors to appreciate that students with neurological or cortical visual impairments are listening and are using auditory information to direct visual functioning and interactions with people and objects in their environment.

Conversational Interaction

The importance of conversational interaction cannot be overstated when discussing the unique listening needs of students who have visual impairments, including students with additional disabilities. An inner receptive vocabulary develops from repeated experiences of exploring objects and their sounds in meaningful contexts through interactions and conversations about the objects with familiar people. Students begin to attach meaning to words; they begin to understand words spoken to them and, importantly, receive information through listening.

Equally important, the conventional paradigm of what constitutes conversation needs to be expanded; that is, in its simplest form, conversation is turn taking, a back-and-forth connection. Engaging in conversation with students with visual impairments and additional disabilities involves proximity and mutual action, as in the following sequence:

▸ joint attention on an object of interest to the student with visual impairments and additional disabilities, sitting in close proximity and handling it together, hand-under-hand, hands touching; shared attention on the object is respectful of the student and follows the student's pace and movement; it is not directive and the student's hands are not manipulated but invited to explore the object

▸ offering an item similar to the first and, by doing so, inviting the student to explore it and compare it to the first one

▸ providing verbal narrative to what the student is experiencing, using clear speech, concrete labels, and judicious use of pauses or quiet, not only to allow the student time to organize a behavioral or verbal response, but also to avoid cluttering the auditory landscape

Continuing the conversation and exchange requires engagement and responsiveness from the student, maintaining the structure of active listening. It requires adults to scaffold auditory responsiveness—they must stretch a student's listening skills from awareness, to attending, to comparing sound, and then to discriminating and recognizing sound, nurturing students' understanding of labels and words and building an inner vocabulary.

Adults need to model listening behavior and provide the narrative in ways that create a meaningful receptive vocabulary for students with visual impairments and additional disabilities. Maximizing conversational opportunities within naturally occurring activities by making the objects and materials used during those activities the topics of conversations offers not only meaningful contexts for providing this vocabulary but also opportunities for repetition. These strategies offer students the opportunity to associate a sound or label with a whole activity, so that sound and labels not only can represent an object but also can be associated with an event that has a beginning, a middle, and an end.

Conversations and interactions initially represent *now*, the experience at that moment. As objects and their labels assume significance, they can represent *what is next*, or the future. Subsequent conversation about the activity using the same objects, symbols, and language allows students with visual impairments and additional disabilities to understand the past and to conceptualize that information and experiences cross time, places, and people.

Infusing conversational opportunities and instruction in listening skills within natural contexts for students with visual impairments and additional disabilities requires attentiveness to and reflection on the existing routines and activities that are often considered basic supports within educational programs for students with significant learning challenges. Calendar systems and experience books are two such supports that can be used to emphasize building understanding, concept development, and attaching meaning to sound. Outcomes with each of these instructional supports draw upon auditory-perceptual skills and the development of listening skills.

Using Calendar Systems

Systematic use of calendar systems (Blaha, 2001; Blaha & Moss, 1997; Crook, Miles, & Riggio, 1999b) to target building understanding and attaching meaning to sound offers students with visual impairments and additional disabilities a routine for having conversations about *now* and *what is next* that, with repeated experience, allows them to conceptualize time and develop anticipation and readiness for something that is going to happen. With judicious instructional support and structured conversation as a personal calendar or schedule is reviewed and acted upon, students have the opportunity to make associations between objects and activities and between objects and their labels—and in doing so attach meaning to sound and build understanding.

The most basic calendar or schedule has two components: an object that the student uses in the activity and an "all done" or "finished" basket of some kind. A basic instructional sequence is the following:

▶ The object becomes the topic of conversation for the adult and the student, their point of joint attention, just before the activity begins.

▶ The student then uses the object in the activity.

▶ At the end of the activity, the finished basket is presented, and the student, jointly with the adult, puts the object inside to signal the end of the activity.

The finished basket containing the communication objects from that day's activities can be reviewed with a student, providing another natural opportunity for joint attention and conversation, emphasizing listening skills, auditory memory, and the development of inner, receptive vocabulary. As the adult and student have the opportunity to reexperience the student's day by together handling one by one the objects in the student's finished basket, the labels attached to the objects are spoken and heard once again. The student has the additional opportunity to make associations between objects and the activity and between objects and their labels. The activity—the conversation between adult and student—both requires listening and uses listening to teach.

Personal calendars can be expanded to be a part-day and then a full-day schedule, set in a designated and consistent location, as students develop associations between objects and labels and the activities they represent, as in the following example:

Objects associated with activities were initially given to Micah when he was in afternoon kindergarten. The cup he used at lunch was given to him at or near the lunch table; the toothbrush for grooming time was handed to him near the sink; the crayon he used at journal time for drawing on paper was given to him at or near the table where he used the crayon. As he began to act on these objects by turning and moving to the locations on his own, he was behaviorally indicating understanding that these items represented the activities of lunch, brushing teeth, and journal writing.

A part-day schedule was developed for Micah for afternoon kindergarten activities, initially with just two activities in sequence at a time: circle time, lunch; brushing teeth/grooming, outside play; journal, bus. As Micah's vocabulary of objects grew and as he internalized the routine of going to the calendar at transitions, the calendar came to reflect the entire afternoon. Over time, his schedule became more symbolic as the objects were paired with photographs of the objects. Finally, use of the objects was faded and photographs were used to cue activities and to inspire Micah's listening skills and use of words and labels on his own.

Previewing and having a conversation with students about their part-day or full-day schedule offers an additional opportunity for social interaction as well as development of vocabulary tied to meaningful experience. When Micah was cued to check his calendar, he and a teacher together talked about the object, with the teacher providing the meaningful label and waiting for Micah's response. The adult can enrich the conversation by adding detail about the activity, perhaps lunch, by stating "I am glad it is lunchtime. I am hungry."

Hana has a similar need for attaching meaning to words and building meaningful vocabulary:

This year, Hana has been using a written schedule, as her calendar is called, written in braille. Hana writes words and has strong name-calling skills; that is, she decodes and correctly reads aloud individual written words. However, even as she reads the word lunch and chants, "Lunch, lunch," she does not move toward the classroom door or add words associated with lunch to what she is saying. She calls out the word but is not attaching significance or meaning to the word either as she reads it or as she says it aloud. As she and her teacher preview her schedule each morning, her teacher adds detail to the written word, pacing his conversation with Hana so she will respond. The interaction is structured to attach meaning to words, to build listening skills and meaningful use of spoken language. With increasing comprehension, Hana may also hold in memory the sequence of the day.

As students acquire literacy skills, personal schedules or calendars can be in written form, as Hana's is. Regardless of the form—objects or written words—when the personal schedule or calendar is read, is reviewed, and functions as a topic of conversation with an adult, it continues to be used as a means of developing and honing listening skills. It continues to provide structure for the following:

▸ auditory memory

▸ sound-symbol association, auditory discrimination

▸ sight-word vocabulary

▸ conversation about what will occur on a given day and closure to a day

Using Experience Books

Experience books are based on an event or routine in which a student has participated, representing a record or diary of the event, sequenced as the student experienced it. Like calendar systems or personal schedules, experience books offer routines for embedding and reinforcing listening skills and for attaching meaning to objects and artifacts adults and students gather and use in their creation (Crook & Miles, 1999; Lewis & Tolla, 2003). As the experience book is read again, reviewed, and used as an opportunity for conversation and joint attention by the student and an adult, the event is reexperienced. Reading the experience book offers meaningful engagement with opportunities to embed attention to sound and meaning of sound as the adult offers labels and a description while together the adult and student explore the objects in the book. Experience books allow students to conceptualize that information can cross not only time but also place and person, as it is jointly read and reexperienced with familiar people at school and with family members at home.

Lewis and Tolla (2003) described a basic sequence for creating an experience book for students who have visual impairments and are acquiring early literacy skills and concepts related to understanding words and labels:

▸ Identify an activity or routine that is meaningful for the student. The activity can be one that happens regularly or a particular event. For example, an experience book could be made around a natural routine, such as a grooming routine in the morning, or it could record a particular event that took place in the community, such as going to a particular fast-food restaurant for lunch.

▸ The method of illustrating the book is based on the extent to which the student requires concrete referents, as well as on the student's visual functioning, and might include objects from the activity in which the student participated, parts of objects, or photographs taken during the activity or routine.

▸ One object from the activity or event is secured to a page, and simple text in braille, large print, or both is written at the bottom. Use of multiple literacy modes allows the experience book to be shared with individuals whose learning modality differs from the student's (Crook & Miles, 1999; Lewis & Tolla, 2003), and the consistent location of the text means the student can learn where to look for the print or braille that accompanies the illustration as he or she acquires concepts related to literacy—that print has meaning, that it is read left to right, that there are words and spaces (Lewis & Tolla, 2003). Also, the addition of text allows different individuals in the student's world to read the book in joint attention with the student and use consistent, meaningful vocabulary to label the object.

Students with visual impairments, particularly students with additional disabilities, need to be actively involved in the creation of an experience book so it attains relevance and becomes a meaningful record of their experience of the event. For some students, participation may consist of collecting the objects that will be used in the experience book. For example, they may choose or follow indirect cues to collect a party napkin, balloon, ribbon, and other concrete items from a birthday party where they encountered them. The items can be reviewed in a fashion similar to reviewing the finished basket of a student's day at school prior to sequencing the story and attaching the items to a page. Students can glue items or attach them with Velcro, which offers the option of removing the item from the page for more active exploration of the item in its three-dimensional form (Lewis & Tolla, 2003). Students who are not able to secure the items on their own can assist in this process, giving items to the adult or using hand-under-hand assistance from an adult.

Mutual-action and co-active reading of an experience book provide a meaningful context for embedding listening skills: auditory attention and memory, development of receptive vocabulary and language usage, social behavior and turn taking in conversation. They can be used as topics of conversation as an adult and a student explore the illustrations together, read the line of text on each page, and reexperience the routine or event. Additionally, experience books about a routine at home can be read at school; one about a school routine or event can be read at home, allowing students to learn that information can cross time and place.

As students acquire literacy skills, experience books can evolve to include a greater emphasis on symbolic representation—not only listening and speaking but also reading and writing. Students can be supported in dictating the content per page, can copy from a model as they acquire writing skills, and can use the content for sight-word vocabulary, identifying a word by initial letter sound, and as an initial tool for making predictions, drawing upon memory of the event and opportunities to have read and shared the experience book.

Auditory Comprehension and Spoken Language

Emerging skills to encourage or reinforce auditory comprehension and spoken language include the following:

- ▶ communicates personal choice during structured activities
- ▶ matches a familiar object or communication object to a word card
- ▶ offers a greeting in response to the greeting from someone else
- ▶ answers a question, such as "What is your name?" when asked
- ▶ engages in conversation with a familiar adult and remains on topic for two conversational exchanges
- ▶ confirms a communication partner's response (such as a customer's order or a next activity) in a structured routine
- ▶ uses an "I" message during a conflict
- ▶ follows a one-step direction given to the group
- ▶ responds to questions posed by a teacher during small-group activity
- ▶ identifies neighborhood sounds while on "listening walk"
- ▶ waits for a break in conversation without interrupting
- ▶ retells a story read aloud in the correct sequence
- ▶ predicts the end result when participating in the development of a social story

As students with visual impairments and additional disabilities develop understanding of verbal language, they are crossing the threshold from responding to sound and its nuances to symbolic understanding. Sounds become discrete words, their meanings attached to referents that may not be present, and evolve into vocabulary that relies less on labeling and includes subtleties of action, feeling, and prediction. Listening to and understanding spoken language reflect comprehension—"symbols are converted to meaning" (Harley, Traun, & Sanford, 1997, p. 225).

Students with visual impairments and additional disabilities who have listening skills that include auditory comprehension and spoken language are learning to follow verbal directions, engage in increasingly detailed conversations with another person, participate in verbal exchanges on a topic, and learn from verbal information given to a group. Activities described in other chapters of this book for developing comprehension of spoken language for students with visual impairments have relevance for students with visual impairments and additional disabilities acquiring these same listening skills, with prudent use of modifications discussed in this chapter that accommodate the unique interplay of visual impairment and additional disabilities for an individual student. Other activities that can be used to build comprehension of spoken language and auditory memory and hone the skills of listening for detail or meaning for students with visual impairments and additional disabilities are presented here as expansions or increasingly sophisticated applications of instructional strategies and activities for other functions of listening.

Strategies for developing oral language rely largely on creating and maintaining language-rich environments, structured to be responsive to students' communicative efforts, with feedback to students that contains redundancy of vocabulary and paraphrasing as well as descriptive language that enhances meaning and supports concept development (Crook, Miles, & Riggio, 1999b; Erickson & Hatton, 2007). As models of listening behavior and effective communication partners, educators, parents and caregivers, and paraeducators and other service providers are also establishing language environments (Miles, 1999) that can be rich in comments and description, paced to invite conversation from students with visual impairments and additional disabilities, and structured to expand their use of language to include functions of greetings, sharing, and commenting.

Calendar systems and experience books offer a natural context in which to introduce awareness of letters and sounds in words, build a sight-word vocabulary, and scaffold listening skills from listening and speaking to reading and writing. Social stories, simple stories written from a student's perspective, usually intended as a means of reinforcing positive behavior in a social situation (Crozier & Sileo, 2003), provide an additional tool for integrating experiential learning and listening skills that strengthen the relationship between language and thought. Each of these instructional supports can be aspects of comprehensive educational and behavioral plans for students with visual impairments and additional disabilities. For individual students, they offer meaningful routines that not only draw upon listening skills but also offer opportunities to creatively embed instruction in listening skills into ongoing activities and routines.

Guided reading of experience books and social stories embed auditory attention, auditory discrimination, and auditory memory skills into the activity, just as reviewing a personal calendar with supported discussion of the events with an adult does. The adult and student read the story together, and the adult pauses at keywords in the story, allowing the student to draw from auditory memory and fill in the space with the appropriate word. The keyword may be the label for the object on the page of the experience book; it may be the label attached to an illustration in the social story. With careful attention to the stages of auditory skill development and to existing routines and curricular and behavioral supports, listening skills can be infused and emphasized within meaningful activities.

Using Social Stories

Like calendar systems and experience books, social stories can be used as an activity to target students' auditory comprehension and spoken language skills. Social stories can be generic stories related to general social situations a student with visual impairments and additional disabilities encounters or can be targeted for situations that are problematic for a student. For example, a social story can reflect general behavior and activity in the cafeteria. Or it can target a specific behavior for a student, such as eating the food on his lunch tray only, not the food of classmates seated near him.

Crozier and Sileo (2003) identified six steps necessary for the use of social stories as part of an effective behavioral intervention:

1. identifying the target behavior
2. conducting a functional analysis to gain a baseline of the targeted behavior and its trigger or cause
3. identifying what might be changed and what behavior to teach
4. writing the story
5. introducing the social story to the student
6. evaluating its effectiveness in reinforcing appropriate behavior

Whether social stories created for students with visual impairments and additional disabilities reflect general participation in activities or serve as part of a behavioral intervention, they need to reflect the comprehension level of the student. Crozier and Sileo (2003) pointed out that they need to be organized with one concept per page, with the text limited to "one directive sentence per page and one to three descriptive or perspective sentences" (p. 28).

The descriptive sentence offers information about the setting or what is happening during an event, while a directive statement reinforces how the student needs to behave. Perspective sentences offer information about how other people think or feel about the activity or the student's behavior. Students who have visual impairments and additional disabilities often miss social cues and other nonverbal communicative behaviors, limiting their appreciation for the perspectives of others and for the social climate. Social stories can enhance students' awareness of and consideration for

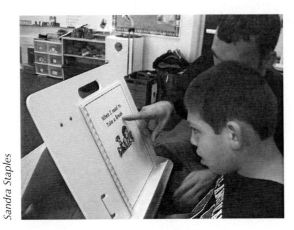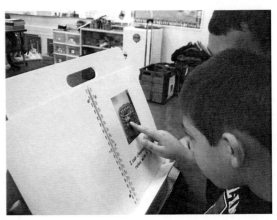

Sandra Staples

This student and his teacher are using a guided reading strategy with one of the student's social stories. The adult points to the words as he reads them aloud, pausing to let the student fill in the name of the item pictured on the page.

others as well as providing a means of reinforcing and shaping their social behavior. Illustrations can also support emerging literacy. They can include a photograph, line drawing, or an object or part of an object, depending on the student's picture interpretation skills, need for additional cues to the story, and the extent to which the illustration supports rather than detracts from the key concept.

When an adult and student share a social story, the adult reads the words on the page while pointing to draw and maintain the student's visual attention. The adult can pause in the reading, giving the student time to fill in the pause with the label of the main item illustrated on the page, drawing on auditory memory and listening skills. Micah, a student encountered in previous vignettes, provides an example of an instance in which social stories functioned both as an effective behavioral support and a meaningful activity for teaching listening skills.

> *Micah often cried and hit other people at school, saying "No!" emphatically to supports that had been effective in calming him in the past. A functional analysis of the behavior led the team to conclude that he needed communication strategies to label what he was feeling and express a choice for what he was going to do as a means of shaping his behavior and building in appropriate choice making. They had concluded that this behavior was not reflecting a drop in blood sugar or another basic need but related more to frustration or fatigue and a desire to escape whatever he was currently asked to do. They created a social story for Micah titled "When I Need to Take a Break," and each page contained one sentence and one photograph to mirror his language and listening skills.*

Descriptive sentences included "Sometimes I am happy"; "Sometimes I am sad"; "Sometimes I am mad." Directive sentences included " When I am mad, I can choose to go for a walk to calm down"; "When I am mad, I can choose to sit on the beanbag to chill out"; "When I am mad, I can choose to play with fidgets to feel quiet"; "When I feel better, I can check my schedule." A perspective sentence at the end was "My teacher is happy when I make a choice."

Micah's social story was the first of many, and they form a basis for his functional literacy program at school. With a favorite paraeducator, Micah selects a social story, and he and the familiar adult jointly read that day's choice using a guided reading strategy. Micah fills in the meaningful word at pauses, drawing on auditory memory, and points to that label in the photograph that it illustrates. Thus, listening skills have been embedded within a behavioral support—the social story—reinforcing desired behavior while simultaneously placing listening skills in a meaningful context.

Eccentric Language

For many students with visual impairments and additional disabilities, the path listening takes toward understanding and using spoken language may be longer than that for other students with visual impairments, with plateaus and deviations that require educators, parents and caregivers, paraeducators, and other service providers to exercise creativity and give careful consideration to alternative communication strategies and supports. Students with visual impairments and additional disabilities often display eccentric patterns of language use. Some of these patterns are not uncommon in young children, such as confusion regarding pronoun usage, particularly in young blind children for whom appreciating perspective and understanding the referents "I" and "you" are hampered by lack of visual experience. However, many eccentric patterns linger over time for students with visual impairments and additional disabilities (Fazzi & Klein, 2002; Warren, 1994).

In addition to atypical use of pronouns, these eccentric language patterns may also include prolonged use of echolalia, or the repetition of statements made by other people; excessive use of questions, often unrelated to the topic of conversation; a prevalence of verbalisms, or words and language unconnected to meaningful experience or comprehension; and language that perseverates on topics or phrases uniquely interesting to the student (Fazzi & Klein, 2002; Silver, 2003; Warren, 1984; Warren, 1994). Students with visual impairments and additional disabilities may parrot phrases and questions they have heard, such as "Do you want to go to the swing?" as an attempt to communicate the statement "I want to swing," combining both confusion with pronouns and echolalia. They may repeatedly ask "Where is . . . ?" even when holding the item in question. Or, like Hana in the previous vignette, students repeat or recite language for which they lack experience or a concrete referent. Hana repeated "Check your schedule, check your schedule" in an agitated manner without acting on those words, suggesting she had no meaningful interpretation of those words at that time. When her transition object was paired with spoken language, she quieted and acted on that message—she moved toward her schedule. The concrete referent had meaning for her. Students with visual impairments and additional disabilities may have deceptive language, saying phrases and words correctly but in contexts unrelated to the topic of conversation. Their impressive auditory memory skills and often lengthy and accurate recitations of chants, songs, or sections of film dialogue or radio programs suggest attention to auditory information but without attachment to real experience; what they are reciting lacks meaning.

Literature suggests that to some extent these idiosyncratic language patterns are related to the impact of blindness on language development. Warren (1994), in a review of literature related to language development and blind children, noted that with respect to referential language and the use of pronouns to refer to oneself or to another person, vision acts as an "extralinguistic source" (p. 147) of information and eases the integration of referential language concepts for students who are sighted. The referent for the pronoun someone may use in conversation, for example, *she*, is immediately accessible to students with vision. When one person comments on what another person in the room is doing by saying "She is reading a book," vision allows the sighted student to attach meaning right away to the pronoun *she* in a way that is not available to a student who is visually impaired.

Similarly, straying from the topic of conversation during an exchange with an adult has roots in the impact of visual impairment on maintaining joint attention that might otherwise keep the conversation going. Students who have visual impairments, particularly those with additional disabilities, require not just proximity to their communication partner but also judicious use of touch to signal and sustain attention. Looking at one another during a conversation, using vision, offers nonverbal cues that support reciprocity and understanding of whose turn it is to speak (Warren, 1984). Students with visual impairments do not have this same incidental access to a language partner and miss gestures or subtle clues to turn taking in a conversation.

In other circumstances, eccentric language reflects students' attempts to contribute to a conversation drawing upon the language models that are available to them. Some studies suggest that excessive use of questions by students with visual impairments may evolve from attempts for assurance about who or what is in their environment (Fazzi & Klein, 2002) as well as parroting the language used by parents and teachers (Bruce, Godbold, & Naponelli-Gold, 2004). Adults, parents of young children who are blind, and teachers of students with visual impairments and additional disabilities in those studies tended to use questions and commands, and there was a low level of communication around objects beyond offering labels. Students hear questions; their attempts to communicate may draw upon the language models and functions they hear. Again, experience with Hana illustrates this type of communication:

> When Hana started to board the bus each day to go home, if the driver was not Ms. Ruthie, she chanted, "Where is Ms. Ruthie? Where is Ms. Ruthie?" during the entire bus ride home. The educational team determined that her question was Hana's attempt to know who was there, a desire for reassurance about who the driver was that day. The team scripted and modeled an exchange for Hana in which she paused at the door of the bus every day and said "My name is Hana. What is your name?" Hana was satisfied with knowing the substitute driver's name and no longer asked about Ms. Ruthie if there was another driver. She was afforded control by listening to the way to get information about who was in her environment, which was modeled for her.

Many of these idiosyncratic language patterns have their basis in lack of visual experience, and experiential learning in language-rich environments can positively shape the development of oral language for younger children who are blind (Erickson & Hatton, 2007). Modeling descriptive language, providing feedback and descriptions as students explore, and engaging in activities with real objects as supports can be effective in shaping language while developing concepts and experiences that can anchor language. For example, as an adult and a student share attention on an object, in addition to simple labels, the adult can model descriptive comments on a feature of the object ("The chains on the swing rattle when we shake them, don't they? I like shaking them too.").

Eccentric language patterns linger and are more pronounced for some students who have visual impairments and additional disabilities. The interplay of their visual impairment and additional disabilities uniquely affects their environmental and social awareness and their ability to integrate sensory information and attach meaning to sound. Each student's understanding of how sound, language, and experience needs to be appreciated as uniquely his or her own. Adults need to enter that world, attempt to take the student's perspective, and carefully consider the function of the student's communicative efforts so they can respond in a manner that will be meaningful to the student, furthering the communication exchange as well as the student's listening skills.

Developing listening skills that include auditory comprehension and spoken language for students with visual impairments and additional disabilities who have eccentric language patterns requires a balance of structure and spontaneity (Olsen,

Miles, & Riggio, 1999). Adults need to embed listening skills and opportunities to understand and use spoken language within natural contexts and daily routines, as well as in structured lessons that refine specific skills and introduce new concepts.

Using Natural Routines

The following are strategies and suggestions that take advantage of natural contexts and daily routines to create opportunities to understand and use spoken language:

▸ Adults need to be mindful of the need to be models of listening behavior. Effective communication partners can ensure that the learning environment is rich in language. Adults tend to use directives and questions when speaking to students with visual impairments and additional disabilities (Bruce, Godbold, & Naponelli-Gold, 2004), limiting not only opportunities for students to hear and then express themselves using language but also students' perception of themselves as communication partners.

▸ When interacting with students who have eccentric language patterns but whose language use lacks meaning, adults need to use combinations of touch and sound to gain and maintain the students' attention. (Refer to assessment information to verify the quality and location of touch that the student will tolerate.) Often, a hand resting calmly on a student's shoulder is adequate tactile input to establish an interpersonal connection. Students may pause or stop moving and reach up to touch their hand to the adult's before responding to any spoken language or greeting.

▸ Adults need to paraphrase statements students make that include confusion with pronouns or echolalic yet intentional communication. For example, if a student uses echolalic language to communicate a desire, such as the earlier example of "Do you want to go to the swing?" an adult can rephrase it in a way that models appropriate language, adding repetition and description or comment to expand the exchange and offer alternative ways to communicate. One option might be "Let's go to the swing. I want to go to the swing."

▸ Adults need to pause and allow students time to process the auditory information and organize a response. Students may not reply, they may initially parrot their original phrase, they may behaviorally communicate their desire to continue by orienting toward the swing, for example, or they may repeat the last phrase said to them—which in this case reflects appropriate language use.

▶ Adults need to avoid ending exchanges with a question. For some students the last part of the string of auditory information may be the phrase that is remembered and repeated, continuing the cycle of confusion with pronouns and inadvertently building students' repertoire of echolalic expressions. For example, if the earlier example closed with "Do you like to swing?" that may be the phrase that resonates with students and the expression that they continue to parrot.

▶ Adults need to attach meaning to the exchange by attempting to respond with the action appropriate to the student's communication—in the previous example, going to the swings. Swinging may not in fact have been the student's intention, and therefore the amount of time spent swinging will be short because the student did not really want to swing. However, to convey that spoken language does have meaning and allow students to realize that their communication has power, completing the communication exchange with the appropriate action adds functionality and closure. If the student's comments are on the swing, together go to the swing.

▶ Adults need to be sensitive to the manner in which language is simplified when communicating with students who have visual impairments and additional disabilities or whose language patterns are eccentric. It is important to use vocabulary that the student understands and sentence structure that is meaningful (and possibly short), and to consider the pace of a communication exchange, but adults need to use intonation and a quality of voice that is natural. It is equally important to ensure that communication is respectful, conveying desire for interaction and an interest in the student's response (Crook & Miles, 1999).

▶ Many students with eccentric language patterns use vocabulary or repeat phrases and sentences that are remarkable for their sophistication, suggesting a level of comprehension that students may not possess. They may be drawing upon eccentric skills in auditory memory and are reciting information that they have heard but to which they lack an experiential connection. Adults can paraphrase the information, using simplified vocabulary and repetition within the exchange (as previously explained) to determine the extent to which students understand what they have said, while also modeling alternative ways to think and talk about that topic. In some situations, adults can follow up by considering ways to provide experience that can create a foundation or connection for that language. In other situations, directing the student's attention and conversation to the current experience—the activity at the moment and the individuals with whom the student is interacting at the moment— can anchor communication and listening opportunities.

▶ Many students need to handle a concrete object or tactile communication symbol to attach meaning to and process spoken language. It may be necessary for adults to carry duplicates of the communication objects or tactile symbols that might further communication during an activity in a particular environment. This was an effective means of anchoring spoken language for Hana, in the earlier vignette when she transitioned from one activity to the next. She chanted, "Check your schedule! Check your schedule!" but did not attach meaning to that language or respond with language that had intent until she handled the transition object that cued her to check her schedule.

Using Structured Situations

Structured lessons can target specific skills and introduce new concepts. The following are some structured instructional strategies and activities that are particularly adaptable for developing auditory comprehension and spoken language:

▶ Adults can structure opportunities for students to deliberately "eavesdrop" on an appropriate conversational routine between two adults. To ensure that students follow the conversation and understand who is speaking, they will need to be in close proximity to the speakers, and depending on their visual functioning and environmental awareness, may need tactile contact with the speakers. The exchange can be scripted and include language that might occur within naturally occurring conversational exchanges for the student, such as a greeting. With the appropriate combination of touch and language, the models of proper pronoun use can be provided, and with repetition, the student may internalize the script. Simple examples include greetings and farewells.

For a student who repeats the last thing said to her whenever there is a pause in the conversation, tending to repeat "Good-bye, Mykala" when someone says good-bye to her—two adults can script an exchange around good-byes. The teacher who is leaving might say, "It's time for me to leave now. Good-bye, Ms. Terry. Good-bye, Mykala." Ms. Terry responds, "Good-bye, Mr. Ortega," and touches the student's shoulder while pausing for the student to repeat this: "Good-bye, Mr. Ortega." Ms. Terry can continue by stating, "We said good-bye to Mr. Ortega. He is walking out of the classroom and will be back after lunch." The structured exchange models and cues the appropriate response for the student. Positioning the adults so that Ms. Terry is slightly behind the student, so that her reply to Mr. Ortega is in the same direction as the student's, lends additional support to the turn taking and appropriate response.

▸ With a small group of students, a teacher can establish a structured routine of sharing an object or sharing news. This structured routine limits the topic of conversation and provides an opportunity to facilitate conversational exchanges with a central focus (Diaz-Rico & Weed, 1995b). The teacher joins the news circle as a participant, modeling both listening behavior and use of language to ask questions or make comments to the person sharing his or her object or news. Establishing the routine may require two adults: one to facilitate the group conversation and one to model listening as a student needs to and asking questions as a student might.

▸ A teacher can establish a routine for reviewing students' daily schedule with them, expanding conversation around the events, building vocabulary and comprehension (Crook & Miles, 1999). The schedule may be prearranged for the student, and each item in the schedule can be previewed and discussed in turn. As a student internalizes this routine, it can be expanded to an empty schedule, with the icons, objects, pictures, or word cards for that day in a separate basket or set out on the table. An adult can talk about what will be happening first, not only the label or name of the activity, but also what the activity might entail and others who might be involved. The student can look for the appropriate item and place it in the first spot in the schedule. The entire schedule can be reviewed at the end of the process, with descriptions and comments repeated as ways to build vocabulary and use increasingly complex language connected to meaningful experiences in which the student will be engaged.

▸ Adults can encourage interactions between one student and another. Initially, the interaction will need to be simple, such as sending one student with a message to deliver to the other.

LISTENING SKILLS FOR RECREATION AND LEISURE

Recreation and leisure activities are an extremely important area of the expanded core curriculum for students who have visual impairments and additional disabilities. Because listening skills are required for meaningful participation in these activities, focus on listening within this area will greatly enhance the quality of students' lives (Hatlen, 1996; Sapp & Hatlen, 2010). Students with visual impairments may not understand options available to them for filling free time due to lack of visual experience. Also, students with visual impairments and additional disabilities often require adult facilitation to participate in activities, both at school and at home, and when that support is unavailable they have periods of time throughout the day that are not productively filled. They need to be exposed to a variety of recreation and leisure activities so they can develop preferences for filling free time at school and at home.

Many recreational and leisure activities from which students might choose draw upon listening skills and behaviors. Like activities in other curricular domains for students with visual impairments and additional disabilities, recreational skills involving listening need to be taught systematically and supported in natural contexts so students acquire meaningful skills. The activities and learning environment need to be structured and materials modified to reflect the sensory functioning of the student—the student's experience, learning characteristics, and environmental awareness.

Embedding listening skills within leisure activities not only ensures students' active engagement within the activity but also offers a springboard for acquiring listening skills in activities that are often highly motivating for students who have visual impairments, including those with additional disabilities. Refining listening skills and honing auditory-perceptual skills in leisure activities may offer a springboard to generalizing listening skills to other areas of the expanded core curriculum as well as to other aspects of the core educational curriculum.

Some recreational or leisure activities, such as aural reading or enjoying music, are independent pursuits. Others leisure activities that involve listening include group skills, such as learning to listen to others and taking turns during structured games. Each type of recreational and leisure activity offers opportunities for using listening skills in meaningful contexts as well as establishing a foundation for auditory attention, auditory memory, and higher-order listening skills, such as listening for detail. Examples of each type of leisure activity are considered here: listening independently to recorded stories or music and group activities involving music and turn taking.

Independent Recreational Listening: Aural Reading and Listening to Music

The following are emerging listening skills to teach or reinforce within activities targeting aural reading and listening to music:

> ▸ indicates awareness of sound by change of expression when music or a recorded story is turned on

- ▸ indicates awareness of sound by change of expression when music or a recorded story turns off
- ▸ demonstates auditory attention by listening to a recorded story or music without interrupting the activity
- ▸ after listening, retells personal experience or story read aurally (with words, icons, illustrations, etc.)

To ensure that independent leisure activities that draw upon listening skills are meaningful and that students with visual impairments and additional disabilities are actively engaged, both the materials selected and the instructional sequence need to be carefully considered for each student. Students with visual impairments and additional disabilities need to be involved in each step of the listening routine to conceptualize the activity and act rather than be acted upon. Without deliberation and attentiveness to the process of active learning, a student's experience risks becoming an isolated one, with sound that lacks relevance and meaning. Educators, parents and caregivers, and paraeducators and other service providers need to maintain a focus on students and their experience during an activity and ensure that recreation or leisure routines are independent pursuits that support attentive, pleasurable listening to meaningful auditory content.

Listening activities involving recorded stories or music need to be structured to include sound and touch in ways that allow students to understand the source of the sound and its location—that the reader or narrator they hear is not a live person sitting with them and while the music may be the same music they hear at home or in the car, the source differs. Students need to have the opportunity to participate in and conceptualize the entire activity. They need to handle and maintain contact with the player and speaker so they have access to any vibrotactile feedback and can appreciate that this mechanism is part of the listening experience.

Adults need to also be mindful of the extent to which the environment and location in the environment enhance students' understanding of not only where they are in space but what the expected activity is and what they might be expected to do. Recreational or leisure listening activities become more meaningful when offered in an area that is dedicated to that activity, where materials are stored in consistent locations, and where the physical space is organized for the student's access and comfort. Sidebar 7.6 offers specific suggestions and strategies for targeting listening skills using recorded stories and music.

Experience books and social stories, discussed in earlier sections of this chapter, offer options for independent reading of print books. Audible books offer opportunities for aural reading for purposeful listening and, with judicious consideration of the

Strategies for Targeting Listening Skills Using Recorded Stories and Music

Many students with visual impairments and additional disabilities will require playback devices with modifications ranging from marked "on/off" or "play" buttons to tools that can be handled and operated with a switch or minimal assistance. Digital media, such as MP3 files, may be more accessible if burned to a compact disc (CD) and accessed through the various devices in which they play. The follow strategies reflect use of a CD and CD player:

- Gain students' attention and use their preferred mode of communication to let them know they will be participating in a recreational or leisure listening activity. The icon in their schedule or the concrete object used to communicate this idea must reflect some aspect of the activity that the student experiences. If students typically handle the music player or remove the CD from the case, those items can serve as meaningful communication objects. If students depress the marked "play" button, a button removed from a nonworking player and marked the same way can be used.

- Allow students opportunities to select the story or music. Cases containing recordings can be identified by marking them with a distinct texture or with an object, depending on the content of the story. For example, a recording of the sounds of going to the car can be labeled with car keys (if the student has had the experience of handling car keys when going to the car; if not, then keys would not be meaningful, while a piece of a seat belt might be).

- Assist students in the process of opening the case, removing the CD, inserting it in the player, and pushing a marked "on" button. For students with physical impairments or low strength, a push-style button can be extended with something simple such as a Popsicle stick, creating a lever and reducing the energy needed to depress it.

- Students also need access to the sounds from the player without the confusion of competing background noise. Initially, recreational listening ought to be scheduled when the classroom is quiet.

- The recreational listening activity needs to be experienced with a familiar person mutually enjoying the listening activity to support its importance as a purposeful activity; the student and adult must be in close proximity, and if the student is resting a hand on the speaker of the player, the adult does so as well, to both model listening behavior and to communicate "I am listening too."

- As a student indicates pleasurable responses to recreational listening activities, the use of a pillow speaker can be introduced. The adult needs to make sure that the student still has contact with the player as well as the pillow speaker, to create a link between the running player and the sound source now closer to the student's ear level but farther away from the player.

- A headset can be substituted as the student indicates responsiveness to the pillow speaker; the headset can be rested in the same spot previously occupied by the pillow speaker.

- Introduce actual wearing of the headset gradually. This can be accomplished in various ways, depending on the sensory functioning of the student:
  ‣ The adult can model wearing the headset and invite the student to visually and tactilely inspect the headset as the adult puts it on.

> ▸ The adult can invite and assist the student to imitate the action so the adult and student each wear a headset. Some students may imitate the adult's actions after visually observing them. Other students with additional disabilities will require assistance to tactilely observe them before imitating them. The adult can provide touch cues, such as lightly resting hands on the student's ears, and verbal labels to indicate what will happen. Then, using hand-under-hand guidance, the adult invites the student to place his or her hands on the adult's and together put the headset on.
>
> ▸ It is important to make sure the volume on the headset is adjusted to a comfortable level before a student wears it.
>
> ▸ As the student behaviorally indicates that he or she is finished tolerating the headset, provide the appropriate communication cues, co-actively remove the headset, and place it at its former resting position until the story or tape is finished, allowing the recreation activity to continue to its natural conclusion, when the student turns the player off and puts the tape or CD away.
>
> ▸ Gradually increase the amount of time the student tolerates the headset by offering tactile input and mutual hand-to-hand interaction as both encouragement and distraction.
>
> ▸ Adult facilitation can be faded at any step in the sequence as students with visual impairments and additional disabilities integrate the process and become engaged in the recreation-leisure listening activity.

recorded material and systematic introduction to students with visual impairments and additional disabilities, can offer meaningful and pleasurable ways for students to occupy their leisure time. The content of the recorded material will vary depending on the extent to which a student requires concrete referents for the auditory information and language to be meaningful. Educators, parents, and caregivers need to consider the interests of students, as well as their experiences and connections to the environment and to people, when they are creating a library of audible books for a particular student.

The content of commercial recordings of stories is often not accessible for students with visual impairments and additional disabilities. The stories often refer to events that are highly visual in nature and familiar to the listening audience through incidental learning rather than real experience. For example, a story might be about farm animals that many students listening to the recording have seen only in picture books or on television, without having had an opportunity to see, hear, or touch them in real life. Nonetheless, they, as sighted students, have some understanding of what a cow or a chicken is because they have looked at pictures in other books or watched a TV program in which there were cows or chickens. As they listen to the recording, they have those images to draw upon and enhance their understanding of the story. For students with visual impairments and additional disabilities, who often lack the opportunity for such incidental learning and who have challenges conceptualizing sound, commercial recorded stories involve language that is unconnected to their experiences (such as the word "cow" or "chicken") and sound without meaning for them (a moo or a cluck). In addition, commercial audible books that contain simple language and whose length accommodates the attention span of many students with multiple disabilities are generally intended for younger children and do not reflect the chronological age of older students.

Creative homemade or teacher-made recordings of a student's personal experiences offer meaningful opportunities for recreational listening that can reinforce auditory memory and auditory attention skills and also offer exposure to higher-order listening skills such as listening for detail and sequence, as they draw upon the memory of that recorded experience. Auditory recordings of a student's participation in an activity are akin to a photo album—they provide the opportunity to recall and reexperience an event from the distance of time and place. Sidebar 7.7 provides suggestions for creating a library of recorded stories and music that will be meaningful to students.

Group Recreational Listening: Music and Taking Turns

The following are emerging listening skills to teach or reinforce in group recreational listening activities:

- ▶ listens for music and responds by standing when the music begins and sitting when the music ends
- ▶ follows directions to walk, reach, wave, clap, sway, and so forth during music activity
- ▶ orients to the speaker during a turn-taking game

Games that involve taking turns provide opportunities for shaping social awareness and the back-and-forth interaction inherent in listening and speaking. Music activities often provide a means of introducing turn-taking skills that can then be taught in other recreational or interactive contexts. Music activities and games are effective as tools for teaching listening skills and concepts for students with visual impairments and additional disabilities for many reasons (Bevans, 1992), among them:

- ▶ Music has an inherent structure, with repetition of words and melodies.
- ▶ Music activities invite self-expression.

Creating an Audible Book and Music Library to Support Listening Skills

The options for creating an audible library include both audible books—including auditory recordings of various types—and music. To avoid the possibility that a student's independent recreational activity extends beyond the student's attention span, use information gathered through assessment and ongoing evaluation to determine the length of a music tape or audible book/experience tape and ensure that the routine remains purposeful and meaningful.

The following are suggestions for types of recordings that students might enjoy:

STORIES

- An auditory recording of an activity the student with visual impairments and additional disabilities regularly enjoys narrated by a familiar support person who usually facilitates that activity. This might be the grooming routine in the morning, an art activity, going from the classroom to recess and then swinging, ending recess, and going back inside class. The narration should include words that are familiar to the student and pertinent to the activity being recorded, with a balance that provides sufficient description to build spoken vocabulary and add richness to the recording while not overriding other auditory aspects of the experience.

- A recording of a pleasurable event, such as fun Friday pizza at school or a birthday party, that has descriptive adult narration to ensure the content has meaning and is not just an unconnected sequence of sounds.

- An environmental recording or a soundscape recording of a regularly occurring event that the student experiences that has distinct sound effects, such as leaving the house or classroom and getting into a car. Such a recording could include the sound of jingling car keys, footsteps walking to the door, the door opening, footsteps walking through the doorway, the door closing, footsteps on the sidewalk, the car door opening, sounds of entering the car and snapping the seat belt, the sound of the door closing from the inside, the keys being inserted and turned, the engine starting, and the car driving.

- An auditory recording of a familiar person or family member and the student reading one of the student's experience books together.

- An auditory recording of students reading their own experience books.

- An auditory recording of a social story, as read by the student; social stories are in first person, so maintaining proper perspective is an important consideration.

MUSIC

- Recorded music that the student's family or typical peers enjoy, if a student is not yet expressing a preference for style of music.

- A recording of special music selections made for a particular student; in this case, leave several seconds of quiet between selections to offer contrast and ensure that the student does not habituate to the music—that is, to offer a break in the auditory background that will offer contrast and maintain the student's attention and interest. Constant music, constant sound, conversely, can become background and discourage active listening.

▸ Music activities are not threatening to students who may have struggled and experienced failure in other educational areas.

▸ Music provides a common frame of reference or topic for students with visual impairments and additional disabilities and many individuals with whom they may interact.

Music activities can be modified to reflect the chronological ages of students by the music selections chosen and by structuring the listening activity so it is dependent on taking turns. These listening activities can be as simple as moving and dancing when music begins and stopping when it ceases, or as complex and sophisticated as comparing pitch or identifying instruments or the artist. Within music activities, students can learn the use of voice for whispering words, speaking words, or singing words as well as repeating chants that encourage spoken language. Students can listen for and match the beat, or add their own creative movement and movement interpretation to the tone or language of the song. Students can be cued to listen for specific words or word phrases in chants of songs, or participate in adapted versions of "Name that Tune." Such games offer social interaction, listening to others, and taking turns and reinforce listening skills that include auditory memory, auditory discrimination, and language usage. Activities such as these that draw upon recreational music can be used to introduce higher-order listening skills of word associations and listening for detail in pleasurable learning and listening experiences.

It is often necessary to introduce activities individually to students with visual impairments and additional disabilities or with one other student before they can participate in the activity in a situation that involves taking turns. The visual props and cues that support social awareness and a sense of connection to others in a group—including facing the speaker to indicate attention or turning toward or gesturing to someone to indicate that it is their turn next to speak—are frequently not available to students with visual impairments and additional disabilities. Such skills and social behaviors as attending to another speaker while waiting for a turn is a skill that needs to be taught within meaningful routines and with concrete supports.

Introducing the social art of taking turns can begin with a group of two students and a concrete object that is passed from one student to the other when it is the next student's turn to speak or take part in a listening activity. The student holding the item is the one who responds, sings, performs, or shares a comment, while the other student listens and waits for his or her turn in whatever listening game they are playing. They are sharing a single topic, the game, and the activity therefore lends itself to facilitated review and discussion at the game's conclusion, drawing upon auditory memory, spoken vocabulary, and staying on topic for a certain number of exchanges. The music activity can then be expanded to include a group of three students. Over time, the concrete object signifying the person whose turn it is to speak or perform can be faded as students with visual impairments and additional disabilities gain the listening skills and social awareness to maintain attention to others and wait for their turn through listening alone.

Structuring listening activities using recreational music provides a social context for listening to music, which often serves as a passive listening activity or filler during free time for many students with visual impairments and additional disabilities. Music may represent a preference, or it may, by default, be the only option for filling free time with which students with disabilities are familiar. These students sometimes idiosyncratically offer statements about music unconnected to the topic of conversation going on around them, reflecting two areas of need for students with visual impairments and additional disabilities: broader exposure to recreational activities and the skills to initiate a conversation about areas of interest and engage in a back-and-forth discussion with someone else. Structured activities that involve social listening, turn taking, and recreational music may enrich conversational opportunities for students with disabilities who otherwise have fewer personal interests and experiences to share.

As noted at the beginning of this section, students who have visual impairments and additonal disabilities often require adult facilitation to participate in activities, both at school and at home, and when that support is unavailable they have periods of time throughout the day that are not productively filled. Recreational skills involving listening must be systematically taught and supported in natural contexts so students acquire meaningful skills. This section of the chapter offered strategies for structuring activities and the environment as well as modifying materials to reflect the student's preferences and experience to ensure that the student is actively engaged, building active listening skills with recreational activities that include music and recorded stories.

CONCLUSION

Because of the complex ways in which learning can be affected when students have a visual impairment and additional disabilities, this chapter began with a consideration of various types of additional disabilities that may affect students with visual impairments, their learning characteristics, and needed supports, and then discussed strategies for teaching listening skills to each.

It falls to educators, caregivers and parents, and paraeducators and other service providers to design and offer meaningful learning experiences for students with visual impairments and additional disabilities that foster the development of listening skills as signals to change, inspiration for movement and discovery, and nourishment for spoken language and understanding. In general, instructional strategies for supporting listening skills have at their foundation the following:

▸ The value of contingency learning, in which continuation of an activity depends on the student's response or behavior, ensures that students with visual impairments and additional disabilities are engaged and have opportunities to act, rather than to be acted upon.

▸ For students with visual and additional disabilities who have emerging connections with people and with the environment, sound may not have sufficient relevance or meaning on its own. Activities to teach the awareness of sound require judicious pairing of sound and touch.

▸ Activities that emphasize meaningful engagement and interaction with other people are central to the development of listening skills.

▸ Activities need to be individualized to accommodate and respect the unique interplay of visual impairment and additional disabilities of each student.

▸ Listening skills cannot be separated into isolated categories but need to be embedded within natural routines so that they are both functional and relevant to students.

▸ Supporting listening skills for students with visual and additional disabilities requires the partnership of educators, parents and caregivers, and paraeducators and other service providers.

REFERENCES

Aarnoutse, C. A. J., van den Bos, K. P., & Brand-Gruwel, S. (1998). Effects of listening comprehension training on listening and reading. *Journal of Special Education 32*(2), 115.

American Speech-Language Hearing Association. (2005). *Acoustics in educational settings: Technical report.* Retrieved August 13, 2007, from www.asha.org/docs/html/TR2005-00042 .html.

Anthony, T. L. (2004). Individual sensory learning profile interview. In I. Topor, L. P. Rosenblum, & D. D. Hatton, *Visual conditions and functional vision: Early intervention issues.* Session 4: Functional Vision Assessment and Developmentally Appropriate Learning Media Assessment, Handout K. Chapel Hill: Early Intervention Training Center for Infants and Toddlers with Visual Impairments, FPG Child Development Institute, University of North Carolina at Chapel Hill.

Anthony, T., & Lowry, S. S. (2004). Sensory development. In T. Anthony, S. S. Lowry, C. Brown, & D. Hatton (Eds.), *Developmentally appropriate orientation and mobility* (pp. 125–240). Chapel Hill: Early Intervention Training Center for Infants and Toddlers with Visual Impairments, FPG Child Development Institute, University of North Carolina at Chapel Hill.

Bevans, J. (1992). Developmental music. In C. Cushman, K. Heydt, S. Edwards, M. J. Clark, & M. Allon. *Perkins activity and resource guide,* Vol. 2 (pp. 11.4–11.85). Watertown, MA: Perkins School for the Blind.

Blaha, R. (2001). Daily calendars. In R. Blaha, *Calendars for students with multiple impairments including deafblindness* (pp. 53–82). Austin: Texas School for the Blind and Visually Impaired.

Blaha, R., & Moss, K. (Winter 1997). Let me check my calendar. *See/Hear*. Retrieved from www.tsbvi.edu/seehear/archive/Let%20Me%20Check%20My%20Calendar.htm.

Brown, C., Anthony, T. L., Lowry, S. S., & Hatton D. D. (2004). Session 4: Motor development and movement. In T. L. Anthony, S. S. Lowry, C. Brown, & D. Hatton, *Developmentally appropriate orientation and mobility* (pp. 347–462). Chapel Hill: Early Intervention Training Center for Infants and Toddlers with Visual Impairments, University of North Carolina at Chapel Hill.

Brown, D. (2001). Follow the child—Approaches to assessing the functional vision and hearing of young children with congenital deaf-blindness. *reSources, 10*(9), 1–3.

Bruce, S. (2005). The application of Werner and Kaplan's concept of "distancing" to children who are deaf-blind. *Journal of Visual Impairment & Blindness, 99*(8), 464–477.

Bruce, S., Godbold, E., & Naponelli-Gold, S. (2004). An analysis of communicative functions of teachers and their students who are deafblind. *Re:view, 36*(2), 81–90.

Cass, H. (1998). Visual impairment and autism. *Autism, 2*(2), 117–138.

Chen, D. (1995). Understanding and developing communication. In D. Chen & J. Dote-Kwan (Eds.), *Starting points: Instructional practices for young children whose multiple disabilities include visual impairment* (pp. 57–72). Los Angeles: Blind Children's Center.

Chen, D. (1999). Interactions between infants and caregivers: The context for early intervention. In D. Chen (Ed.), *Essential elements in early intervention: Visual impairment and multiple disabilities* (pp. 22–53). New York: AFB Press.

Crook, C., & Miles, B. (1999). Developing basic language forms. In B. Miles & M. Riggio (Eds.), *Remarkable conversations: A guide to developing meaningful communication with children and young adults who are deafblind* (pp. 180–213). Watertown, MA: Perkins School for the Blind.

Crook, C., Miles, B., & Riggio, M. (1999a). Assessment of communication. In B. Miles & M. Riggio (Eds.), *Remarkable conversations: A guide to developing meaningful communication with children and young adults who are deafblind* (pp. 94–123). Watertown, MA: Perkins School for the Blind.

Crook, C., Miles, B., & Riggio, M. (1999b). Developing early communication and language. In B. Miles & M. Riggio (Eds.), *Remarkable conversations: A guide to developing meaningful communication with children and young adults who are deafblind* (pp. 146–179). Watertown, MA: Perkins School for the Blind.

Crozier, S., & Sileo, N. (2003). Encouraging positive behavior with social stories: An intervention for students with autism spectrum disorders. *Teaching Exceptional Children, 35*(3), 26–31.

Cushman, C. (1992). Teaching children with multiple disabilities: An overview. In C. Cushman, K. Heydt, S. Edwards, M. J. Clark, & M. Allon. *Perkins activity and resource guide,* Vol. 1 (pp. 1.2–1.15). Watertown, MA: Perkins School for the Blind.

Diaz-Rico, L., & Weed, K. (1995a). Content area instruction. In L. Diaz-Rico & K. Weed, *The crosscultural, language, and academic development handbook: A complete K–12 reference guide* (pp. 114–143). Boston: Allyn and Bacon.

Diaz-Rico, L., & Weed, K. (1995b). English language development. In L. Diaz-Rico & K. Weed, *The crosscultural, language, and academic development handbook: A complete K–12 reference guide* (pp. 71–113). Boston: Allyn and Bacon.

Dote-Kwan, J. (1995). Instructional strategies. In D. Chen & J. Dote-Kwan (Eds.), *Starting points: Instructional practices for young children whose multiple disabilities include visual impairment* (pp. 43–56). Los Angeles: Blind Children's Center.

Dote-Kwan, J., Chen, D., & Hughes, M. (2001). A national survey of service providers who work with young children with visual impairments. *Journal of Visual Impairment & Blindness, 95*, 325–337.

Downing, J., & Chen, D. (2003). Using tactile strategies with students who are blind and have severe disabilities. *Teaching Exceptional Children, 36*(2), 56–61.

Downing, J. E., & Demchak, M. (1996). First steps: Determining individual abilities and how to support students. In J. E. Downing (Ed.), *Including students with severe and multiple disabilities in typical classrooms* (pp. 35–61). Baltimore: Paul H. Brookes.

Downing, J., & Eichinger, J. (1996). Educating students with diverse strengths and needs together: Rationale and assumptions. In J. E. Downing (Ed.), *Including students with severe and multiple disabilities in typical classrooms* (pp. 1–14). Baltimore: Paul H. Brookes.

Dunn, W. (1996). The sensorimotor systems: A framework for assessment and intervention. In F. Orelove & D. Sobsey (Eds.), *Educating children with multiple disabilities: A transdisciplinary approach* (3rd ed.) (pp. 35–78). Baltimore: Paul H. Brookes.

Erickson, K. A., & Hatton, D. (2007). Expanding understanding of emergent literacy: Empirical support for a new framework. *Journal of Visual Impairment & Blindness, 101*(5), 261–277.

Erin, J. (2000). Students with visual impairments and additional disabilities. In A. Koenig & M. C. Holbrook (Eds.), *Foundations of education* (2nd ed.), Vol. 2: *Instructional strategies for teaching children and youths with visual impairments* (pp. 720–748). New York: AFB Press.

Fazzi, D., & Klein, M. D. (2002). Cognitive focus: Developing cognition, concepts, and language. In R. L. Pogrund & D. Fazzi (Eds.), *Early focus: Working with young children who are blind or visually impaired and their families* (2nd ed.) (pp. 107–152). New York: AFB Press.

Ferrell, K. A., with Shaw, A. R., & Dietz, S. J. (1998). *Project PRISM: A longitudinal study of developmental patterns of children who are visually impaired.* Greeley: University of Northern Colorado.

Gense, M. H., & Gense, D. J. (2005a). Autism spectrum disorders: An introduction. In M. H. Gense and D. J. Gense, *Autism spectrum disorders and visual impairment* (pp. 15–24). New York: AFB Press.

Gense, M. H., & Gense, D. J. (2005b). Challenging behaviors. In M. H. Gense and D. J. Gense, *Autism spectrum disorders and visual impairment* (pp. 175–190). New York: AFB Press.

Gense, M. H., & Gense, D. J. (2005c). Program planning and core instructional principles. In M. H. Gense and D. J. Gense, *Autism spectrum disorders and visual impairment* (pp. 47–75). New York: AFB Press.

Harley, R., Truan, M., & Sanford, L. (1997). Developing listening skills. In R. Harley, M. Truan, & L. Sanford (Eds.), *Communication skills for visually impaired learners: Braille, print, and listening skills for students who are visually impaired* (2nd ed.) (pp. 217–233). Springfield, IL: Charles C Thomas.

Hatlen, P. (1996). The core curriculum for blind and visually impaired students, including those with additional disabilities. *Re:view, 28*(1), 25–32.

Hatton, D. D. (2001). Model registry of early childhood visual impairment: First-year results. *Journal of Visual Impairment & Blindness, 95,* 418–433.

Heller, K. W., Alberto, P. A., Forney, P., & Schwartzman, M. N. (1996a). Introduction to physical and health impairments and members of the educational team. In K. W. Heller, P. A. Alberto, P. Forney, & M. N. Schwartzman, *Understanding physical, sensory, and health impairments* (pp. 3–11). Pacific Grove, CA: Brookes/Cole.

Heller, K. W., Alberto, P. A., Forney, P., & Schwartzman, M. N. (1996b). Learning and behavioral characteristics. In K. W. Heller, P. A. Alberto, P. Forney, & M. N. Schwartzman, *Understanding physical, sensory, and health impairments* (pp. 35–42). Pacific Grove, CA: Brookes/Cole.

Heller, K. W., Alberto, P. A., Forney, P., & Schwartzman, M. N. (1996c). Multiple disabilities. In K. W. Heller, P. A. Alberto, P. Forney, & M. N. Schwartzman, *Understanding physical, sensory, and health impairments* (pp. 351–369). Pacific Grove, CA: Brookes/Cole.

Jalongo, M. R. (1995). Promoting active listening in the classroom. *Childhood education, 72*(1), 13–18.

Jamieson, S. (2004). Creating an educational program for young children who are blind and who have autism. *Re:view, 35*(4), 165–177.

Jan, J. E., Groenveld, M., Sykanda, A. M., & Hoyt, C. S. (2006). Behavioral characteristics of children with permanent cortical visual impairment. In E. Dennison & A. H. Lueck (Eds.), *Proceedings of the summit on cerebral/cortical visual impairment: Educational, family, and medical perspectives, April 30, 2005* (pp. 51–59). New York: AFB Press.

Lawson, G. D., & Wiener, W. R. (2010). Audition for students with vision loss. In W. R. Weiner, R. L. Welsh, & B. B. Blasch (Eds.), *Foundations of orientation and mobility* (3rd ed.), Vol. 1, *History and Theory* (pp. 84–137). New York: AFB Press.

Lewis, S., & Tolla, J. (2003). Creating and using tactile experience books for young children with visual impairments. *Teaching Exceptional Children, 35*(3), 22–28.

Liefert, F. (2003). Appendix A: Common causes of vision loss in children and implications for assessment. In S. Goodman & S. Wittenstein (Eds.), *Collaborative assessment: Working with students who are blind or visually impaired, including those with additional disabilities* (pp. 353–374). New York: AFB Press.

Lueck, A. H. (2010). Cortical or cerebral visual impairment in children: A brief overview. *Journal of Visual Impairment & Blindness, 104,* 585–592.

Mar, H., & Cohen, E. (1998). Educating students who have visual impairments and who exhibit emotional and behavioral problems. In S. Sacks & R. Silberman (Eds.), *Educating students who have visual impairments with other disabilities* (pp. 263–302). Baltimore: Paul H. Brookes.

McHugh, E., & Lieberman, L. (2003). The impact of developmental factors on incidence of stereotypic rocking among children with visual impairments. *Journal of Visual Impairment & Blindness, 97*(8), 453–474.

Miles, B. (1999). Conversation: The essence of communication. In B. Miles & M. Riggio (Eds.), *Remarkable conversations: A guide to developing meaningful communication with children and young adults who are deafblind* (pp. 54–75). Watertown, MA: Perkins School for the Blind.

Miles, B., & McLetchie, B. (February 2008). Developing concepts with children who are deaf-blind. In *The national consortium on deaf-blindness* (pp. 1–8). NCDB. Monmouth, OR: Retrieved August 14, 2011, from www.nationaldb.org/documents/products /concepts.pdf.

Nelson, P. B., Soli, S. D., & Seltz, A. (2002). *Classroom acoustics II: Acoustical barriers to learning.* Melville, NY: Acoustical Society of America.

Nielsen, L. (1992). Educational and psychological statements concerning the usage of the "little room." In L. Nielsen, *Space and self* (pp. 53–62). Copenhagen: SIKON.

Northern, J., & Downs, M. (2002). Auditory development and early intervention. In J. Northern & M. Downs, *Hearing in children* (5th ed.) (pp. 126–157). Philadelphia: Lippincott Williams & Wilkins.

Olsen, K., Miles, B., & Riggio, M. (1999). Environments that encourage communication. In B. Miles and M. Riggio (Eds.), *Remarkable conversations: A guide to developing meaningful communication with children and young adults who are deafblind* (pp. 76–93). Watertown, MA: Perkins School for the Blind.

Orelove, F., & Malatchi, A. (1996). Curriculum and instruction. In F. Orelove & D. Sobsey (Eds.), *Educating children with multiple disabilities: A transdisciplinary approach* (3rd ed.) (pp. 377–409). Baltimore: Paul H. Brookes.

Orelove, F., & Sobsey, D. (1996). Communication skills. In F. Orelove & D. Sobsey (Eds.), *Educating children with multiple disabilities: A transdisciplinary approach* (3rd ed.) (pp. 253–299). Baltimore: Paul H. Brookes.

Palisano, R. (1992). Assistive positioning as a control parameter of social-communicative interactions between students with profound multiple disabilities and classroom staff. *Physical Therapy,* September 1.

Perfect, M. (2001). Examining communicative behaviors in a 3-year-old boy who is blind. *Journal of Visual Impairment & Blindness, 95*(6).

Roman-Lantzy, C. (2007a). Medical and other causes of cortical visual impairment. In C. Roman-Lantzy, *Cortical visual impairment: An approach to assessment and intervention* (pp. 11–19). New York: AFB Press.

Roman-Lantzy, C. (2007b). Program planning and intervention. In C. Roman-Lantzy, *Cortical visual impairment: An approach to assessment and intervention* (pp. 113–151). New York: AFB Press.

Rosen, S. (1998a). Educating students who have visual impairments with neurological disabilities. In S. Sacks & R. Silberman (Eds.), *Educating students who have visual impairments and other disabilities* (pp. 221–262). Baltimore: Paul H. Brookes.

Rosen, S. (1998b). Educating students who have visual impairments with orthopedic disabilities or health impairments. In S. Sacks & R. Silberman (Eds.), *Educating students who have visual impairments and other disabilities* (pp. 187–220). Baltimore: Paul H. Brookes.

Rowland, C. (1983). Patterns of interaction between three blind infants and their mothers. In A. Mills (Ed.), *Language acquisition and the blind child: Normal and deficient* (pp. 114–132). San Diego, CA: College-Hill Press.

Sacks, S. (1998). Educating students who have visual impairments with other disabilities: An overview. In S. Sacks & R. Silberman (Eds.), *Educating students who have visual impairments with other disabilities* (pp. 3–38). Baltimore, MD: Paul H. Brookes.

Sapp, W., & Hatlen, P. (2010). The expanded core curriculum: Where have we been, where are we going, and how we get there. *Journal of Visual Impairment & Blindness, 104,* 338–348.

Silberman, R., Sacks, S., & Wolfe, J. (1998). Instructional strategies for educating students who have visual impairments with severe disabilities. In S. Sacks & R. Silberman (Eds.), *Educating students who have visual impairments with other disabilities* (pp. 101–138). Baltimore, MD: Paul H. Brookes.

Silver, M. (2003). Speech and language assessment. In S. Goodman & S. Wittenstein (Eds.), *Collaborative assessment: Working with students who are blind or visually impaired, including those with additional disabilities* (pp. 196–236). New York: AFB Press.

SKI-HI Institute. (1989). Communication program. In S. Watkins (Ed.), *The INSITE model: A model of home intervention for infant, toddler, and preschool aged multihandicapped sensory impaired children,* Vol. 1 (pp. 117–298). Hyrum, UT: HOPE, Inc.

Smith, M. (2010). *Dens.* Retrieved on November 12, 2010, from www.tsbvi.edu/component /content/article/64-mivi-general/1732-d.

Smith, M., & Levak, N. (1996a). Biobehavioral state management for students with profound impairments. In M. Smith & N. Levak, *Teaching students with visual and multiple impairments: A resource guide* (2nd ed.) (pp. 251–265). Austin: Texas School for the Blind and Visually Impaired.

Smith, M., & Levak, N. (1996b). Students with deafblindness and multiple impairments. In M. Smith & N. Levak, *Teaching students with visual and multiple impairments: A resource guide* (2nd ed.) (pp. 299–351). Austin: Texas School for the Blind and Visually Impaired.

United States Access Board. (2007). *Implementing classroom acoustic standards: A progress report.* Retrieved on August 18, 2007, from http://tna.europarchive.org/20081201235917 /access-board.gov/acoustic/.

van Dijk, J. (1991). Education strategies. In J. van Dijk, *Persons handicapped by rubella: Victors and victims: A follow-up study* (pp. 127–162). Amsterdam: Swets and Zeitlinger.

Warren, D. H. (1984). Language development. In D. H. Warren, *Blindness and early childhood development* (2nd ed.) (pp. 195–224). New York: American Foundation for the Blind.

Warren, D. H. (1994). Language, concept formation, and classification. In D. H. Warren, *Blindness and children: An individual differences approach* (pp. 134–154). Cambridge: Cambridge University Press.

((Appendix 7A
Listening Skills Embedded into Alternative Functional Goals That Align with a Standards-Based Core Curriculum

The following tables show how listening skills and behaviors can be embedded into alternative functional goals for students with moderate and severe disabilities that align with a standards-based core curriculum in English language arts (ELA) and the additional curricular areas of performing arts (dance) and health. Each of these areas of core curriculum contains standards that draw upon and enhance the development of listening skills for all students. Like the charts in the Listening Skills Continuum in Appendix A at the end of this book, this listing of skills does not represent a prescribed scope or sequence of either listening skills or functional skills but is a tool for attaching functionality to listening skills. It is intended to assist readers in the development of educational programming for students with visual impairments and additional disabilities. IEP goals follow the table as examples illustrating the implementation of the contents of the table for each of the students in the vignettes in Chapter 7, as well as those that follow Chapter 8.

ENGLISH LANGUAGE ARTS CONTENT STANDARDS

I. Listening

TRADITIONAL ELA STANDARD: UNDERSTANDS AND FOLLOWS ONE- AND TWO-STEP ORAL DIRECTIONS

Alternative Standard: Indicates awareness of an environmental sound source . . .

Functional behaviors	by quieting or stilling when his or her name is called
	by a change of facial expression when music is played
	by a change of facial expression when music is turned off
	by repeating his or her own movement or action that creates the sound

Alternative Standard: Localizes environmental sound source and demonstrates auditory discrimination and differentiation . . .

Functional behaviors	by orienting in the direction of the speaker
	by orienting toward the speaker when his or her name is called

Alternative Standard: Demonstrates auditory attention and auditory memory and possesses receptive vocabulary to follow simple directions . . .

Functional behaviors	by imitating or repeating an action of a communication partner that creates sound in a resonance or turn-taking activity
	by listening for music and responding by standing or sitting when the music begins or ends
	by following a one-step direction given directly to him or her
	by following a one-step direction given to a group

Alternative Standard: Demonstrates auditory attention and auditory discrimination and possesses receptive vocabulary to perform an action to comply with one- and two-step directions . . .

Functional behaviors	by raising a hand when his or her name is called
	by activating a switch when a specific auditory cue is given

TRADITIONAL ELA STANDARD: LISTENS ATTENTIVELY

Alternative Standard: Indicates awareness of environmental sound; attaches meaning to sound; and demonstrates auditory attention, discrimination, and differentiation . . .

Functional behaviors	by stopping an activity
	by repeating an action that creates sound
	by going to the source of a voice or to a communication partner
	by identifying neighborhood sounds while on a "listening walk"

Alternative Standard: Indicates auditory attention and discrimination and responds to voice . . .

Functional behaviors	by attending to the speaker
	by waiting for a break in the conversation without interrupting
	by listening to a story without interrupting

II. Speaking Applications

TRADITIONAL ELA STANDARD: STAYS ON TOPIC WHEN SPEAKING

Alternative Standard: Demonstrates auditory attention, language usage, and responsiveness to a speaker . . .

Functional behaviors	by answering a question, such as "What is your name?" when asked
	by giving a yes or no response to a question
	by offering a greeting in response to a greeting from someone else

Alternative Standard: Demonstrates auditory attention, responsiveness to speaker, language usage, and turn taking in a conversation with another person . . .

Functional behaviors	by engaging in conversation with a familiar adult, remaining on topic for two conversational exchanges
	by correctly responding to questions posed by a teacher during a small-group activity
	by communicating a personal choice during structured activities
	by confirming a communication partner's response (such as a customer's order, a next activity) in a structured routine

TRADITION ELA STANDARD: RECOUNTS EXPERIENCES IN A LOGICAL SEQUENCE

Alternative Standard: Demonstrates auditory attention and memory and language usage to identify the next event in a sequence . . .

Functional behaviors	by indicating the correct schedule item when asked "What comes next?" at transitions between activities

Alternative Standard: Demonstrates auditory attention and language usage to respond to questions about experiences . . .

Functional behaviors	by providing an accurate response (object, icon, word) to a question or in a conversation about daily activities
	by sharing information about an event with family members, using a communication book, drawings, and writing as communication supports
	by sharing information about a field trip using a communication book, drawings, and writing as communication supports, when asked

III. Reading/Word Analysis

TRADITIONAL ELA CONTENT STANDARD: MATCHES ALL CONSONANT AND SHORT VOWEL SOUNDS TO APPROPRIATE LETTERS

Alternative Standard: Attaches meaning to and discriminates sounds and associates sound with an object . . .

Functional behaviors	by orienting to the sound of a door closing or a telephone ringing
	by picking up or giving a named familiar communication object or icon
	by categorizing environmental sounds (for example, indoors, outdoors, cafeteria)
	by categorizing types of music (such as an instrument by its sound, a radio station, bells that signal passing periods)
	by identifying sounds of lawn equipment or household equipment or the playground

Alternative Standard: Sequences sound and communicates the sound of letters . . .

Functional behaviors	by singing a phonics song
	by choosing an object that matches its initial letter

IV. Sight-Word Reading

TRADITIONAL ELA STANDARD: MATCHES ORAL WORDS TO PRINTED WORDS

Alternative Standard: Demonstrates understanding of spoken vocabulary, listening for details to identify a written name or word when expressed by another . . .

Functional behaviors	by finding his or her own labeled desk (by written name, icon, textured symbol, or the like) upon staff request
	by identifying the written name (icon, textured symbol, or the like) of a classmate when specified by staff
	by identifying daily activities or a schedule when expressed by another
	by pointing to a named icon on his or her schedule

V. Reading Comprehension

TRADITIONAL ELA STANDARD: ASKS AND ANSWERS QUESTIONS ABOUT ESSENTIAL ELEMENTS OF A TEXT

Alternative Standard: Demonstrates auditory memory, listening for details to respond to simple questions about a text after listening to a short passage . . .

Functional behaviors	by selecting the correct answer from a field of three
	by answering simple yes or no questions

Alternative Standard: Demonstrates auditory memory and listening for details and sequence to recall events with a beginning, a middle, and an end after listening to a story . . .

Functional behaviors	by retelling a personal experience in sequential order
	by retelling a story read aloud in the correct sequence

TRADITIONAL ELA STANDARD: IDENTIFIES THE MAIN EVENTS OF THE PLOT, THEIR CAUSES, AND THE INFLUENCE ON FUTURE EVENTS

Alternative Standard: Demonstrates auditory attention, listening for sequence and word meaning to sequence a story line after listening to a short passage . . .

Functional behaviors	by retelling the story read (with words, icons, illustrations, and so forth)
	by retelling the events of the school day using a communication book

Alternative Standard: Demonstrates auditory attention, listening for comprehension to tell what comes next after given short story or social situation . . .

Functional behaviors	by predicting the outcome
	by predicting the end result when participating in the development of a social story

DANCE

Alternative Standard: Demonstrates auditory attending and memory performing simple movements in artistic perception in response to oral instructions . . .

Functional behaviors	by imitating or repeating an action of an adult that creates sound in a resonance or turn-taking activity
	by following directions to walk, reach, wave, clap, sway, and the like during a music activity

Alternative Standard: Responds spontaneously to different types of music, rhythms, and sounds during creative expression . . .

Functional behaviors	by adding original movement to songs, music, or poems

HEALTH CONTENT STANDARDS
Interpersonal Relationships

Alternative Standard: Demonstrates auditory localization during leisure activity to establish a positive relationship . . .

Functional behaviors	by orienting toward the speaker or communication partner
	by moving toward the speaker (using an ambulatory device such as a wheelchair, as needed)
	by orienting toward the speaker while making a request

Alternative Standard: Demonstrates auditory localization, auditory discrimination, and differentiation during leisure activities with peers . . .

Functional behaviors	by imitating or repeating an action of a communication partner that creates sound in a resonance or turn-taking activity
	by orienting to the speaker during a turn-taking game
	by orienting to a speaker calling his or her name

Alternative Standard: Demonstrates listening for meaning and language usage, and turn taking during guided conflict resolution with a peer . . .

Functional behaviors	by using an "I" message during a conflict
	by sharing an item with someone else

Sources: California County Superintendents Educational Services Association and Special Education Administrators of County Offices, *Curriculum Guide for Students with Moderate to Severe Disabilities* (Lakeshore Learning Materials, 2005); R. Swallow & A. Connor, "Aural Reading," in S. Mangold (Ed.), *A Teacher's Guide to the Special Educational Needs of Blind and Visually Handicapped Children*, pp. 119–135 (New York: American Foundation for the Blind, 1982); and R. K. Harley, M. B. Truan, & L. D. Sanford, "Developing Listening Skills" in *Communication Skills for Visually Impaired Learners: Braille, Print and Listening Skills for Students Who Are Visually Impaired*, 2nd ed., pp. 217–233 (Springfield, IL: Charles C Thomas, 1997).

SAMPLE ALTERNATIVE FUNCTIONAL IEP GOALS THAT EMBED LISTENING SKILLS

The following are examples of IEP goals created for the students presented in the vignettes in this chapter. Listening skills and behaviors are embedded in these alternative functional goals for students with moderate and severe disabilities that align with the standards-based core curriculum, showing how these students might apply the listening skills in question.

The particular alternative standard selected for each student was chosen based on assessment and ongoing evaluation information and individualized to reflect the student's sensory functioning and contexts that are meaningful to him or her. Note that IEP goals contain the following required components: the name of the student, measurable behavior, conditions or setting, mastery, level of criteria, a reporting date, and how it will be measured.

Sample Goal That Embeds Listening in the Area of Listening: Auditory Awareness

This is a projected goal in which listening skills are embedded for Yi, the student whose additional disabilities include physical impairment. The particular alternative standard selected for Yi was chosen based on assessment and ongoing evaluation information, and individualized to reflect her sensory functioning and contexts that are meaningful to her.

> By _____, during a play activity involving facilitation by a familiar adult, Yi will demonstrate auditory localization by first stilling and then orienting toward the adult with body movement when the adult calls her name within a communication bubble* of about 2 feet, in 4 of 5 interactions during 8 of 10 trial days, as measured by charting and teacher records.

Sample Goal That Embeds Listening in the Area of English/Language Arts, Reading/Word Analysis: Attaches Meaning to and Discriminates Sounds

The following is a projected goal in which listening skills are embedded for Micah, the student whose additional disabilities include health impairment and cortical abnormalities:

---

* One of the strategies for establishing meaningful listening environments for students who are deaf-blind involves identifying a student's "communication bubble" (Griffin, Davis, & Williams, 2004, p. 153), the area within the student's field of vision and hearing range in which a student can get information from the environment or communicate with someone else. See Chapter 8.

By _____, Micah will associate sound with objects and will discriminate sounds by picking up the named familiar communication object or icon and repeating its label when he is presented with a communication icon (photo or object) simultaneously labeled by the adult as a cue to his destination or next activity and offered at least 5 seconds to process the information and respond, in 4 of 5 interactions during 8 of 10 trial days, as measured by charting and teacher records.

Sample Goal That Embeds Listening in the Area of English/Language Arts, Listening: Understands and Follows One- and Two-Step Commands

The following is a projected goal in which listening skills are embedded for Hana, the student whose additional disabilities include challenging behavior:

By _____, when in a small group of no more than 3 students (2 others besides Hana) in a familiar structured activity and when the teacher has the group's attention but is not specifically speaking to any one student or using any student's name, Hana will demonstrate auditory attention, auditory memory, and receptive vocabulary by following a simple one-step direction given to the small group in 4 of 5 interactions during 8 of 10 trial days, as measured by charting and teacher records.

Sample Goal That Embeds Listening in the Area of English/Language Arts, Speaking Applications: Recounts Experiences in a Logical Sequence

The following is a projected goal in which listening skills are embedded for Eli, the student whose additional disabilities include deaf-blindness, who is described further in Chapter 8:

By _____, when wearing his hearing aids and asked "What comes next?" at transitions between activities by familiar adult standing at his personal schedule with him, Eli will demonstrate auditory memory and language usage to identify the next event in a sequence by indicating the correct schedule item, by saying the name of the activity while pointing to it or picking it up, 4 of 5 interactions during 8 of 10 trial days, as measured by charting and teacher records.

Chapter 8

Students with Hearing Impairments: Making the Most of Listening

Sandra Staples

To know a child's etiology is not to say you know the child. Every child is unique, and many etiologies present skills and levels of disability across a broad spectrum.

—M. Belote, *Fact Sheet: Points to Consider about Etiologies*, n.d.

CHAPTER PREVIEW

- ▸ Listening and Hearing Impairment
- ▸ Students with Visual Impairment and Hearing Loss
- ▸ Addressing the Basics
- ▸ Hearing and Amplification
- ▸ Unique Considerations for Students Who Are Deaf-Blind
- ▸ Supporting Amplification

The potential impact of a visual impairment on children's awareness and understanding of their world, incidental learning, curiosity about people and objects beyond arm's reach, and readiness for interaction is discussed throughout this book. As described in Chapter 1, in order to develop comprehension of their environment in the face of limited or absent vision, students with visual impairments need opportunities to become aware of, understand, and respond to information they obtain from their other senses, particularly information they hear. In the presence of a visual impairment, hearing can become a critical avenue for the gathering of data about the surrounding environment. Sounds beckons; sounds of familiar people talking inspire reaching and moving; sounds offer an opportunity to anticipate interaction; sounds provide cues to the familiar upon which new experiences can be layered, and learning and understanding can thus occur. The importance of access to auditory information is no less true for students with visual impairments and hearing loss than it is for other students with visual impairments, including those with additional disabilities. For all students who are visually impaired, auditory input can be an important learning channel that needs to be optimized to the greatest possible extent.

LISTENING AND HEARING IMPAIRMENT

The term *deaf-blind* is sometimes used to refer to children who have a hearing as well as a visual impairment. Most children who experience sensory losses of this kind retain some degree of vision and some degree of hearing. Deaf-blindness, the condition in which both a loss of vision and a loss of hearing are present, adds yet another layer of variability to the wide range of disabilities that can have an impact on the functioning of students who are visually impaired. In this case, both primary distance-learning channels, visual and auditory, are affected, but in ways that are unique for each student who is deaf-blind. Not only does functional vision vary from one student to another, but so does functional hearing. The age of the student at the onset of each of the sensory losses is an additional variable affecting how the student responds to and interprets visual images and sound. Furthermore, the effects of the sensory losses experienced are cumulative in that their interactive influences can complicate their impact on a child's concept and language development and overall learning.

Dalby et al. (2009) noted that students with both a visual and a hearing impairment can be considered in two groups: students whose onset of visual impairment and hearing loss occurred after the age of 2 years, and students whose deaf-blindness occurred prior to that. The early experiences of infancy and toddlerhood, which contribute significantly to the development of concepts about the world, social connection and communication, differ for these two groups. Their interactions with other people, objects, and their environment differ, as do their understanding and memories of visual impressions and sound. For example, a student may have congenital vision loss (a visual impairment prior to age 2) and an acquired hearing loss (hearing loss after age 2—for our example, perhaps at age 7); he may use a long cane and read using low vision devices or braille. Because of his acquired hearing loss, he may need to learn a new set of skills related to using amplification, or hearing aids, and also need to re-learn or finely tune listening skills. Another student may have a congenital hearing loss and acquired vision loss; she may have already used hearing aids before the on-set of her visual impairment and relied on subtle nonverbal or visual cues to support her understanding of sound and spoken language. With her change in visual functioning, she may perceive a loss of hearing since she may now have difficulty using nonverbal cues to what others are saying and may have difficulty interpreting environmental cues. She, too, will need to refine her listening skills and her understanding of spoken language and sound. Another student may have both acquired hearing loss and acquired vision loss and require extensive support and instruction in all com-pensatory skill areas. Still another may have congenital vision and hearing losses and need to learn that there is a world beyond his or her body, develop awareness of and responsive-ness to sound, and undergo experiences with people and objects that build both attach-ment to others and a connection of meaning to what is heard. For each of these students, deaf-blindness has a unique impact on com-munication and on accessing, interpreting, and acting on sound. Each student needs to have opportunities to develop an awareness of sound and a means of communicating that awareness. Obtaining these opportunities typically involves the provision of proper sound amplification, with the student learn-ing to tolerate wearing amplification devices and to identify differences in sound when doing so.

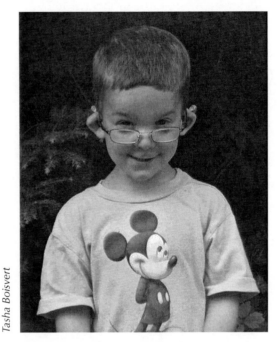

Tasha Boisvert

Access to auditory information is no less important for students with visual impairments and hearing loss than it is for other students with visual impairments.

This chapter focuses on the listening needs of students who are visually impaired and also have hearing losses, in other words, who are deaf-blind. It highlights factors unique to these students that caregivers, educators, and other professionals need to respect, acknowledge, and support when creating environments and experiences that facilitate the process by which these students learn to listen. It is intended to be a complement to each of the other chapters in this book focusing on young children, stu-dents in elementary grade level classrooms, students in middle and high school, and students who have additional disabilities, enhancing their discussions of listening skill development and strategies for targeting specific listening skills. It contains specific considerations for students with visual impairments and hearing loss, with similar need to develop and refine listening skills. A vignette of a student who is deaf-blind introduces specific sections highlighting communication forms and amplification in the classroom.

STUDENTS WITH VISUAL IMPAIRMENT AND HEARING LOSS

Eli, a high school student with visual impairment and hearing loss who was introduced in Chapter 7, enters the classroom from an outdoor hallway, pausing at the doorjamb while he visually adjusts to the dimmer classroom lighting. He walks to his personal study area, a modified U-shaped "den," where he places his baseball cap on a set of shelves to the right and parks his long cane at the corner of this bookshelf and a partition with sound-absorbing qualities. There is another set of bookshelves on the left holding special objects Eli has chosen. A large beanbag-style chair and his desk with a traditional chair are between the sets of shelves and against the partition. One of Eli's favorite leisure activities is looking at albums with photographs of his family while fully reclining in the beanbag, one leg crossed over the other. Eli has poor vestibular function, and "slouching," as his family refers to it, offers him full-body support and allows him to concentrate on looking at the photograph on each page and the label of the event or name of the person in the photo in bold large print.

Eli is sixteen years old and is congenitally deaf-blind. He has reduced visual acuity and nystagmus as well as restricted visual fields and was prescribed his first glasses when he was a year old. Later that same year, Eli's hearing loss was identified. He was fitted with hearing aids for a moderate-severe sensorineural hearing loss in his right ear and a severe sensorineural hearing loss in his left ear. Eli's visual functioning and hearing have remained stable, and the cause of his deaf-blindness is not known.

When he is wearing his hearing aids and when background noise is minimized, Eli can hear speech. He tends to understand speech more easily when the vocabulary, communication partner, and context are familiar. Eli links two or three words together in spoken language, most often in response to direct or indirect comments from a familiar communication partner, tending to begin with "Ummm . . ." almost as a jump start. He rarely initiates interaction or conversation with others. Without his hearing aids, Eli does not hear voices and does not turn to someone within 2 feet calling his name. He does hear lower-frequency environmental sounds, such as traffic, which he labels "cars," and prefers to remove his hearing aids when he is outdoors on community-based instruction, on an orientation and mobility lesson in the community, or riding in a vehicle.

The world of students who have congenital vision and hearing loss is often fragmented, sometimes extending only as far as their bodies reach. The experiences of many of these students are limited to what they can touch and what touches them (Chen & Downing, 2006; Miles & Riggio, 1999). The interplay of two primary sensory losses can have a unique influence on the development of attachment to significant others (van Dijk, 1991), on communication (Miles, 1999), and on movement (Gee, Harrell, & Rosenberg, 1987). Adults who live and work with students with both visual and hearing impairments accordingly need to structure learning experiences for these students that accommodate the unique impact of these impairments and provide opportunities for them to learn through touch and to learn to listen as well. Many strategies for undertaking these efforts are described in Chapter 7. For many students who are deaf-blind with acquired hearing loss, activities and strategies to teach listening and develop listening skills can be considered and implemented as described in previous chapters. However, supporting the development of listening skills for many students with vision impairment and a hearing loss will also require thoughtful deliberation regarding the environment, the learning experience, and the instruction. These additional considerations include the following:

▸ addressing the basics:
  • modifying and managing the student's environment so it is an acoustically friendly and supportive listening environment
  • collaborating with families, care providers, and service providers to ensure that a hearing loss is identified and monitored and that amplification is prescribed
▸ understanding unique considerations relating to the student when addressing his or her listening skills in the classroom
▸ working effectively with the student's communication systems and the student's "communication bubble" (Griffin, Davis, & Williams, 2004, p. 153)
▸ supporting the student's personal amplification systems

ADDRESSING THE BASICS

Many students who have visual impairments and hearing loss may exhibit little reaction to sound. In some cases, they may have lacked opportunities to learn the significance of sounds because of issues related to an absence of personal amplification systems (or hearing aids) or the use of improper amplification. Both of these are critical factors when considering the communication and listening needs of students who have a visual impairment and a hearing loss. Basic factors to address include controlling ambient noise in a student's surrounding environment while creating supportive listening environments for him or her and ensuring that any possible hearing loss is identified and that proper amplification is prescribed. Once these factors are addressed, formal attention needs to be paid to the art of listening with the student and helping him or her become aware of, understand, and respond to environmental sound and spoken language.

Creating Supportive Listening Environments

Chapter 7 discusses the importance of creating acoustically friendly classroom environments for students who have visual impairments, drawing on justifications for "quiet learning spaces" identified by Nelson, Soli, and Seltz (2002, p. 2):

▸ Students through adolescence are developing language and require appropriate listening environments to understand spoken communication.

▸ Many students are learning in a language that is not spoken in their home, and listening in a nonnative language is complicated by interfering background noise.

▸ Students with specific disabilities such as auditory processing disorders (see Chapter 9) as well as students with additional disabilities that include health, behavioral, or significant learning challenges have a particular need for learning environments that allow "clear listening" (p. 2).

▸ Students with hearing loss for whom sound is quieter and harder to discern as well as distorted have a similar need for learning environments that offer clear listening and clear communication. Hearing aids, if recommended for a student, may amplify all sound in the environment, making it difficult to sort out background noise from important sound or communication. They do not correct distortion, and while students may be more aware of sound and spoken communication, that sound may lack clarity.

Educators therefore need to be mindful of factors that contribute to unnecessary background noise and strategies for minimizing their effects. Chapter 7 describes strategies that can be implemented to minimize unnecessary noise, smooth the acoustic climate, and address arousal levels within the classroom. Simple strategies can include low-technology solutions, such as

▸ carpet to soften footfalls and sounds of chairs being moved

▸ curtains or drapes to both absorb sound and filter light

▸ use of partitions or acoustic panels that have sound-absorbing qualities to define activity spaces

▸ turning off radios or music playing in the background for ambience and not for instructional purposes

Strategies can also include class management options that can modify the arousal and activity levels of students in the classroom by considering how students are grouped, the sequence or scheduling of activities, and managing transitions from one activity to another. Attention to classroom design and the arrangement of furniture can also simplify the environment or create activity or work areas.

Students who have visual impairments, and particularly those who are deaf-blind, depend on adults not only to manage a classroom environment that is acoustically friendly and to structure learning experiences that are meaningful as they learn to listen, but also to serve as models of listening behavior and as responsive communication partners. Strategies for modeling listening behavior and acting as effective communication partners are described in Chapter 7 and discussed further in this chapter. They require a shared perspective and collaborative approach among educators and caregivers to support students who are deaf-blind as they acquire listening skills.

Identifying a Hearing Loss

Members of the educational team for a student who has a visual impairment need to work in collaboration not only regarding the management of the listening environment but also regarding the student's hearing. Students with visual impairments, including those with additional disabilities, need to have both proper medical referral regarding the health of their hearing system and regular hearing evaluations (Lawson & Weiner, 2010). Adults need to appreciate the ways in which students use hearing, ensure that an undiagnosed hearing loss is identified, and make sure that every avenue for enhancing hearing is pursued. Also, students with additional disabilities that affect movement and limit their opportunities to change their body positions are at increased risk for middle ear disease related to a chronic buildup of fluid in the middle ear (Northern & Downs, 2002d). Additionally, audiological testing is important for students whose medical diagnosis entails a high risk of an accompanying hearing loss.

Often, only one of the sensory impairments is initially identified for students who are deaf-blind (Anthony & Lowry, 2004). If the visual impairment is identified first, identifying the hearing loss can be delayed because of the following factors:

▸ Parents and educators are not aware that audiologic testing can be conducted on students of any age (Anthony & Lowry, 2004), including those with additional disabilities (Northern & Downs, 2002c).

▸ Routine medical care does not regularly include simple hearing evaluations that might identify children with suspected hearing loss (Northern & Downs, 2002c).

▸ Managing day-to-day health care for students who also have complicated medical conditions can be overwhelming and may crowd out any questions about whether hearing loss might be an additional impairment (Miles & Riggio, 1999).

Deaf-blindness can result from complications of prematurity, childhood infection, near drowning or asphyxia, or prenatal exposure to maternal infection and can be associated with certain chromosomal abnormalities and syndromes (Belote, n.d.; Smith & Levak, 1996). In some cases, the cause of deaf-blindness is not known. Some of the conditions associated with deaf-blindness include Alport's syndrome, CHARGE Association, Cockayne's syndrome, Crouzon's syndrome, cytomegalovirus (CMV), Down syndrome, Duane's syndrome, encephalitis, Goldenhar's syndrome, Hurler's syndrome, Klippel-Feil syndrome, meningitis, neurofibromatosis, Norrie's disease, prematurity, Refsum's disease, congenital Rubella syndrome, Tay-Sachs disease, toxoplasmosis, traumatic brain injury including stroke, Treacher-Collins syndrome, Usher's syndrome, and Van Buchem syndrome.

If a student with a visual impairment has a medical diagnosis that includes one of these etiologies, educators, parents, and caregivers need to direct their attention to the student's hearing and gather informal information that can complement and perhaps drive formal audiologic testing. Completing a sensory learning profile, as described in Chapter 7, can be part of that process. Parents, caregivers, paraeducators, and educators can share information and their perspectives regarding a student's hearing and can document their observations, focusing on questions such as the following (Crook, Miles, & Riggio, 1999):

▶ What types of sounds can the student hear? How loud do they need to be? At what distance?

▶ How does the student respond to the sound?

▶ Does the student enjoy sound? Are new sounds frightening? What response does he or she make that lets you know this?

▶ Does the student respond to voices of favorite people? From what distance does he or she respond? How loud do the voices need to be?

▶ Do background noises distract the student?

▶ Has the student had a formal audiologic evaluation in the past? How long ago?

▶ Does the student have a history of ear infections?

HEARING AND AMPLIFICATION

If a hearing impairment is suspected, an audiologist—a health care professional specializing in identifying, diagnosing, and treating disorders of the hearing system—needs to be consulted. Northern and Downs (2002b) noted that the usefulness of audiology services is largely dependent on the extent to which families and, by extension, educators understand the information that is shared with them. It is of particular importance, therefore, that educational teams, in partnership with families and caregivers, have a basic framework for understanding the implications of particular hearing loss, the types of audiologic testing that might be conducted, and the proper use and care of any amplification system that is prescribed for a student.

There is tremendous variability with regard to the type and degree of hearing loss and the extent to which amplification enhances access to sound. Students who are deaf-blind can have a conductive hearing loss and use bone-conduction hearing aids; they can have a sensorineural hearing loss and have both a behind-the-ear hearing aid and a personal FM system (a radio frequency–modulated transmission system that broadcasts sound directly to a receiver worn by the student, as discussed in more detail later in this chapter). A student with deaf-blindness may have a progressive hearing loss and may become a candidate for a cochlear implant. Appreciating the implications of a particular hearing loss, what benefits hearing aids and other listening devices offer, and the experience for the student wearing them can be enhanced by a basic understanding of the hearing system, hearing loss, and types of amplification systems.

The Hearing System

The hearing system can be structurally and functionally divided into three sections (see Figure 1.1 in Chapter 1) (Lawson & Weiner, 2010):

- the outer ear, which includes the pinna, or earlobe, and the ear canal
- the middle ear, with the tympanic membrane (or eardrum) and an air space with ossicles (three small bones, the malleus, the incus, and the stapes)
- the inner ear, which includes the cochlea and the auditory nerve; the vestibular mechanism responsible for maintaining balance is also in the inner ear

There are two physiological pathways for sound: an air-conduction route and a bone-conduction route (Northern & Downs, 2002c). In the air-conduction route, sound gets transmitted through the entire hearing system: the outer ear, the middle ear, and the inner ear. Sound waves enter the outer ear and are conducted through the ear canal to the tympanic membrane, causing it to move back and forth. The back-and-forth vibrations of the tympanic membrane are transmitted to the ossicles, and as the third of these small bones vibrates, the vibrations move fluid in the cochlea, the auditory portion of the inner ear. The vibrations of the fluid in the cochlea stimulate changes in the sensory cells, activating neural impulses that travel through the auditory nerve to the brain, where they are processed and interpreted, "creating the sensation we recognize as 'hearing'" (Northern & Downs, 2002c, p. 5).

In the bone-conduction route, sound bypasses the outer and inner ear and is transmitted to the cochlea through the bony parts of the skull. Vibrations are conducted or transmitted through the mastoid, the bony area behind the ear, to the inner ear, where they move the fluid in the cochlea, much as vibrations of the bones in the middle ear do. The moving fluid similarly stimulates changes in the sensory cells, creating neural impulses that travel through the auditory nerve to the brain, where they are processed and interpreted. As Northern and Downs (2002c) noted, the brain interprets sound transmitted by either air-conduction vibrations or bone-conducted vibrations as "precisely the same sound" (p. 6).

Types of Hearing Loss

Types of hearing loss are generally classified as follows (Lawson & Weiner, 2010; Northern & Downs, 2002c):

▶ *Conductive hearing losses* result from the following: abnormality of some part of the outer or middle ear; a tear in the tympanic membrane; fluid in the middle ear; or an obstruction that interferes with the transmission of sound to the inner ear. Sound is not transmitted or is poorly transmitted through the outer and middle ear. This type of hearing loss can often be corrected by surgery, medication, or amplification.

▶ *Sensorineural hearing losses* are usually caused by infection, heredity, trauma, genetic abnormalities, or syndromes that result in damage to the hair or nerve cells in the cochlea (the sensory component of the inner ear) or that affect the auditory pathway (the neural component of the inner ear). The outer and middle ears transmit sound to the inner ear, but due to the damage to the cochlea or damage to the auditory nerve, either the nerve cells do not get stimulated to create neural impulses or the neural impulses are inadequately transmitted along the auditory pathway. Many students with sensorineural hearing losses can benefit from amplification. Sensorineural losses cannot be corrected by surgery or medication.

▶ *Mixed hearing loss* occurs when there is a combination of conductive and sensorineural hearing loss.

▶ A *central auditory processing disorder*, an additional dysfunction of the auditory system (described in more detail in Chapter 9), occurs when the auditory pathway or auditory cortex is damaged. With central auditory processing disorders, there is no loss of sensitivity to sound, but the information received by the cortex is processed poorly or not at all (Northern & Downs, 2002c).

Audiological Testing

Audiologists determine the type of hearing loss a student has by using several diagnostic measures, the most common of which include the following:

▶ air-conduction testing, which evaluates the entire hearing system (outer, middle, and inner ear)

▶ bone-conduction testing, which bypasses the outer and middle ear to test the functioning of the inner ear alone

▶ tympanometry, which tests the movement of the tympanic membrane and helps identify whether a hearing loss involves the outer or middle ear

Sound is classified by two characteristics: frequency, or pitch, measured in Hertz (Hz), and intensity, or loudness, measured in decibels (dB). During audiometric testing for either air-conduction or bone-conduction testing, the audiologist presents a single tone of a single frequency, at gradually increasing levels of intensity (loudness), to determine the threshold at which a student responds to that frequency of sound. The results are recorded on a graph known as an audiogram. The student's responses can be verbal (students announce that they heard the tone); an action (raising a hand; an alerting, a movement, or a change in facial expression, which the audiologist interprets as a reaction to hearing a sound); or a conditioned response that is patterned and taught. For example, in play, an adult and child may each be holding a block. When a tone is presented, the adult may say "I hear something!" and drop his block in the container, which the child imitates. This response, drop-the-block-when-I-hear-something, becomes a reliable conditioned response for audiometric testing, taught in play.

However, many students with additional disabilities do not respond to a testing environment requiring behavioral responses. The out-of-context setting and the audiologist as an unfamiliar person may be confusing or alarming, particularly if the student has a history of medical testing and medical procedures. Alternatively, students may not respond to the presentation of sound if they are intent on the testing materials and equipment, or they may not understand what is being asked of them. Other types of nonbehavioral or physiological testing may need to be utilized to gather useful and accurate information regarding a student's hearing, the appropriate type of amplification, and the extent to which amplification can be helpful.

Physiological testing does not require students to actively respond and can be an alternative to traditional behavioral testing of hearing (Northern & Downs, 2002d). In testing situations for students with additional disabilities who may not understand the testing situation and may not be able to passively cooperate by remaining still, the tests are administered when the student is sedated. Physiological tests might include the following:

▸ *Auditory brainstem response* (ABR) assesses the auditory function of the hearing system through interpretation of brain-stem responses to auditory stimuli.

▸ *Otoacoustic emissions* (OAE) *testing* measures the response of the cochlea to sound and reflects the integrity and functioning of the sensory hair cells in the cochlea.

▸ The *acoustic immitance battery* evaluates middle ear function, including the mobility of the eardrum and the ossicles, middle ear pressure, and acoustic reflex.

A hearing loss is identified by type (conductive, sensorineural, or mixed), as well as the degree or severity of loss and whether it involves one ear or is bilateral.

▶ *Typical* hearing has an average hearing level on an audiogram at 0 to 15 decibels (dB).

▶ *Mild hearing loss* has an average hearing level on an audiogram at 25 to 30 dB; vowel sounds may be heard clearly, but individuals may miss some consonant sounds.

▶ *Moderate hearing loss* has an average hearing level on an audiogram at 30 to 50 dB; individuals may not hear all speech at levels of typical conversation; people who know them may best understand their speech.

▶ *Severe hearing loss* has an average hearing level on an audiogram at 50 to 70 dB; without amplification, individuals are unlikely to hear speech sounds at typical conversation levels; they can hear loud environmental sounds and may be able to hear their own vocalizations.

▶ *Profound hearing loss* has an average hearing level on an audiogram at 70 dB or greater intensity; individuals do not generally hear sound.

A combination of terms, such as mild-moderate, is used if the hearing loss is on the border of two categories (Northern & Downs, 2002c).

Working with the Audiological Team

Professionals involved with examinations and testing of the auditory system include an ear, nose, and throat specialist, a medical doctor whose specialty is also called otolaryngology; an audiologist, who is professionally trained and licensed to assess hearing and to determine an individual's ability to use hearing and benefit from personal amplification systems and assistive listening devices, and who obtains medical clearance before hearing aids are selected; and a dispenser of hearing aids based on a prescription from a physician or audiologist. Audiologists and otolaryngologists may also dispense hearing aids.

While it is important for educators and other specialists to be able to read audiograms and tympanograms, much of the diagnostic testing for students who have additional disabilities may be physiologic, and understanding the results will require collaborating with members of the audiologic team. Crook, Miles, and Riggio (1999) suggested that educators solicit information from an audiologist to further their understanding of how a student might be able to use sound and gather information that can support developing listening skills within the home and school environments using questions such as the following:

▶ How loud does a sound need to be for the student to hear it?

▶ What sounds can the student hear or not hear?

▶ Can the student hear speech sounds? Are there some speech sounds the student misses? High-frequency sounds? Low-frequency sounds?

▶ What kind of benefit can the student receive from personal hearing aids? From an FM system?

▶ Has the student's family or caregivers been trained in the care and use of the student's hearing aids or assistive listening device?

▶ Is the hearing loss correctible through surgery or medication? (This may be true of a conductive hearing loss—and the ear, nose, and throat specialist would identify the medical intervention that might correct a conductive loss.)

▶ Is the hearing loss progressive?

Amplification

The basic goal of amplification is to provide an individual with hearing loss with as many acoustic cues as possible at a safe and comfortable listening level. The amplification system—a personal hearing aid possibly combined with an FM system—which depends on the type, severity, and onset of the hearing loss, needs to strike a balance that includes making close soft sounds audible and environmental sounds comfortably loud, accessing the best amplified signal with clarity and quality of sound, utilizing high technology when appropriate, keeping the cost from being prohibitively expensive, and maximizing individual benefit (Northern & Downs, 2002a).

One of the primary considerations for providing amplification is ensuring that students have binaural amplification—that is, a hearing aid for each ear. Binaural amplification provides several advantages:

▶ Sound presented through both ears simultaneously is perceived as louder than sound presented to one ear alone, allowing the volume control to be set lower, reducing the likelihood of feedback, and preserving the battery.

▶ Binaural hearing aids avoid depriving the unaided ear of sound and allow a student to learn to detect sound to both sides.

▸ Presenting sound to both ears offers increased speech recognition in the presence of background noise.

Northern and Downs (2002a) wrote, "Other advantages attributed to binaural hearing aids include increased auditory localization abilities, improved sound quality (fidelity), spatial balance, and ease of listening" (p. 313). Access to sound and the importance of localizing sound are discussed in Chapters 6 and 7.

Types of Amplification

The basic components for any hearing aid are the microphone, which picks up sound waves and changes them into electrical signals; an amplifier to enhance the signal; a receiver that converts the amplified electrical signal back into an acoustic sound wave, which is directed to the tympanic membrane through the earmold; and a battery compartment.

Air-Conduction Hearing Aids

Air-conduction hearing aids come in one of two styles: *ear-level* hearing aids and *body-type* hearing aids. There are three models of ear-level hearing aids: behind the ear (BTE), in the canal (ITC), and in the ear (ITE). They can use either analog or digital amplifiers and can have directional microphones that are able to pick up sound from in front of the hearing aid while dampening the sound from behind, decreasing the impact of background noise and increasing clarity (Northern & Downs, 2002a). Because the microphone is at ear level, hearing reception is at a natural position. BTE and ITE hearing aids have switch options for microphone or telephone coil, allowing their use with assistive listening devices such as a frequency-modulated (FM) system, discussed later in this chapter.

Body-type hearing aids are less commonly recommended although they are durable. Major components of a body-type hearing aid are housed in a case that is carried in a harness or in a pocket. Hearing reception is at the level of the case, where the microphone is, and it often picks up and amplifies the rustle of clothing.

Bone-Conduction Hearing Aids

Two other types of personal amplification systems are bone-conduction hearing aids and cochlear implants, both of which bypass the outer and middle ear and send signals to the cochlea. Bone-conduction hearing aids are often prescribed on a temporary basis, but a cochlear implant is permanent.

Bone-conduction hearing aids are prescribed and fitted for students with conductive hearing losses. They provide vibrotactile information directly to the mastoid, or bony part of the skull behind the ear, through an oscillator. The bones in the skull vibrate, and they, in turn, vibrate and stimulate the sensory cells in the cochlea. As mentioned, bone-conduction hearing aids are intended to be temporary and are often prescribed for young children with congenital abnormalities affecting the outer and middle ear, such as missing pinna or earlobe or a very small ear canal, while the family and child await surgery and fitting with any needed air-conduction hearing aids (Northern & Downs, 2002a).

Cochlear Implants

A cochlear implant is a sophisticated, surgically implanted device that electrically stimulates the cochlea and the auditory nerve. Its internal components include a very small receiver implanted behind the ear with electrodes that are surgically inserted into the cochlea, "replacing defective hair cells of the inner ear" (Northern & Downs, 2002a, p. 332). The external components are a BTE aid with a microphone to pick up sound, a speech processor worn on a belt or in a pocket, which filters and digitalizes the sound from the microphone, and a transmission coil that attaches to the mastoid. The system is designed to convert acoustic sound waves in the air to digital and then to FM signals that the electrodes of the cochlear implant ultimately apply to intact auditory nerve fibers as electrical stimulation. The brain interprets these induced neural signals as sound. An audiologist using a sophisticated computerized system needs to program the speech processor and the implanted electrodes to fit the specific hearing loss of the student. This activation and the ongoing programming of the system involve teaching the student who has the cochlear implant to respond to the electrical stimulation of the electrodes (Northern & Downs, 2002a).

The decision to pursue a cochlear implant for their child is a complicated one for families and caregivers. The surgery results in complete loss of hearing in the implanted ear; the surgery is permanent and not without risks; it requires a significant family commitment both before and after the surgery for post-implant programming and auditory training. A cochlear implant team at an approved implant center performs the surgery and evaluates minimum requirements that need to be met for a child to be considered for a cochlear implant, including profound sensorineural hearing loss, lack of auditory development despite proper amplification and training, and viable, intact auditory nerve fibers (Northern & Downs, 2002a). The benefit varies from increased awareness of environmental sound to understanding spoken language and depends on many factors, including the age of onset for deafness and understanding of sound prior to hearing loss and implanting the cochlear device.

The extensive follow-up required both medically and for auditory training involves not only the members of the implant team and family but also the educators and specialists within the school environment. The effectiveness of a cochlear implant is dependent on a host of factors, two of which are the amount of time the device is used each day and the extent to which its use is integrated into meaningful listening activities for that student (Bashinski, Durando, & Thomas, 2010; Northern & Downs, 2002a).

The requirements for an individual to be considered for a cochlear implant do not include vision, and a student who is deaf-blind and who otherwise meets the established requirements may be considered for a cochlear implant. In a survey of families whose child with deaf-blindness who has cochlear implants, Bashinski, Durando, and Thomas (2010), noted that "children need to be taught how to use auditory skills in authentic environments" and "must have opportunities to hear meaningful speech and language within the context of meaningful interactions" (p. 88).

UNIQUE CONSIDERATIONS FOR STUDENTS WHO ARE DEAF-BLIND

The impact of deaf-blindness is very much interactional—much more than blindness plus deafness—particularly since "when a person is missing both hearing and vision, it is highly likely, though not necessarily the case, that there will be additional medical and neurological involvement that will affect his or her overall developmental growth" (Miles & Riggio, 1999, pp. 34–35). Many of the genetic syndromes and medical disorders that cause congenital deaf-blindness affect neurological function, metabolism, and cardiac function or include other health or physical impairments. For some students, the medical needs are so complex that managing health care becomes the overwhelming concern for the family and educational team and obtaining additional medical information regarding vision or hearing has not been a priority. The thought of additional medical testing may be unwelcome, and the possibility that it might identify additional disabilities may be overwhelming (Miles & Riggio, 1999).

However, knowing what a student can see or can hear, or how the student responds to touch, allows family members, caregivers, and educators the opportunity to appreciate the student's experience and, in partnership, develop a means to "connect with her and help her connect with the world around her" (Miles & Riggio, 1999, p. 35). This requires, as stated in Chapter 7, that educators and caregivers understand and appreciate each student's general functioning and responsiveness, sensory functioning, and basic biobehavioral state. Medical and clinical evaluations can add important information to the ongoing functional assessments that are part of the educational process. They may identify treatments that can improve visual functioning or hearing and may yield information that will be useful in understanding a particular student's development, sensory function, related health conditions, and learning and behavioral challenges.

The constellation of effects that can be associated with deaf-blindness compounds the challenge of establishing effective and rich communication environments, including an environment that supports learning to listen, as well as developing a meaningful way to tell a student what is going to happen. This includes creating communication systems that allow a student who is deaf-blind to receive a message and provide him or her with a means of sharing information in response. It also involves creating environments that provide meaningful information about where the student is and what he or she might do or might choose to do.

Working with the Student's Communication Systems

Combinations of spoken language, gestures and sign language, drawings, written words that are part of his sight-word vocabulary, and objects are used together to support meaningful communication with Eli. Both manual sign language and spoken language have been embedded in Eli's educational program since he was in preschool, both at home and at school. Eli does occasionally use formal signs that touch his body, such as "eat" or "home," but he has significant difficulty imitating and remembering handshapes and their orientation for manual signs. As with speech, Eli tends to understand sign language when the vocabulary, the communication partner, and the context are familiar. Eli often fingerspells single words, such as names of favorite people or memorable events, like a trip to Disneyland. He turns his hand to first form letters to himself and then turns his hand back toward his communication partner. Eli does understand these same familiar words fingerspelled to him but looks around for additional cues or vocalizes confusion unless other communication supports, such as an icon or photograph, object, or spoken word, are paired with less familiar words.

After putting his cap and cane in his study area, Eli visually locates his personal schedule on the desk, a left-to-right set of eight small boxes. His schedule uses various literacy or written communication modes: 3- by 5-inch index cards with a single word in very large bold print; a card containing a bold line drawing or icon and the written word associated with it; a card with a bold line drawing or icon alone; or a real object used in any activity for which Eli does not yet have a sight word or icon. Eli checks or reads his schedule, returns to the first activity, and removes a card with a bold line drawing of a BTE hearing aid. After he inspects it for several seconds, he carefully puts it back in its spot in the schedule, opens his backpack, and removes a hearing aid case.

Mr. Ortega, the paraprofessional who most often works with Eli to facilitate interaction with others and active participation in daily school activities, waits nearby while Eli goes through the steps of his familiar morning routine. As Eli places the hearing aid case on his desk, Mr. Ortega enters the study space and, while standing at arm's length, gently places his hand next to and touching Eli's hand. Eli visually traces Mr. Ortega's arm to his face. He smiles at Mr. Ortega and vocalizes a greeting.

Mr. Ortega identifies himself as he speaks and signs, "Good morning, Eli. I am Mr. Ortega." He points slowly to Eli's hearing aid case so that Eli can visually follow. Eli reaches for the case, picks it up, and opens it. Eli gives one hearing aid to Mr. Ortega, who checks the voltage on the battery and ensures that the tubing is clear and the hearing aid is off. He and Eli together place the earmold in Eli's ear and the hearing aid behind his ear, one hearing aid at a time. Mr. Ortega checks the settings on each so the microphone is on and the volume control is set properly. Then, standing between 2 and 3 feet in front of Eli and speaking clearly and at a moderate rate, Mr. Ortega again states, "Good morning, Eli," and waits for Eli to reply or gesture a response. Mr. Ortega continues to use spoken and sign language. "What is in your schedule today?" Eli shakes his head and replies in distinctive but understandable speech, "Umm, I don't know," and turns back to his schedule. He first picks up the card with the bold line drawing of the BTE hearing aid and, after looking closely, puts it in a different basket for activities he has completed. He turns back to the beginning of his schedule and picks up the card from the second box. He and Mr. Ortega talk about each activity in sequence before going back to the second activity in Eli's schedule, the morning meeting. During this routine activity, the five other students in the classroom and the adults gather in a small area with a rug, sofa, and comfortable chairs so they can greet one another, socialize with communication support as needed, and know who is at school that day.

The "Communication Bubble"

One of the strategies for establishing meaningful listening environments for students who are deaf-blind involves identifying a student's "communication bubble" (Griffin, Davis, & Williams, 2004, p. 153), the area within the student's field of vision and hearing range in which a student can get information from the environment or communicate with someone else. This is of particular importance for communication from one person to another, for building conversations between a communication partner and the student who is deaf-blind (Crook & Miles, 1999). Adults need to consider the student's visual functioning and functional hearing, as well as the extent to which the student uses other sensory information, such as smell, to identify people, and appreciate that someone outside this space may not exist for the student. Adults need to maintain appropriate tactile, auditory, and visual contact so they behaviorally communicate to the student their attention and their message. When adults enter this identified communication space and pause for the student to become aware of them before proceeding with any action or conversation, it ensures that the student is ready for interaction and has the opportunity to be actively engaged.

In the previous vignette, Mr. Ortega approached Eli in a manner that reflected Eli's communication bubble—the range in which Eli uses functional hearing and functional vision for communication, for interacting with others and with his environment. When wearing his hearing aids, and in the absence of competing background noise, Eli can hear Mr. Ortega's voice. Eli has low visual acuity and also has significantly restricted visual fields. Mr. Ortega approached Eli and stood at a 2- to 3-foot distance to balance accommodating Eli's hearing and visual range so that he would not crowd Eli and fill his visual field. Eli did not alert to his presence since he was not yet wearing his hearing aids and Mr. Ortega was standing to the side, outside of Eli's visual field. When, from arm's length or still about 2 feet away, Mr. Ortega placed his hand next to Eli's and held it there, offering a touch cue, he gave Eli a target—his arm—to visually trace upward to Mr. Ortega's face. Eli received communication that someone was there and a means to identify who was trying to interact with him.

Methods of Communication

Sign language, a formal language, is often offered alone or without first layering informal and concrete language systems to students who are congenitally deaf-blind (van Dijk, 1991). However, "conversational interaction precedes language" (Miles, 1999, p. 57). Before attempting to teach formal language to students who have both visual and hearing impairments, adults need to consider creative and meaningful ways to communicate with them and be attuned to any signals from the student that suggest awareness and response. This interaction establishes a foundation of communicative behavior that over time can assume the functions of anticipating and preparing for actions or events, sharing a message with someone else, and taking turns in a conversation. These, in turn, are aspects of meaningful listening behavior and listening instruction.

Effective communication supports for formal language, whether it is speech or sign language, include the use of touch cues, object cues, bold line drawings, or icons. Students who are deaf-blind may depend on several of these forms of communication simultaneously (Chen & Downing, 2006). For example, to offer a message to a student, an adult may use spoken language, a touch cue, and sign language, making sure they are in the student's communication bubble—that is, within the student's field of vision and hearing range. Students may also use multiple forms of communication to express a response. They may move, vocalize or say a word, and gesture. The forms or combination of forms used may vary depending on the sensory functioning of the student, context, experience, and communication partner.

Touch Cues

Chen and Downing (2006) describe a touch cue as a clear physical signal, a touch on the student's body, that is intended to communicate a specific message. It is a means of building receptive communication for students who are acquiring awareness of their environment and who do not understand words. Touch cues are used before an action that is going to involve the student, allowing the student to know someone is there and to prepare for what is going to happen. Adults provide the touch cue, maintain contact with the student so the interaction is sustained, while pausing to allow the student time to process the cue—the touch—and indicate responsiveness. Touch cues are used within naturally occurring routines and help connect a student with deaf-blindness with other people and with his or her environment (Chen & Downing, 2006). Touch cues are based on context: resting one's hand next to but touching a student's hand communicates "Someone is here to interact with you"; touch on the ear may communicate "Ready for your hearing aids?"; touch under the arms may communicate "I am going to pick you up"; touch on the shoulder with a slight downward movement might communicate "It's time to sit down." Touch cues need to be individualized to reflect each student's perspective and the actions or routines that are part of that student's experience.

Families and educational teams can work in partnership to develop a matrix or grid that records each touch cue, its associated activity, and any speech and manual signs that are paired with the touch cue so that communication remains consistent across partners. Combining forms of communication, such as touch cues and speech, with careful attention to where a student tolerates touch, the length of time the touch needs to be sustained to elicit a student's response, and the student's communication bubble is a basic component when supporting a student's awareness of sound and attention to sound as it builds anticipation and readiness for interaction.

Object Cues and Object Symbols

Objects are a concrete form of communication that often starts with the real object used as a cue in a familiar and naturally occurring activity. With consistent use over time, the student begins to associate the two and to attach meaning to the object as a representation of the activity (Smith & Levak, 1996). The object communicates what is going to happen (the activity) and where that might take place (if the environment is consistent and structured, with specific activities taking place in specific areas). The object cue needs to be selected based on the student's experience during an activity: For example, if the student does not use a spoon at meals, a spoon would not be a meaningful object to cue lunchtime. If she always drinks milk from the carton using a straw, however, a straw might be a meaningful object cue.

Initially, the object can be offered to the student at the area where the activity takes place; then, as the student indicates by her behavior that she understands the meaning of the object, it can be presented at a distance further removed. As a student acts on the communication offered by the object by moving toward the activity or area it represents, the student is demonstrating that the object has symbolic significance. For example, if a straw is handed to a student and she moves to the snack table, then that straw handed to her out of context (away from snack), symbolizes meal or snack time.

The use of objects for communication can take on a more symbolic form as the student associates the real object with the activity (Crook, Miles, & Riggio, 1999; Smith & Levak, 1996). A duplicate of the object can be attached to a communication card; for example, a straw can be glued to a piece of heavy cardboard, transitioning from the three-dimensional object as communication to a less salient representation or form. The process of making a transition from a concrete real object to an object symbol needs to be individualized for a student and depends on the student's sensory functioning and experience.

Objects cues are initially used so students receive a meaningful message. They can be used to build the concepts of time and sequence by using them in a student's calendar or personal schedule (as discussed in Chapter 7) as they become associated with routines and activities. An object cue or object symbol may also assume an expressive function. A student may hold and explore an object, then give it to someone to communicate a desire for that activity or initiate a conversation about that object (Crook, Miles, & Riggio, 1999).

As with touch cues, families and educational teams can work in partnership to develop a matrix or grid that records the object cues or object symbols, their associated activities, and speech and manual signs with which they are paired so communication remains consistent across partners. Combining forms of communication, such as object cues and object symbols, with speech (with careful attention to the student's communication bubble of functional vision and functional hearing) supports the development of listening skills, including auditory discrimination and auditory memory, that enable students to recognize and respond to familiar sounds and words.

Other Symbolic Forms of Communication

Other symbolic forms can be used to expand communication opportunities for students who are deaf-blind while also introducing literacy options. Textured symbols, drawings, pictures, and photographs can offer an alternative means of communication, particularly for events for which there isn't a logical concrete referent or for which the student lacks vocabulary. Like any symbol system, including ink or braille print, these need careful consideration of students' sensory functioning as well as how students process or interpret sensory information; symbolic forms of communication need to be systematically taught and their use supported in natural contexts. The process of using some of these symbolic forms includes the following:

▶ A simple and familiar object can be traced co-actively to introduce the concept that lines can have meaning (Erin, 2000). Over time and when taught in the natural situation in which the object symbol has been used, students may attach meaning to that tracing, that line drawing of that object.

▶ When the outline of the object itself is not sufficiently distinct for a student with additional disabilities who has low vision, adding simple, clear internal detail enhances the line drawing and distinguishes it from the background (Smith & Levak, 1996).

▶ An adult and a student who is deaf-blind can have a conversation supported by a simple drawing of the two of them. For example:

Mr. Ortega used simple drawings to communicate to Eli that he would be driving him to the audiologist. He drew stick figures to represent himself and Eli. He pointed to the drawing of himself and said his name, then pointed to himself and repeated "Mr. Ortega." He repeated this process for the figure representing Eli, and used touch cues to prompt Eli to touch the figures in the drawing and repeat their names. Then Mr. Ortega drew the shape of a car around the figures and paused. Eli said "Mr. Ortega and Eli go in car." Mr. Ortega then copied the drawing from Eli's communication card for hearing aid. He said, "Go in car to check hearing aid." Eli pointed to the line drawing of the car, touched his hearing aid, and said "We go." This process added visual support to spoken communication.

Students can select the marker, remove the cap, and give the marker to the adult, and the two share joint attention on the process of making the line drawing, allowing the student to attach meaning to drawing and learn that drawing, or writing, has significance.

▶ Pictures and photographs can be enhanced or modified for visual access. In addition to factors such as contrast, size, glare (matte finish versus glossy), issues related to detail and background need to be considered. Pictures and photographs used in communication systems need to be of a single object if possible, have little or no clutter, and have a plain, contrasting background (Erin, 2000; Smith & Levak, 1996). While for some students color cues can support their interpretation of a picture, other students do not perceive color. Black-and-white pictures or photographs may be more meaningful for them; they also provide enhanced contrast.

Pictures as supports for communication need to be used along with speech and sign. As Crook, Miles, and Riggio (1999) wrote, though a student who is deaf-blind may not expressively use or produce sign or speech, "she can benefit from them receptively" (p. 175). The pairing of visual communication with speech and judicious attention to a student's communication bubble is a basic component of strategies that target the development of listening skills that reflect attaching meaning to words and building meaningful receptive vocabulary.

The earlier vignettes of Eli illustrated the various ways listening skills are supported and developed through ongoing routines and activities for a student with deaf-blindness. Multiple forms of communication were in place for Eli. Information was shared with him using combinations of picture communication, in this case simple bold line drawings, along with touch cues, speech, and manual sign language. Mr. Ortega was cognizant of the communication bubble in which Eli functioned as well, allowing time for Eli to process the communication and respond. In this manner, Mr. Ortega not only supported Eli's responsiveness to sound and to spoken communication but also modeled effective and attentive listening behavior for both Eli and others in Eli's world.

SUPPORTING AMPLIFICATION

As noted earlier, students who are deaf-blind need to have proper amplification, learn to tolerate wearing the prescribed amplification system, and learn how sound differs when the hearing aid is worn. Members of the educational team for a student who is deaf-blind need to work in collaboration regarding the management of hearing aids and developing listening skills.

Hearing Aids

Educators, paraeducators, parents, caregivers, and other service providers need to work together to ensure that students whose disabilities include deaf-blindness get maximum benefit from amplification, regardless of the type, and have the opportunity to develop listening strategies. The first steps in this process are making sure that the hearing aid is working correctly, that it is put on correctly, and that the student learns to tolerate wearing it for increasing periods of time. The most common personal amplification system is BTE hearing aids (Northern & Downs, 2002a), and most of the discussion in this chapter regarding handling and maintenance of hearing aids has BTE aids as the focus.

Adults involved with students who have personal amplification systems need to understand how the hearing aids are used and how to care for and maintain them. Students might be wearing their hearing aids, but that does not necessarily mean that they are working properly. As Olsen, Miles, and Riggio (1999) pointed out, "Any day that a child does not use her hearing aids—because of dead batteries or being left at home or sent out for repairs—is a day the child does not have access to the amount and level of sound she should" (p. 89).

Checking Hearing Aids

Family members, caregivers, and the audiologist need to share information regarding settings for a student's hearing aids and when each might be used. The typical switch settings on a BTE hearing aid are "O" (off); "M" (microphone or on); "T" (telephone coil, often used with FM systems, discussed later in this chapter); and "MT" (for both telephone coil and microphone, in which a student hears not only the sound from an FM system, for example, but also his or her own vocalizations or background sounds).

Families and educators need to ensure that hearing aids worn in school are functioning properly. Basic steps for checking hearing aid function include the following (Northern & Downs, 2002a; SKI-HI Institute, 1989):

- Check the earmold for rough spots and cracks, and ensure that it is clean of earwax.
- Use a battery tester to check the voltage of the battery, and replace it if the reading on the battery tester is low (less than 1.0).
- Check the case for cracks, and ensure that the microphone is clean.
- On an ear-level hearing aid, check the tubing for cracks and check that the connections at either end—to the earmold and to the hearing aid— are good.

- Put the microphone/telephone switch on "M," put the volume on the lowest setting, and turn the hearing aid on.

- Hold the earmold close to your ear and slowly turn the volume louder while saying sounds that cross the frequency range ("oo," "ah," "ee," "sh," and "s").

- Cover the opening of the earmold and turn the dial to the highest amplification setting. If there is feedback, usually a high whistle, check for leakage of sound or a gap between the tubing/earhook and the case.

- If the hearing aid, regardless of type, loses power or has static, call the audiologist and get a replacement on loan while the broken aid is being repaired.

- Turn off the aid and make sure the settings for gain and volume are returned to the way the student wears them.

Putting on a BTE Hearing Aid

Many times, students do not wear their hearing aids on their trip to school, particularly if they ride a school bus. The rumble of the engine, the noise of other students, the rattle of the seats, and the shaking of the frame of the bus are all sounds that would be amplified if the hearing aids were worn on the ride. Being bombarded with all of that noise might exhaust students prior to their arrival at school. Families and caregivers can share information regarding the particular details of the handling and fitting of an individual student's hearing aids.

Putting hearing aids on, for those students who are not doing so for themselves, is another event in which adults can inadvertently do actions to a student rather than involving the student in the actions. Creating a routine for the process that includes the student's active participation provides both the pacing to ensure the student's readiness and embeds communication and listening into a naturally occurring activity. In the previous vignette, Eli and Mr. Ortega followed a routine for putting on Eli's hearing aids that was structured to offer Eli combinations of visual and auditory cues and paced to ensure his readiness and participation.

A general routine that can serve as a framework when assisting a student as he or she puts on hearing aids might include the following steps (Northern & Downs, 2002a; SKI-HI Institute, 1989):

- If it is the first time that day that the hearing aids are being worn, first do a general check of the hearing aid.

- Check that the tubing between the hearing aid and earmold is secure and that there are no twists or bending.

▸ Make sure the hearing aid is off.

▸ Provide appropriate visual or touch cues so the student can prepare for his or her ears being touched.

● Show the hearing aids to the student if he or she can take advantage of visual cues, followed by a touch cue to fully communicate that this device will be placed in and around the student's ear. (The student's experience needs to be considered in devising the touch cue. Touching the student's ear may be meaningful.)

● Pause to allow the student to respond.

● Offer hand-under-hand cues so students can mimic or repeat the action.

▸ Place the earmold in the student's ear (lifting the ear upward can facilitate this).

▸ Place the hearing aid behind the pinna or earlobe.

▸ Switch the microphone on (the "M" setting) and turn the volume to the recommended setting. (If there is feedback, turn the volume down and check that the earmold is resting in the ear canal properly.)

▸ Be mindful of the need to include the student in the routine, offering cues and communication in his or her learning modalities, and pausing for the student's response before proceeding.

▸ Provide similar touch cues as communication supports when removing the hearing aid.

Introducing Hearing Aids

If hearing aids are newly prescribed for a student whose additional disabilities include deaf-blindness, educators and family members will be collaborating on the process of teaching the student to tolerate wearing hearing aids. This process has two parts: learning to tolerate the hardware—the hearing aid itself; then becoming aware of and tolerating a change in sound when the hearing aid is turned on. Communication with students is critical during this process, both to provide an opportunity for the student to prepare for being touched and having something novel on their bodies, and to offer an invitation to participate.

The INSITE model (SKI-HI Institute, 1989) described strategies that can be effective when introducing hearing aids, including the following:

▸ Establish routines regarding putting hearing aids on. Use the same locations and the same times in the student's schedule.

▸ Make sure the student is positioned for comfort and security—optimally, already connected or in touch with a familiar person.

▸ Introduce one hearing aid at a time.

▸ Provide a touch cue as a communication support for what is going to happen. Consider the student's perspective when choosing touch cues. For example, if the student has a BTE hearing aid, his experience is feeling the earmold in his ear and the hearing aid behind the earlobe, so provide touch cues that circle his earlobe, and encourage his reach or his hand on an adult's to mimic the cue. Offer visual cues as well if the student has functional vision and anticipates actions based on visual information.

▸ Put the earmold in the student's ear, making sure the hearing aid is off, one hearing aid at a time.

▸ If the student starts to move his hand toward the hearing aid to remove it, redirect his reach by offering hand-under-hand guidance and engage in a game he likes using hands, exploring a favorite object together, or using movement, still hand under hand.

▸ Once the student tolerates the tactile sensation of wearing the hearing aid, turn the aid on.

▸ Leaning toward the side of the student with the hearing aid, use your voice to offer a greeting; use a natural volume but with the intonation and pauses to add emphasis and interest. For young children, an adult's voice, preferably the parent's or caregiver's voice accompanied by close body contact to add additional sensory input, can be the first sound the student detects.

▸ After vocalizing, stop and give the student time to locate the direction the voice came from.

▸ Carefully observe the student for signals that he needs time to process information or has had as much auditory stimulation as he can handle—perhaps by a head turn or a change in affect or expression.

▸ Provide the same touch cue for *hearing aid*, turn it off, and remove it before the student has an opportunity to do so.

This routine can be implemented in positive social interaction with familiar people during preferred activities. Document the length of time the student tolerates wearing the hearing aids, gradually extending that amount of time, making sure that the student is wearing hearing aids while engaged in activity, with social interaction, both to make positive associations for wearing hearing aids and to have experience with the differences in sound when wearing them.

FM Systems

An FM amplification system that articulates with Eli's personal hearing aids is used during instruction at school that takes place outside of Eli's hearing range of about 3 feet or when he is engaged in an activity in an environment with poor acoustics. The teacher or other communication partner, most often Mr. Ortega, wears a wireless microphone and transmitter that sends high-fidelity signals to Eli's hearing aid when it is switched on and when the switch on the back of the hearing aid has been set to FM reception. The communication partner with the microphone has to monitor his position carefully, staying within Eli's field of vision so Eli can attach listening with the speaker. When the interaction with Eli has ended or if it is interrupted, the partner turns to Eli, points to the microphone and transmitter, and tells Eli that the microphone is being turned off. After Eli indicates he understands, the transmitter and microphone are given to Eli to hold until the communication partner returns or puts it away in its special place on one of the shelves in his personal study space.

Not only is courtesy and respect for Eli built into the routine, but it ritualizes the transition from using the FM system to turning it off for each individual involved in the conversation. Eli understands what is happening and is actively involved in the process, and Eli's communication partner is less likely to inadvertently walk away with the microphone still on. Should that happen, the microphone unit will continue to transmit what the speaker is saying even from across the room, leaving Eli unable to visually locate his communication partner and confused by what he is hearing.

Recently, Eli retrieved the FM transmitter and microphone from the shelf on his own initiative and gave it to Mr. Ortega, behaviorally communicating discontent with background noise and with the quality of the sound he was receiving. His team has implemented a strategy within familiar routines by offering indirect comments, such as that it is noisy, loud, or hard to listen, as cues to reinforce Eli's initiative and continue to build his awareness that he can control his environment.

Hearing aids alone can often be insufficient as a means of accessing, attending to, and understanding sound. For some students, use of an additional assistive listening device in conjunction with their personal hearing aids, such as an FM system, is of benefit. Personal hearing aids, regardless of type, do not amplify just the voice of a communication partner close to them or the sounds of an interesting object the student is handling. As described earlier in this chapter as well as in Chapter 7, a host of factors affect the listening environment: general classroom acoustics, ambient noise and reverberation, and general sounds of other students engaged in learning activities. These same factors affect the quality of sound that is amplified by personal hearing aids. Students' hearing may be enhanced, but their personal listening environment and opportunity to learn to listen with attention and understanding may not be improved.

While adults can position themselves within a student's functional hearing and vision range as a means of enhancing the signal of their voice over background noise, when they move, the signal of their voice degrades and blends into the background noise. Even when interacting with adults who maintain their position in the student's communication bubble, many students whose additional disabilities include deaf-blindness are not yet skillful perceivers and have difficulty attending to relevant auditory information, such as the adult's voice or the sound of an object, even within the proximity for functional access to sound.

Using an FM System

Assistive listening devices, such as an FM system, used in conjunction with a personal hearing aid are a means of providing enhanced quality of sound to a student. FM systems (radio frequency–modulated transmission units) used in a classroom situation functionally amplify the voice of a communication partner while minimizing background noise. FM amplification systems have two sets of components: a microphone and transmitter for the adult and a receiver that couples with the student's hearing aid. As Northern and Downs (2002a) noted, the use of an FM system reduces the distance of the signal from the adult to the listener, so that it "becomes effectively no more than 6 inches, the distance between the microphone and the speaker's mouth" (p. 329).

While an FM amplification system provides enhanced sound for the student, it poses challenges when it is used with students whose additional disabilities include deaf-blindness. That perceived listening distance of 6 inches remains the same regardless of the location of the speaker within the range of the FM system—a 650-foot radius for many systems. The adult can be sitting next to the student or standing across the room—the sound of the speaker's voice, the volume, and the quality of the background remain the same.

For students who are sighted and have hearing aids and an FM system, the perceived distance of the speaker's voice and the speaker's actual position do not pose a conflict or create confusion. Students can visually locate the speaker around the room, follow any nonverbal communication or gestures, and appreciate that the speaker may point to or momentarily direct attention to a classmate. Students who are deaf-blind do not have that same level of access to the speaker. They may be disoriented when an FM system is not used with judicious consideration for their unique challenges in accessing and understanding their environment and people in it. As Olsen, Miles, and Riggio (1999) pointed out, adults can "be giving a child incomprehensible extraneous input that will confuse more than help" (p. 89). Educators, paraeducators, other specialists, and parents and caregivers not only need to be trained in the use and care of an FM system; they also need to understand the unique challenges of connecting sound with sound source for students whose additional challenges include deaf-blindness and, when they are using an FM system, be mindful of their positions and interactions when engaging in listening activities with students.

Components

A personal FM system has the following components:

▶ a microphone that is a close as possible to the speaker's mouth

▶ an FM receiver coupled to binaural hearing aids

▶ switch positions on the hearing aids that allow for hearing options: hearing aids alone (often the "M" or microphone position); FM alone (often the "T" or telephone coil position); or FM and microphone together, so the individual can hear both the speaker and any background the hearing aid picks up, including his or her own voice

Many receivers couple with a student's personal hearing aid through electrical, induction, or acoustic techniques (Northern & Downs, 2002a). Older styles of FM systems use a body-type receiver and either use direct audio input plugging into the student's hearing aid or connect via an induction loop. Collaboration among the audiologist, parents, caregivers, and educators can ensure that all adults are familiar with the proper settings and coupling for a particular FM unit and the student's hearing aids.

Strategies for Introducing an FM System

Using an FM system, adjusting the settings, and putting on the receiver if an older-style body-type FM is used are also situations in which adults may inadvertently do actions to a student rather than involving the student in the actions. As with the process of putting on hearing aids, creating a routine that includes the student's active participation provides both the pacing to ensure the student's readiness and embeds communication and listening into a naturally occurring activity (SKI-HI Institute, 1989). The following are some strategies that educators and families can implement when supporting students whose listening supports include FM systems (Northern & Downs, 2002a; SKI-HI Institute, 1989):

▶ Before introducing an FM system, wait until the student tolerates his or her own ear-level hearing aids.

▶ If an older body-type receiver is used, allow the student to become used to simply wearing the unit before using it to enhance sound. If the student uses visual information, present the device and allow the student to handle it before putting it in a body harness or clipping it to the student's belt. For a student who uses tactile information, provide touch cues to the location of the receiver and pause, encouraging and cuing hand-under-hand repetition of the cue.

▶ Initially use the system in social interactions with a familiar person, engaging in preferred activities involving co-active touch or joint attention on an item the student enjoys.

▶ Adjust the student's hearing aid to the FM-only setting (usually "T") so the student can hear the adult's voice without being distracted by background sound.

▶ Set the volume controls to the lowest setting initially, gradually increasing the volume until the recommended setting is reached.

▶ When speaking, adults need to use a natural volume but with intonation and pauses that add emphasis and interest.

▶ Use hand-under-hand guidance to offer the student the opportunity to touch the speaker's chin or feel the adult's breath on his or her hand so that the student can begin to understand that the sound—the voice— is connected to the person with whom he or she is interacting.

▶ Once the student tolerates the FM-only setting, his or her hearing aids can be set for microphone and FM system ("MT") so the student can also hear his or her own voice and background sounds.

▶ Until the student understands distance, the adult using the FM unit needs to be in physical contact with the student during their interactions or in the student's visual field but still within close proximity; otherwise, the sound becomes auditory input that is unconnected to the student's experience.

▶ Adults wearing the FM microphone need to be mindful that their every word is transmitted to the student. If they need to speak to someone else, they need to inform the student that the unit will be turned off before doing so or they need to make sure the student knows that a sidebar conversation will be taking place.

▶ Students who are socially and environmentally aware can take advantage of the use of an FM system in a small group. The microphone unit can be passed from one speaker in the group to another, or an adult using the unit can facilitate communication among members of the group by voicing what someone says and by pointing to or moving next to a speaker (adjusting the pace and distance to allow a student with low vision to visually track the adult's movement).

▶ Students with social and environmental awareness can also use the FM system for recreational listening. They can place the microphone unit close to a TV or CD player and listen to the recorded sound, alone or with others, without the interference or distraction of ambient noise. They can set (or can ask someone else to set) their receiver for FM only if there is a lot of background noise.

As mentioned earlier, students who are deaf-blind may have little opportunity to learn the significance of sound, to learn to listen, because of a lack of amplification, improper amplification, or improper use of amplification. Educators and families must work in partnership to ensure that a student's hearing aids are in working order; that they are worn, and that routines for putting on and removing hearing aids involve the student, as the student learns to tolerate wearing them and learns to respond to and understand sound. Similar routines and specific issues of listening etiquette must be considered when an FM system is an additional element of amplification for a student. In addressing listening skills, adults must first ensure the basics, which include caring for, introducing, and supporting the use of any amplification prescribed for a student.

SUMMARY

This chapter has focused on unique considerations related to the listening needs of students who are deaf-blind. Deaf-blindness adds yet another layer of variability to the wide range of disabilities that can affect functioning for a student with visual impairments. Both primary distance-learning channels, vision and hearing, are affected, but in ways that are unique for each student who is deaf-blind. Not only does functional vision vary from one student to another, but so does functional hearing. The onset of each of the sensory losses is an additional variable affecting how a student responds to and interprets visual impressions and sound.

In order to establish routines that support development of listening skills and communication, adults need to appreciate the ways in which a student who has both a visual impairment and a hearing loss uses hearing. The nuances of sound and the unique learning characteristics of students who are deaf-blind require that adults be cognizant of a student's "communication bubble" and carefully consider and combine visual, touch, and auditory cues to create meaningful listening experiences.

In addition to supporting methods of communication for students who have both visual and hearing losses, adults who live and work with them need to ensure that any hearing loss is properly identified, that avenues for enhancing hearing are pursued, and that they know how to manage the use of hearing aids and frequency-modulated (FM) systems.

The vignettes of Eli, a student whose additional disabilities include deaf-blindness, were included in this chapter to give form to the explanations and strategies offered throughout the chapter. Appendix 7A at the end of Chapter 7, which provides alternative functional goals that include listening skills, includes a sample goal reflecting listening skill development for Eli.

Dame Evelyn Glennie, a percussionist who is deaf, perhaps summed up the experience of listening and communicating for students who are deaf-blind as she discussed the magic of sound (quoted here in a transcription of her speech):

> Hearing is a form of touch, something that is so hard to describe because in a way, sound that comes to you. You can feel as through you can literally almost reach out to that sound and feel that sound. You feel it through your body and sometimes it almost hits your face. You hear less through your ear but feel more through the body. Silence is probably one of the loudest and heaviest sounds that you are likely to experience. (Riedelsheimer, 2005)

REFERENCES

Anthony, T., & Lowry, S. S. (2004). Sensory development. In T. Anthony, S. S. Lowry, C. Brown, & D. Hatton (Eds.), *Developmentally appropriate orientation and mobility* (pp. 125–240). Chapel Hill: Early Intervention Training Center for Infants and Toddlers with Visual Impairments, FPG Child Development Institute, University of North Carolina at Chapel Hill.

Bashinski, S., Durando, J., & Thomas, K. (2010). Family survey results: Children with deaf-blindness who have cochlear implants. *AER Journal, 3*(3), 81–90.

Belote, M. (n.d.) *Fact sheet: Points to consider about etiologies.* San Francisco: California Deaf-Blind Services, San Francisco State University. Retrieved July 31, 2007, from www.cadbs.org/english/.

Chen, D., & Downing, J. (2006). *Tactile strategies for children who have visual impairments and multiple disabilities: promoting communication and learning skills.* New York: AFB Press.

Crook, C., & Miles, B. (1999). Developing basic language forms. In B. Miles & M. Riggio (Eds.), *Remarkable conversations: A guide to developing meaningful communication* with children and young adults who are deafblind (pp. 180–213). Watertown, MA: Perkins School for the Blind.

Crook, C., Miles, B., & Riggio, M. (1999). Developing early communication and language. In B. Miles & M. Riggio (Eds.), *Remarkable conversations: A guide to developing meaningful communication with children and young adults who are deafblind* (pp. 146–179). Watertown, MA: Perkins School for the Blind.

Dalby, M. D., Hirdes, J. P., Stolee, P., Strong, J. G., Poss, J., Tjam, E. Y., . . . Ashworth, M. (2009). Characteristics of individuals with congenital and acquired deaf-blindness. *Journal of Visual Impairment & Blindness, 103*(2), 93–102.

Erin, J. (2000). Students with visual impairments and additional disabilities. In A. Koenig & M. C. Holbrook (Eds.), *Foundations of education* (2nd ed.), Vol. 2, *Instructional strategies for teaching children and youths with visual impairments* (pp. 720–748). New York: AFB Press.

Gee, K., Harrell, R., & Rosenberg, R. (1987). Teaching orientation and mobility skills within and across natural opportunities for travel: A model design for learners with severe multiple disability. In L. Goetz, D. Guess, & K. Stremel-Campbell (Eds.), *Innovative program design for individuals with dual sensory impairments* (pp. 127–157). Baltimore, MD: Paul H. Brookes.

Griffin, H., Davis, M. L., & Williams, S. (2004). CHARGE syndrome: Educational and technological interventions. *Re:view, 35*(4), 149–157.

Lawson, G. D., & Wiener, W. R. (2010). Audition for students with vision loss. In W. R. Weiner, R. L. Welsh, & B. B. Blasch (Eds.), *Foundations of orientation and mobility* (3rd ed.) Vol. 1, *History and Theory* (pp. 84–137). New York: AFB Press.

Miles, B. (1999). Conversation: The essence of communication. In B. Miles & M. Riggio (Eds.), *Remarkable conversations: A guide to developing meaningful communication with children and young adults who are deafblind* (pp. 54–75). Watertown, MA: Perkins School for the Blind.

Miles, B., & Riggio, M. (1999). Understanding deafblindness. In B. Miles & M. Riggio (Eds.), *Remarkable conversations: A guide to developing meaningful communication with children and young adults who are deafblind* (pp. 20–37). Watertown, MA: Perkins School for the Blind.

Nelson, P. B., Soli, S. D., & Seltz, A. (2002). *Classroom acoustics II: Acoustical barriers to learning.* Melville, NY: Acoustical Society of America.

Northern, J., & Downs, M. (2002a). Amplification. In J. Northern & M. Downs, *Hearing in children* (5th ed.) (pp. 303–339). Philadelphia: Lippincott Williams & Wilkins.

Northern, J., & Downs, M. (2002b). Auditory development and early intervention. In J. Northern & M. Downs, *Hearing in children* (5th ed.) (pp. 126–157). Philadelphia: Lippincott Williams & Wilkins.

Northern, J., & Downs, M. (2002c). Hearing and hearing loss in children. In J. Northern & M. Downs, *Hearing in children* (5th ed.) (pp. 1–31). Philadelphia: Lippincott Williams & Wilkins.

Northern, J., & Downs, M. (2002d). Physiologic hearing tests. In J. Northern & M. Downs, *Hearing in children* (5th ed.) (pp. 209–257). Philadelphia: Lippincott Williams & Wilkins.

Olsen, K., Miles, B., & Riggio, M. (1999). Environments that encourage communication. In B. Miles and M. Riggio (Eds.), *Remarkable conversations: A guide to developing meaningful communication with children and young adults who are deafblind* (pp. 76–93). Watertown, MA: Perkins School for the Blind.

Riedelsheimer, T. (Director). (2005). *Touch the sound: A sound journey with Evelyn Glennie* [Motion picture]. United States: Docurama.

SKI-HI Institute (1989). Hearing program. In S. Watkins (Ed.), *The INSITE model: A model of home intervention for infant, toddler, and preschool aged multihandicapped sensory impaired children,* Vol. 1 (pp. 299–397). Hyrum, UT: HOPE, Inc.

Smith, M., & Levak, N. (1996). Students with deafblindness and multiple impairments. In M. Smith & N. Levak, *Teaching students with visual and multiple impairments: A resource guide* (2nd ed.) (pp. 299–351). Austin: Texas School for the Blind and Visually Impaired.

van Dijk, J. (1991). Education strategies. In J. van Dijk, *Persons handicapped by rubella: Victors and victims: A follow-up study* (pp. 127–162). Amsterdam: Swets & Zeitlinger.

Chapter 9

Listening and Understanding: Language and Learning Disabilities

Laura Anne Denton and Marsha A. Silver

I'm reading with my ears you know I'm reading what I hear
The words I read fulfill my need they make ideas clear
I'm grateful for the faculty communication here,
I'm reading what I'm hearing yes I'm reading with my ears.

—Excerpt from a song by Jeff Moyer, 1996

CHAPTER PREVIEW

- ▶ Factors Affecting Listening
- ▶ Visual Impairment and Concomitant Learning Disabilities
- ▶ Organization of This Chapter
- ▶ Role of the Teacher of Students with Visual Impairments
- ▶ Assessment and Visual Impairment
- ▶ Attention, Self-Regulation, and Listening
- ▶ Listening Disorders Related to Auditory Processing
- ▶ Listening Disorders Related to Phonological Awareness
- ▶ Listening Disorders Related to Semantics and Language Comprehension

▸ Appendix 9A: Avenues for Intervention for Students with Concomitant Language and Learning Disabilities

▸ Appendix 9B: The RTI Process

The importance of listening for students with visual impairments or blindness cannot be overestimated. Good listening skills can compensate for limited vision in so many crucial ways. The auditory sense, together with input from tactile, kinesthetic, and proprioceptive channels, is the major avenue for receiving information to compensate for blindness or to augment limited visual information in the case of compromised vision. Inefficient listening skills affect the ability of a student with a visual impairment to travel independently, to learn, and to communicate with others.

When the visual channel is unavailable or inefficient, any weakness or deficit in the process of listening can significantly affect learning and understanding. Since concept and language development are cumulative processes, built by the interaction of a child's thinking and his or her multiple experiences with the environment, students with visual impairments who have concomitant listening difficulties often have significant language delays or gaps in knowledge that go beyond those associated with visual impairment alone. Service providers rely on the way in which auditory and visual information supplement and reinforce each other when teaching students with a weakness or sensory loss in either area. Students with language disorders—those who have difficulties with either understanding or expressing language—are often supported with visual information; that is, the use of visual cues and graphics may be purposefully increased to compensate for weaker understanding of language. Conversely, students with visual impairments typically are taught to rely on auditory information or language input as a way to receive information that is not being provided by their visual sense. When both poor listening skills and a visual impairment are present, the student's ability to obtain information and learn may be severely compromised.

FACTORS AFFECTING LISTENING

Listening is a process that begins with an input of information and culminates with comprehension. Many factors can affect that process, including hearing acuity, the physical environment, and the attention and language abilities of the listener. These factors may be related to and have an impact on two subcomponents of the overall process of listening: the processes that affect the *receipt* of an auditory message, both neurological and environmental, and the cognitive processes that relate to *interpreting* the message. (The term *process,* which is often encountered in the allied fields of psychology, education, and speech and language pathology in phrases such as *cognitive processing*, *language processing*, or *auditory processing*, refers to the way that input is acted upon, or processed, by the brain.)

Before the brain can interpret and act upon information, the information needs to be received. The listening environment, as well as the person's attention and focus levels, affects the brain's receipt of the acoustic signal. The major influences on whether an auditory message is received, beyond hearing acuity, are the listener's attention, focus, and neurological capacity for auditory processing. A student who is experiencing difficulty with attention may or may not have a diagnosis of attention deficit/hyperactivity disorder (ADHD).

Once the brain receives sensory input, it acts upon, or processes, that information. It interprets the sensory input by connecting it with other information, manipulating it, comprehending it, or some combination of these processes, before storing it in memory or using it to formulate a response. Auditory processing disorders (including the subtype related to phonological, or sound-unit, processing, discussed later in this chapter) cross categories to affect an individual's ability to interpret as well as receive sensory input. Separately, or in addition to these issues, a student may have a receptive language disorder that affects comprehension.

When these processes are ineffective or disordered and interfere with learning, they are generically referred to as constituting a language disorder, a learning disability, or a language-based learning disability.

This chapter examines characteristics of students with visual impairments who are experiencing difficulties with listening, despite having average cognition, in order to identify the language and language-based learning disabilities that may be contributing to their challenges. Identifying the underlying source of the student's difficulty can assist his or her educational team with instructional planning and may lead the team to recommend that the student receive additional services or be classified in additional special education eligibility areas. In particular, the chapter aims to provide an understanding of these complex and intertwined disabilities for teachers, assessment and educational teams, other staff who work directly with students with visual impairments, and family members or caregivers.

VISUAL IMPAIRMENT AND CONCOMITANT LEARNING DISABILITIES

A visual impairment has significant effects on a student's learning and response to instructional input. It does not necessarily follow, however, that all educational difficulties experienced by a student with a visual impairment are related to the student's visual issues.

Research regarding children with visual impairment and additional disabilities is mixed; however, it is estimated that approximately 60 percent of the population of students with visual impairments have additonal disabilities (Dote-Kwan, Chen, & Hughes, 2001; Ferrell, 1998; Hatton, 2001). The most common causes of visual impairment include cortical visual impairment, retinopathy of prematurity, and optic nerve hypoplasia. Some children with these visual conditions may experience concomitant learning disabilities. In fact, some children with these conditions have received secondary diagnoses of mental retardation, language and learning disabilities, autism spectrum disorders, and attention deficits. Thus, children with visual impairments may experience both language and learning disabilities that create learning difficulties above and beyond those that would be anticipated from the existence of a visual impairment alone.

Language Disabilities

The American Speech-Language-Hearing Association has defined the term *language disorder* as "trouble understanding others (receptive language), or sharing thoughts, ideas, and feelings completely (expressive language)" (American Speech-Language-Hearing Association [ASHA], 2011). The area of language most directly associated with listening relates to the content of language, termed *semantics* by linguists and speech and language pathologists. Semantics, the delivery of meaning, relates directly to the interpretation of the auditory signal. *Phonology*, an understanding of the sound system of language, is a second area of language that relates to interpretation of auditory input. Essentially, phonology is the system that translates sounds into words, which can then be associated with meaning through semantics. Although phonology also affects clarity of speech (articulation), it has a direct link to listening because of its impact on language comprehension.

Learning Disabilities

The term *learning disability* refers to difficulty in an area of learning that is unexpected given a student's average cognitive level. The cause of this difficulty is a processing disorder (documented by psychoeducational assessment) that interferes with a student's ability to comprehend information or demonstrate his or her skills. The processing disorders related to listening that may potentially create a learning disability include those affecting attention, memory, auditory processing, conceptualization, and association. Given this extensive list of cognitive processes, overlap between language and learning disabilities can be expected.

The National Institute of Neurological Disorders and Stroke (2010) estimates that 8 to 10 percent of American children under 18 years of age have some type of learning disability. As already noted, students with a visual impairment may have a coexisting learning disability (Loftin, 2005); one survey of research indicated that between 14 and 65 percent of students with visual impairments also have learning disabilities (Erin & Koenig, 1997). Such a wide range can only document learning disabilities as a secondary impairment for students with visual impairments without pinpointing its prevalence. Therefore, those who are concerned with the learning of students with visual impairments need to be alert to the possibility that difficulties their students experience in school may be compounded by issues beyond those typically attributed to visual impairments.

ORGANIZATION OF THIS CHAPTER

As the complex interplay of cognitive processing and language and learning difficulties is explored in this chapter, the more basic and primary areas that affect learning are discussed first, followed by narrower, more specific cognitive and linguistic areas, as follows:

- attention and self-regulation, including the areas of attention, impulsivity, hyperactivity, and executive functioning
- auditory processing and phonological disorders and their effects on listening and learning to read
- language semantics (meaning), including the acquisition of vocabulary and overall difficulties in listening comprehension

The first two areas concern the receipt of a message on a physical level: Can the student distinguish and mentally separate the linguistic information from other sound data in the environment? Is the message received clearly and completely? Then difficulties related to perception and comprehension, or the meaning of language, are discussed: Can the student interpret the incoming information? Difficulties in phonology or semantics often result in a reading disability or difficulty with all facets of language comprehension, whether presented in oral or written language. Strategies designed to improve listening comprehension are parallel to those for reading comprehension; consequently, their use can serve to help develop all facets of listening-related skills, including listening to audio or digital recordings of written text.

Difficulties in any of these areas adversely affect a student's ability to listen. Typical characteristics for each of the areas are outlined in sidebars to serve as red flags for teachers, other professionals, and family members in the identification of the specific difficulties underlying a student's listening comprehension difficulties. A case study is presented for each disability area to illustrate typical characteristics and behaviors; these have been selected to illustrate some of the subtleties of diagnosis and the complexities of determining effective interventions and to provide a foundation for the more specific discussion of strategies in each section. Each case study includes discussion of the role of the teacher of students with visual impairments and the assessment steps used to identify that student's learning challenges and determine the focus of instruction.

Before addressing these specific conditions, there is a brief discussion of the role of the teacher of students with visual impairments and assessment in working with students who have these types of difficulties, to serve as a foundation for the more specific discussion in each subsequent section.

Certain factors that affect listening and language development are not addressed directly in this chapter. Mild or intermittent hearing loss, dual sensory impairments, and acquisition of a second language are covered in Chapters 8 and 10. However, strategies and interventions discussed in this chapter may be useful to professionals working with students who have hearing impairments or are English language learners.

Throughout the chapter, the reader is encouraged to keep in mind the critical connection between interventions provided to improve attention, auditory processing, or language comprehension and the student's consequent improvement in listening skills and therefore learning. The fundamental relationship between understanding language and being able to listen and process what is being said cannot be overemphasized. Only when we understand what we have heard has true listening occurred. Therefore, early identification of and investigation into the reasons for any listening difficulties a student may have are critical to prevent that student from falling further behind.

ROLE OF THE TEACHER OF STUDENTS WITH VISUAL IMPAIRMENTS

Teachers of students with visual impairments play a critical role in the education of students with visual impairments and the identification of any concomitant disabilities because of their specialized knowledge of the impact of visual impairments on learning. In addition, teachers of students with visual impairments may have more personalized information about their students due to the one-to-one interactions that are typical of their services and opportunities to observe their students' learning strengths and weaknesses, as well as check the effectiveness of accommodations made for visual issues the students may experience. Teachers of students with visual impairments may also be a point of continuity in their students' programs, particularly as they move from grade to grade, changing their classroom teachers. Observations made for the purpose of adapting materials in the classroom may also provide a teacher of students with visual impairments with a chance to notice if a student is experiencing listening challenges beyond those that might be expected for a student with a visual impairment alone. Consequently, it is critical that the teacher of students with visual impairments take an active role in the identification or ruling out of concomitant listening and learning difficulties, particularly during the early school years.

An important part of the role of the teacher of students with visual impairments is to assist those general education teachers and special educators who may not have an in-depth understanding of the impact of visual impairment to understand what the individual student might be experiencing and how he or she takes in information. Additionally, the teacher of students with visual impairments needs to take an active role in the student's assessment, as discussed in the next section.

The teacher of students with visual impairments needs to make clear to the other members of the student's educational team that, particularly for a student with concomitant or multiple disabilities, the most effective adaptations for materials and other accommodations are not necessarily determined at the first pass. It is critical for the instructional team to adapt a practice of routinely reviewing and revising assessment and instructional materials and any adaptations and accommodations made to ensure that the student's best possible performance is accurately determined and understood.

The individual nature of each student requires diagnostic teaching; that is, every teaching encounter needs to be considered an opportunity to evaluate the effectiveness of the instructional approach and materials, in relation to the student's performance. Teachers of students with visual impairments can look at this as a three-step process: implement a teaching technique or use adapted materials, gather data on its effectiveness, and adjust as needed. An exploratory attitude helps all concerned recognize that there is no quick fix for students' learning needs and that continual data gathering on how students perform helps develop the best program for them.

ASSESSMENT AND VISUAL IMPAIRMENT

Assessment is designed to meet two goals: first, to investigate a student's learning profile in order to determine appropriate curriculum, teaching techniques, and essential accommodations; and second, to determine a student's suitability or eligibility for intervention programs, including special education. The goal of identifying students' learning needs is discussed in this section. Understanding the ways in which students can obtain access to interventions to address those needs is also crucial, since classification of disabilities and eligibility requirements may determine the provision of services and educational programming. Determining the eligibility for additional special education services of students with visual impairments who have possible coexisting language or learning disabilities is addressed separately in Appendix 9A. Response to Intervention (RTI), a relatively new process for providing interventions for students who have difficulties with learning and for identifying those with actual learning disabilities, is addressed in Appendix 9B.

Accurate identification of a student's needs is at the heart of effective instruction. To target a student's learning needs and select appropriate strategies for remediation, careful assessment is needed. As already noted, accurate, realistic assessment of a student with visual impairment relies on adequate adaptation of test materials in every area, ranging from initial screenings of a student's knowledge of letters to complex tests of reasoning performed by psychologists. Consequently, the teacher of students with visual impairments needs to be involved in all phases of the assessment process to ensure the use of appropriate materials and to help interpret results.

A multidisciplinary team and collaboration with the teacher of students with visual impairments are essential to accurate assessment. Depending on the suspected areas of coexisting disabilities, the teacher of students with visual impairments may need to consult with all members of the assessment team—speech-language pathologist, psychologist, and special educators. Psychological or academic assessment results may be severely compromised if tests are administered without appropriate accommodations or modifications that address a student's visual needs. Although testing with modifications may break norming protocols and make the use of standard scores invalid, it is more important to determine how the student performs with appropriate accommodations than to avoid using these tools. The teacher of students with visual impairments needs to advocate for the provision of individualized accommodations and modifications to ensure that students have the necessary supports so that they can best demonstrate their abilities and knowledge.

It is critical that the teacher of students with visual impairments be proactive to ensure the use of appropriate materials and to help interpret results, as other assessment personnel are not always aware of the need for their involvement or of how inappropriate testing can affect outcomes. For example, letters that are presented in too small a font size or without adequate contrast may affect a student's performance on a screening for sound-letter correspondence. Placement decisions based on these erroneous test results may lead to inappropriate instruction and, consequently, a misuse of instructional time.

In each of the subsequent sections of this chapter, information is included about assessment of the conditions under discussion. For further information about assessment of students with visual impairments, see *Collaborative Assessment* (Goodman & Wittenstein, 2003). For discussion of assessment within the RTI process, see Appendix 9B.

ATTENTION, SELF-REGULATION, AND LISTENING

As a toddler and preschooler, Jay loved listening to books and could fill in the missing words his parents deliberately omitted. He had a well-developed vocabulary and knew words such as pentagon and octagon before he entered school. It was not until he entered preschool that his parents found out that he had difficulty listening and paying attention within the group setting.

By the time Jay was 7, teachers expressed concerns regarding his ability to follow verbal directions and his negative interactions with peers. Jay often interrupted and talked out of turn in class. Jay's mother described him as sometimes self-absorbed and defiant. She reported that at home, once he set his mind to a task—be it writing, drawing, or playing alone in his tent—he became absorbed and it was very difficult to get him to stop and listen. The teacher of students with visual impairments who worked with Jay expressed to the Individualized Education Program (IEP) team that these behavioral patterns would not be expected as a result of his low vision, and further investigation into their causes would be warranted.

Jay's visual impairment was diagnosed at 1 month of age as bilateral ocular scarring secondary to congenital toxoplasmosis; he received services to address his visual impairment from infancy. Jay's visual acuity at age 7, the time of the assessment, was measured to be 20/450 in his right eye and 20/320 in his left eye.

Gaining a student's attention is a key prerequisite for promoting effective listening and therefore learning. Difficulty maintaining attention is a major stumbling block for some students and affects many aspects of learning, memory, and performance, including following directions, sustaining listening for classroom lectures and discussions, following through on tasks and assignments, and remembering concepts. Attentional difficulties can stem from a variety of causes, including physical conditions such as illness, hunger, or sleepiness; emotional states such as worry, anxiety, or emotional disturbance; lack of motivation and interest; difficulty with auditory processing; difficulty with language comprehension; difficulty maintaining visual focus, including eye fatigue; medical conditions, such as a seizure disorder or diabetes; low cognitive ability; and ADHD. In some cases it is possible to pinpoint the cause of a student's attention difficulties, but not always.

Many students with attention deficits who are not visually impaired use their vision to bring themselves back to focus by following other students' leads or referencing the teacher's notes on the board. Depending on the extent of his or her vision loss, the student with a visual impairment may not have this option. Good attention is the prerequisite to the ability to listen and learn on all levels. Students, such as Jay, who was introduced at the beginning of this section, may not be able to listen, despite adequate cognition and language comprehension, because they cannot regulate their mental or physical energy to do so at will.

Researchers who study the interaction of sensory input and attention postulate that vision plays a key role in the development of an individual's ability to maintain attention with increasing levels of focus and for increasingly long periods of time. In a literature review, Tadic, Pring, and Dale (2009) described the development of joint attention, manifested by gaze-related behaviors in the first year of life (see Chapter 2). In their research, many children with visual impairments were able to attain and maintain control of their attention through other nonvisual modalities, such as sound or touch cues. Some subjects with profound and severe visual impairments were as proficient in maintaining attention as their sighted peers. This finding supports intervention with nonvisual techniques as a means of strengthening overall learning potential. Stronger attentional control and the ability to shift attention were generally associated with higher cognitive ability; however, lower attentional abilities were not strictly associated with cognitive delays. From this it can be surmised that, while strong attentional processes may link with higher ability, the lack of attentional control does not mean teachers need to conclude that students with this deficit have low cognition.

Although the precise causes of ADHD are unknown at this time, the causal factors are thought to be biochemical in nature. Research has provided the strongest evidence to support the hypotheses that explain ADHD through brain functioning and heredity (Barkley, 2000; Hunt, 2006). Environmental toxins may also be factors; specifically, exposure to lead and prenatal exposure to alcohol, tobacco smoke, and drugs (Barkley, 2005; Weiss & Landrigan, 2000).

Attention deficits may result from a variety of causes other than ADHD; other conditions have similar symptoms. Inattention may also be attributed to seizure disorders, emotional reactions to materials or school settings, socio-emotional difficulties, and other conditions. These conditions are not as likely to be improved by the medications used for ADHD; consequently, the environmental modications and instructional accommodations are critical.

While pharmacological intervention can address the symptoms of attention deficit, no medical cures have been discovered. Consequently, ADHD is considered a lifelong disability; the interventions to promote learning and strategies to help a student control his or her attention, to the extent possible, are therefore critical. Additionally, helping a student develop a repertoire of strategies for focusing attention and organization increases the likelihood of successful functioning as an adult.

Assessment

Jay passed the hearing screening for pure-tone thresholds, which ruled out hearing loss as a potential cause for his difficulties in listening within the group setting. Reports from his teachers, coupled with formal and informal tests, showed that Jay's overall cognitive development and his language comprehension and expression were within normal limits, yet his ability to maintain and focus his attention was problematic in all settings. Academic progress was slower than expected and appeared to be affected by his distractibility. He demonstrated a relative weakness in working memory (the ability to hold something in mind while performing an operation on it). Jay had difficulty working with and remembering bits of information. He would forget or "lose track" of how to do something or a task he needed to perform later.

Jay met numerous criteria for ADHD: distractibility, hyperactivity, and impulsivity (acting without apparent forethought), according to guidelines in the Diagnostic and Statistical Manual of Mental Disorders *(American Psychiatric Association, 2000). His difficulty with working memory, poor peer relations, and oppositional and aggressive behavior could all be described as characteristics associated with ADHD.*

Jay's ADHD is not the result of his visual impairment; however, the two conditions may have stemmed from the same cause. One study found that the incidence of hyperactivity was 7.8 percent for children who become infected with toxoplasmosis during the pregnancy or birth, as compared with 2.5 percent in the control group (Barkley, 2000), a statistically significant difference. So it is possible that toxoplasmosis was the source of both Jay's visual impairment and his hyperactivity.

The prevalence of ADHD in school-age children has been estimated at 5–10 percent (Scahill & Schwab-Stone, 2000). The diagnoses need to be made by a psychologist or a physician but require input from teaching personnel. The essential impairment in ADHD is a deficit involving response inhibition, also known as impulsivity (see Sidebar 9.1 for the diagnostic criteria).

When difficulties related to sustaining attention have a major impact on listening and learning, a student may receive a diagnosis of ADHD or be identified as a student with a specific learning disability, with attention noted as the cognitive-processing weakness. This latter situation occurs when a student has attentional deficits that are secondary to emotional difficulties, low processing speed, or health-related sources. Despite the diagnostic label that includes hyperactivity in its name, students with ADHD may be inattentive without hyperactivity.

Red Flags for Attention Problems or ADHD

In general, students who need to be referred for evaluation for an attention disorder are judged as being more disorganized, distracted, and forgetful than others of the same age. Students need to be evaluated in reference to others with similar disabilities; consequently, students with visual impairments need to be compared with other students with visual impairments. It is therefore critical that the teacher of students with visual impairments be consulted when a student with visual impairments is evaluated for an attention disorder to ensure that the symptoms attributed to poor attention are not in fact behaviors that are typical of students with visual impairments.

In watching for signs of attention deficit disorders, teachers need to be alert to the behaviors specified in the diagnostic criteria for ADHD. ADHD needs to be diagnosed by a physician or psychologist based on criteria in the *Diagnostic and Statistical Manual of Mental Disorders* (4th ed., Text Revision) (DSM-IV-TR) (American Psychiatric Association, 2000). Input from school personnel, as well as from family, is essential to determine that the observed symptoms are occurring in more than one environment. Three categories of symptoms are evaluated during the diagnostic process: attention, hyperactivity, and impulsivity. A person may be diagnosed with ADHD, inattentive type; hyperactive-impulsive type; or combined type. The criteria for these diagnoses are as follows:

ADHD, INATTENTIVE TYPE

For a diagnosis of ADHD, inattentive type, a student needs to exhibit six of the eight symptoms in the following list to an extent that is inappropriate for his or her developmental level. These need to have been present for six months or more, in two or more settings, with impairment present prior to age 7 years. Evidence of clinically significant impairment (that is, negative effects) in social, academic, or occupational functions need to be present. Additionally, the exclusionary factors, listed later in this sidebar, must *not* be present.

Attentional difficulties are characterized by the following observable symptoms:

- displays a lack of attention to details, careless mistakes
- has difficulty maintaining attention on work or play activities
- has difficulty with follow-through; fails to finish tasks in a variety of settings, not because of oppositional behavior (refusal); or fails to comprehend directions
- has difficulty organizing tasks
- avoids or dislikes activities that require concentrated attention over a long period of time
- loses materials needed for tasks and activities
- is easily distracted from the task at hand
- displays forgetfulness in daily activities

(Continued)

ADHD, HYPERACTIVE-IMPULSIVE TYPE

For a diagnosis of ADHD, hyperactive-impulse type, in addition to meeting the criteria for inattention, a student needs to exhibit at least six of the following nine symptoms from hyperactivity or impulsivity or both. Again, the exclusionary factors, listed near the end of this sidebar, must *not* be present.

Hyperactivity

- fidgets with hands, feet, or objects; squirms
- leaves seat in situations where remaining seated is expected
- runs or climbs excessively at inappropriate times
- has difficulty playing (or engaging in leisure activities) quietly
- is "on the go" or acts as if "driven by a motor"
- talks excessively

Impulsivity

- blurts out answers before questions are completed
- has difficulty waiting his or her turn
- interrupts or intrudes on others

ADHD, COMBINED TYPE

A student may be diagnosed with ADHD, combined type, if the criteria for both the inattentive type and the hyperactive-impulsive type of ADHD are met.

EXCLUSIONARY FACTORS

Symptoms must *not* occur in conjunction with the following exclusionary factors:

- pervasive developmental disorder
- schizophrenia or other psychotic disorders
- other mental disorders, such as mood disorder, anxiety disorder, dissociative disorder, or personality disorder

UPDATE FOR DIAGNOSTIC CRITERIA

The diagnostic criteria for ADHD are under review in preparation for a new edition of *The Diagnostic and Statistical Manual of Mental Disorders* (DSM-V), slated for release in May 2013. The anticipated revisions, as of this writing, include the following:

- upward revision of the maximum age of symptom onset from age 7 to age 12
- differentiation between the number of symptoms needed for children and the number needed for older adolescents and adults
- combined lists of hyperactive and impulsive symptoms; four more characteristics added within these areas

- more specifically defined symptom descriptions
- clearly defined criteria for the following subtypes: combined; predominately inattentive; predominately hyperactive-impulsive; and inattentive, restrictive

---

Sources: Information summarized from American Psychiatric Association, *Diagnostic and Statistical Manual of Mental Disorders*, 4th ed., Text Revision (DSM-IV-TR) (Washington, DC: American Psychiatric Association, 2000); and American Psychiatric Association, "Attention Deficit/Hyperactivity Disorder," 2010. Retrieved September 10, 2010, from www.dsm5.org/ProposedRevisions/Pages/proposedrevision.aspx?rid=383.

The combination of inattention, distractibility, and impulsivity, with or without hyperactivity, is strongly related to impairments in executive functioning (Barkley, 2005), or the ability to self-direct actions and regulate internal and external resources to accomplish a task. These impairments lead to difficulty in organizing and planning, formulating strategies, and analyzing patterns when faced with uncategorized information.

Often the instructional team is able to provide perspective for parents about the impact of difficulties with attention, hyperactivity, impulsivity, and executive functioning on the student's learning. It is not unusual for parents to recognize that their child is overly active, but not to recognize the potential impact of overactive and inattentive behavior on memory and learning. In some families, active children are considered the norm, and this leads parents to minimize the potential difficulties in the classroom.

The role of the teacher of students with visual impairments in assessment is to provide observational data and adapted or modified assessment materials. He or she needs to consult with other professionals on the team regarding the appropriateness of the assessment content for students with visual impairments. Observation, interview, and behavior rating scales are the primary assessment tools. The teacher of students with visual impairments may be asked to fill out a behavior scale to assist the psychologist or physician with the diagnosis. Although the preferred instrument varies, two of the most prevalent are the Conners–3 (Conners, 2008) and the Behavior Assessment System for Children–2 (Reynolds & Kamphaus, 2004). Additionally, this professional's knowledge and experience of the effects of visual impairments on attention can serve as a point of reference for the other assessment professionals.

It is important to recognize that attention-related problems can stem from a variety of sources, as indicated at the start of this discussion. Regardless of the source of the difficulties, recommended strategies to address attention and the constellation of concomitant challenges will most likely still apply. In other words, a diagnosis is not necessary to implement strategies and classroom accommodations. These strategies, if appropriate to address the student's circumstances, will support the student's ability to listen and learn.

Key Strategies to Support Attention

Jay's family consulted with medical personnel and decided not to medicate him for the time being. Their initial goal was to implement memory and learning strategies suggested by the IEP team, giving these a chance to improve his performance and hoping to continue to avoid medication.

The IEP team turned to research-based attention and focus strategies and collaborated to modify them to meet Jay's vision requirements. The team knew that they might have to try several approaches before they would find the combination that worked for Jay. Two of the initial strategies adopted were a personal task list for Jay and an unobtrusive reminder and cuing procedure. After observation in the classroom, it was recommended that the teacher adopt the following practices to support listening and attention:

▸ *Give directions in clear, straightforward language, number steps, and use sequence words (first, then, and so on).*
▸ *Allow Jay to hold a "fidget toy" during times when extensive listening is required. An intentional fidget object is reported to help persons with ADHD self-regulate their attention in order to focus (Rotz & Wright, 2008).*
▸ *Create opportunities for Jay to take a "movement break," by sending him on errands or giving him a classroom job that allows him to get up and move.*

Jay's teacher of students with visual impairments will support his progress with these strategies by ensuring that his learning media needs are being met and that his teachers understand his visual requirements, such as close proximity to all types of instruction in the classroom and other learning environments. Regular monitoring and collaboration among all the members of his teaching team will be essential. The role of the teacher of students with visual impairments will necessarily change as Jay advances in school. In the trial phase for determining which strategies are most helpful for Jay, the teacher of students with visual impairments will be more active. Over time, the role of the teacher of students with visual impairments may decrease to consultations in the early fall to ensure that the new staff are aware of Jay's needs and to an as-needed basis when new techniques or materials are being implemented.

Students who have difficulty achieving and maintaining attention require a strong external support system. Such supports include

▸ alterations in the environment, including the reactions of others to the student's behavior

▸ adaptations to the curriculum and instruction

▸ strategies that are directed by others

▸ the teaching and guided practice of strategies that a student will eventually learn to apply independently

Often, as students mature and internalize the strategies that promote their success, they become more capable of knowing what their optimal learning or work conditions are, and they develop a repertoire of techniques that support their listening, memory, learning, and performance (task completion).

Environmental Alterations

Students with attention difficulties are reported to learn best in a quiet, nondistractive environment with teachers who are tolerant of movement, calm, flexible, and upbeat (U.S. Office of Special Education Programs, 2004). It is therefore desirable to surround the student who has attention-related difficulties with adults who are confident of his or her ability to be successful and who understand that inattention and high levels of activity are not willful misbehavior.

Observation, evaluation, and adjustment of the learning environment, including the teacher's instructional delivery style, help to ensure optimal conditions for listening. The following are some specific suggestions:

▸ Use of straightforward language and breaking oral directions into parts make a message more accessible to the listener.

▸ The student's position within the classroom can make a substantial difference. The student needs to be seated away from distractions such as a noisy fan or an open doorway through which hallway noise can be heard (see Chapter 8 for a discussion of environments that are conducive to listening).

▸ Generally speaking, positioning a student near the edge of the group allows the teacher easy access to the student for monitoring and prompting, and also reduces the likelihood that the student's movement will distract others in the class.

▸ For many students, being seated near a buddy whose behavior they can observe or who is willing to provide a gentle reminder can help them maintain expected behavior.

Adaptations of Curriculum and Instruction

Students who struggle to achieve, maintain, and shift attention can benefit from direct, explicit, and structured instruction with as much small-group and individual teaching as is feasible. Instruction needs to be designed with the following guidelines in mind:

▸ Decrease the proportion of lecture (passive listening) and increase the variety of other learning modes, such as demonstration, hands-on projects, and computers.

▸ Decrease the proportion of sedentary activities and build in opportunities to move around and be active. For example, some materials might be stored in a location that makes it necessary to get up to retrieve them and later put them away. The student who cannot tolerate sitting for long periods of time can be given classroom jobs that require movement, such as collecting and sharpening pencils, delivering notes, or watering plants.

▸ Provide a highly motivating curriculum.

▸ Make the lesson relevant by linking it to previous knowledge and providing a rationale for learning. Refer explicitly to a previous lesson or experience and remind the student of the purpose for learning the information, for example, "At the store, it's important to check your change quickly."

▸ Follow the precepts of guided learning; that is, provide strong support for the student's initial attempts and continue to support practice until the student is ready to complete a task independently. (Guided listening is discussed in more detail in the language comprehension section later in this chapter.)

▸ Eliminate repetition to the extent possible; provide novelty. Break practice and repetitive tasks into sections. For example, instead of practicing addition facts for 20 minutes, break the practice into two 10-minute sections separated by work in another subject.

▸ Design tasks to minimize potential frustration by ensuring that the student is capable of doing the tasks. Only about 5–10 percent of the assigned work needs to be at the challenge level. Monitor the challenging portions closely to support successful completion.

▸ Modify grading criteria to reflect the percentage correct of the items attempted instead of calculating a score based on all items assigned. Set goals jointly with the student in order to increase productivity. Have a frank discussion with the student; for example, "Yesterday, you worked two addition problems in the 10-minute practice period and got both of them right. Can you try to get three of them done today?"

▸ Schedule difficult tasks for the student's most productive time of the day.

▸ Teach and practice organization skills (discussed later in this section under "Key Strategies to Support Executive Function").

Strategies Directed by Others

Teaching staff also need to provide external supports to promote listening and on-task behavior—techniques and systems that help achieve and maintain a student's attention. As already noted, students with attention-related problems tend to perform best when provided with structured tasks, and they can often benefit from being paired with a buddy whose behavior they can reference and who can provide occasional reminders. The following adaptations are ways to provide external supports that have proven effective for many students with attentional problems:

▸ Define attentive listening and the behaviors that accompany it.

▸ Provide frequent, consistent feedback. Catch the student being attentive.

▸ Get the student's attention before asking questions or delivering directions. Call the student's name before starting or provide a physical or auditory prompt. For example, saying "John" before adding "Who is the main character in our story?" warns the student that he needs to listen carefully and be prepared to answer. In contrast, asking the question and then choosing a student to answer assumes that everyone is listening and prepared. Attempt to set up a system or routine that does not stigmatize any particular student. Many teachers inadvertently use these techniques only for the target student, which makes the student's need for assistance obvious to classmates.

▸ Be sure the student is informed of schedule changes and that clear transitions are provided between tasks.

▸ Include the student in setting goals for increasing his or her attention. Set regular and consistent intervals between meetings to monitor and evaluate his or her performance and to set increasingly challenging goals.

▸ Schedule frequent and regular breaks. If at all possible, have these breaks before the student has become distracted, tuned out, or overwhelmed.

Everyone benefits when strategies to promote attention and listening are incorporated into classroom routines. Even though these strategies are designed for the inattentive student, everyone is inattentive and distracted at times. A whole-class method for promoting attentive listening that avoids singling out any particular student is L.I.S.T.E.N. (Bauwens & Hourcade, 1989). In this strategy, the group is taught the mnemonic *LISTEN*, together with the analogy of driving a car: *L*ook, *I*dle your motor, *S*it up straight, *T*urn to me, *E*ngage your brain, *N*ow . . . and then the teacher gives the direction, for example, "Turn to page 75." These prompts are practiced, linked with their meaning, and rehearsed numerous times with teacher support until the class is able to respond to the cue word alone, "Listen!" In some cases, and when the student's vision allows, cue cards can be developed or a tactile reminder can be constructed. The L.I.S.T.E.N. strategy has been shown to increase overall attention, decrease repetitions of information, and increase the frequency and quality of positive teacher-student interactions.

Strategies for the Student to Internalize

The goal for all students is successful independent functioning in daily life. Listening is a key factor in learning, remembering, performance of required tasks, and communication with others. Although many external strategies can be instituted to support attention, listening, comprehension, and work production, the student will eventually need to develop a system of self-support.

An important feature in developing self-support—that is, internalized strategies—is learning to ask for the listening and learning or working conditions he or she needs to function at an optimal level. To aid a student's self-advocacy, teachers and caregivers need to help the student develop an awareness of which strategies and environmental supports are most effective for him or her. Many students benefit from engaging in continuing conversations with professionals about the ways in which they learn similarly or differently from others and how best to utilize their learning strengths to compensate for areas of learning difficulty. This is done through discussion and joint evaluation of results, either assisted by data collected regarding times when the student was attentive and changes in his or her productivity, or, in a more qualitative way, via less formal evaluation of circumstances surrounding the student's completion of tasks and how effectively he or she made use of time. For example, is the student more attentive at the beginning of the period? After transitions? After a warm-up period? Is the student more attentive when the task is listening or during pencil-and-paper tasks? Teachers can keep quantitative information on tally cards or through point systems, checklists, or lists of work finished. Self-rating systems work for some students. Once the student has recognized the conditions that support his or her success, the student may need practice or scripts for asking for others' assistance.

Because of the executive function deficits that often accompany attention difficulties, a critical factor for students' future independent functioning is the development of organizational skills. Although many of the most prevalent strategies to address executive functioning do not directly address listening, their inclusion in the student's overall program supports the student's availability for listening and learning. These strategies are discussed further under "Key Strategies to Support Executive Functioning," later in this section. Additionally, strategies and techniques that support auditory processing and language comprehension, discussed later in the chapter, would be expected to have the added benefit of providing support for executive functioning.

Key Strategies to Address Impulsivity and Hyperactivity

Many professionals consider impulsivity and hyperactivity as negative influences on learning in general. Aside from their disruptive effects, they are strong contributors to a student's difficulty with attention, listening, and learning. When these elements compound visual impairment, a student may have few resources to counteract their influences. A weak or poor ability to use visual stimuli limits the student to other sensory modes for achieving, maintaining, and shifting attention.

Problems with impulsivity and hyperactivity are frequently addressed with similar strategies. Impulsivity refers to an inability to suppress responses and can be described as *acting without thinking*. The student with impulsive tendencies may blurt out answers or comments without regard for their appropriateness or timing. It is as if the student's internal censor is napping. Impulsiveness can have consequences for the student in terms of safety and social relationships, as well as learning. The effects of impulsivity on listening are related largely to impulsive acts or thoughts that lead the student off topic or off task. For example, following a lecture or discussion requires that the student allow the instructor to control his or her train of thought and accept that his or her own role is to follow along. All active listeners are thinking of associations and forming conclusions as they listen, but they continue to follow the reasoning of the speaker. For the impulsive person, one association leads to another and another, away from the speaker's topic.

Hyperactivity, excessive or unproductive movement, may distract the student, impairing listening and learning, and may be detrimental to the learning of others due to the distraction it causes. Current thinking on hyperactivity is that some students use motion to maintain their focus (U.S. Office of Special Education Programs, 2004; Rotz & Wright, 2008); that is, during routine and boring tasks, when the student may be internally or externally distracted, fidgeting keeps his or her brain engaged. If that is the case, intervention strategies focused on reducing a student's activity may not be entirely productive. It is essential to use trial and error to try strategies to find out whether they are effective; data need to be collected to verify if a newly adopted technique is achieving the desired results. This can be done through charts and checklists, as mentioned earlier.

Strategies to address impulsive and hyperactive behavior include all of the strategies previously mentioned for attention, as well as the following:

▸ Consider working with the student to develop a substitute behavior for blurting out, such as marking a card for "I have an idea," while waiting for an appropriate time to contribute. This provides a substitute behavior for blurting out. The student notes the new idea as a tally mark to be discussed later. A tally card can be created in both braille and print.

▸ Provide acknowledgment for desired behaviors. A system for recording attentive or other positive behaviors can be combined with a criteria system for providing rewards. Goals may be set based on a particular time period or across an entire day. Longer periods of time are not recommended. For example, a student might have a prearranged agreement to earn a short period of free time, a small prize, or the opportunity to play a game with a staff member or another student. The criteria might be three instances of positive behavior out of five check-in times or earning five positive ratings on three consecutive days.

▸ Create as many opportunities for movement as possible. This also creates breaks from times in which concentrated attention is required. It is ill-advised to take away the student's recess break or physical education as a consequence for unacceptable behavior because it tends to make the student less able to be still and concentrate. Other breaks might include running errands, delivering messages, and performing classroom jobs. Have frequent "movement breaks"—opportunities to stretch and change location. Jay's teacher incorporated movement during activity transitions and assigned Jay regularly scheduled errands during longer periods.

▶ Allow a "fidget toy," provided that this does not become an additional distractor. Fidget toys are objects that allow movement, usually hand movement, that focus energy so that a student is better able to concentrate. The benefits of such an object need to be evaluated to ascertain that it promotes focus rather than detracts from it. For example, a student may listen and attend well with a squeeze toy or textured object but may be permitted to use it only when it is held out of view of self and others. Students may need to be explicitly taught how to keep the objects out of view. Certainly, objects that make noise need to be avoided.

Key Strategies to Support Executive Functioning

Executive functions refer to the mental prioritizing, coordinating, and organizing that are essential for learning and daily living. These include the areas of sustaining effort; keeping track of time, materials, tasks, or goals; monitoring behavior; achieving, maintaining, and shifting mental focus; and regulating alertness and emotions. Many of these functions are strongly related to a student's ability to listen, remember, and learn, as well as to demonstrate his or her knowledge through tasks and assignments. Although the strategies suggested here for supporting executive function in students with visual impairments and attention deficits may not appear to be directly related to listening, they are designed to free attention from distractions and disorganization in order to promote effective listening.

It is critical that teachers and caregivers actively address deficits in the area of executive functioning. Students do not "mature into" executive skills; organization and self-management need to be taught and practiced so students learn to compensate for deficits in this area. Some strategies are suggested for organizing materials, time, and ideas.

Organizing Materials

Collaborate with the student to set up a system for organizing materials, recording assignments, and storing completed work. Involving students in developing and individualizing any organization system is essential; their involvement in its development creates a sense of ownership and increases the likelihood of its effective use. It is important to check with the classroom teachers because some teachers have a preferred system that can be adapted for the student; others allow students to develop their own systems. The labeling and identification of sections of papers and tools needs to be individualized based on the student's vision needs. Labels can be created in a variety of ways, using symbols, braille labels, enlarged text, color coding, or textures. At minimum, it is useful to include the following elements:

▶ a tool kit of supplies, including pencils, pens, erasers, a stapler, and any specialized tools needed for certain classes, such as colored pencils or a ruler; these might be stored in a pouch in a student's binder or a box or zippered bag kept in the student's desk

▶ a location, for example, a section in a three-ring binder or a pocket folder, in which to keep assignments: worksheets, partially completed written assignments, or other materials that need doing or completing

▶ a location for announcements and returned work to be stored in order to take it home; this too might be a binder section or pocket folder

▶ a location to store blank paper, such as a binder section, a folder, or a standard location in the classroom and at home

▶ a section in the binder or folder to keep reference materials, such as cue cards for procedures, the schedule, and course-specific reference materials, such as equivalent measures, math facts, commonly misspelled words, formats for writing an essay or report, and so on

▶ a system and location for recording assignments and due dates

Cue cards are an element of a well-organized system. They can serve as references for schedules, procedures, rules, and memory aides. For example, a reference card for the steps in long division or a chart of math facts can help the student with assignments. Jay had a personal version of the daily schedule because he was not able to easily refer to the one written on the board.

Organizing Time

Functional routines and schedules serve an organizing function, as discussed in the section on language comprehension later in this chapter. Consistency and repetition help students anticipate what is happening next, internalize the sequence of steps, and be prepared. These clear expectations promote effective use of time and allow students to feel confident that they are in step and in control.

Electronic devices can serve as tools to organize information and to serve as a reminder for responsibilities. Timers and digital alarms can help a student keep track of time, both to be aware of the remaining time for a task and to monitor whether goals are being achieved. Some students set the alarm on a cell phone or watch as a self-monitoring cue to ask themselves if they are on track to finish the current task in the allotted time period.

Organizing Ideas

The impact of executive functioning deficits also extends to difficulty organizing ideas. Noticing the connections and logical relationships between ideas or between previous knowledge and new concepts does not come naturally to students with attention and organization deficits. The discussions of graphic organizers for vocabulary, comprehension for text read aloud and lectures, and note taking in the semantics section later in this chapter offer strategies designed to assist the student with organizing and connecting ideas.

LISTENING DISORDERS RELATED TO AUDITORY PROCESSING

Maya is a cheerful young girl with exceptional talent in art and poetry who has low vision due to retinopathy of prematurity. She attended a local elementary school, participating in general education with support from the teacher for students with visual impairments, who consulted with her classroom teacher to adapt visually presented materials.

The teachers monitored her progress closely and noted that Maya was struggling to develop her early literacy skills. Maya had achieved developmental milestones on the late side, due to her premature birth, so the assumption was that she might be delayed in acquisition of academic skills. Additional small-group instruction was provided in the last half of first grade. During the early part of second grade, however, her teachers and parents began to recognize that although she was progressing at a good pace in math, her learning of sound-letter correspondence had stalled.

Maya had a history of recurrent middle ear infections and problems with her tonsils and adenoids. She had great difficulty breathing at night and snored loudly. Difficulty with hearing was noted at two hearing screenings, yet Maya passed the thresholds, the minimum level considered as adequate hearing, during subsequent rescreenings. Additionally, her voice quality was denasal, lacking resonance from the nasal cavity and sounding as if she could not breathe through her nose, and her articulation was imprecise, creating some difficulty understanding her speech.

Auditory processing is the ability of the brain to process (interpret or act on) incoming auditory signals. To process sounds, the brain analyzes their distinguishing physical characteristics: frequency (perceived as pitch), intensity (perceived as loudness), and temporal features (perceived as duration or length). Once the brain completes its analysis of the physical characteristics of an incoming sound or message, it then constructs a mental image of the signal and compares it with other stored images. If a match occurs, the message is understood or recognized.

These perceived signals may be word-based messages or sounds with important meanings for our lives, be they sirens, doorbells, crying, or traffic noise. Imagine the discrete analysis of sounds and patterns that a successful traveler who is blind needs to employ to determine how to interact with moving objects in the environment. Difficulties with auditory processing can strongly affect the individual's reception of this critical information. When auditory perception is incorrect or inefficient, the traveler with a visual impairment cannot rely on his or her sense of hearing to provide the much-needed information that compensates for the absence of or limitations in visual information. Similarly, spoken messages may be misinterpreted and listening comprehension compromised.

One of the primary channels for learning is hearing; thus, the level of efficiency that a student with visual impairment attains in auditory processing and listening affects his or her academic and social learning and, ultimately, his or her continued cognitive development. Caregivers and staff who work with students with visual impairments need to monitor their development in reference to the sequence of expected auditory development (Barraga & Erin, 2001), which is described in Chapter 2 and also outlined in Table 9.1, to avoid making the assumption that because the student can hear, his or her listening is efficient for and supportive of academic learning. Because of the importance of the sense of hearing for visually impaired students, it is important to be alert to the symptoms that signal difficulty in this area; these are outlined in Sidebar 9.2. Phonological awareness disorders, a subset of auditory processing disorders, are discussed in a separate section; however, their characteristics are also noted in Sidebar 9.2, to clarify their overlap and their differences. Difficulty with auditory processing is more global in nature, affecting learning and social interaction, while phonological awareness has specific implications for learning to read (listening to sounds in order to link them with the letter forms).

The term *auditory processing disorder* covers a wide range of difficulties with auditory perception, which in turn affect attention and comprehension. According to a technical report from the American Speech-Language-Hearing Association, auditory processing disorder refers to difficulty with the perceptual processing of auditory information in the auditory nervous system (ASHA, 2005b). This may be demonstrated by poor performance in one or more of the following areas:

TABLE 9.1

Sequence of Development for Auditory Skills and Listening

Stage	Awareness Level	Child's Response
1	Environmental sounds (reflexive level—cannot be taught)	• Displays initial responses to sound
2	Specific sounds: • Specific sounds are localized	• Smiles, turns head • Listens intently and silently • Later, attempts to imitate vocally • Manipulates objects to produce sound • Reaches for objects to create sound
3	Sound discrimination: • Source of sound is identified • Distance is perceived	• Moves in relation to sounds • Attempts to find source
4	Recognition and association: • Objects have names • Sounds and actions are described with words	• Imitates sounds • Touches to explore • Repeats names for objects and actions • Independently names objects and actions
5	Comprehension and interpretation of verbal instructions	• Appropriately responds to one-, two-, and three-part directions • Concentrates on message; filters out irrelevant and meaningless sounds • Translates vocal instructions into purposeful activity

Source: Adapted from N. C. Barraga & J. N. Erin, *Visual Impairments and Learning*, 4th ed. (Austin, TX: Pro-Ed, 2001).

▶ auditory discrimination, recognizing the difference between similar sounds and fine-tuning that recognition

▶ auditory pattern recognition, the perception of the timing aspects of listening to speech

▶ recognition of boundaries between words and pauses that signal the end of sentences

▶ auditory performance in the presence of noise and other degraded acoustic signals, including auditory closure, the ability to synthesize meaningful words from incomplete or distorted sound patterns

Red Flags for Auditory Processing and Phonological Disorders

Auditory processing disorders and difficulty with phonological awareness have many characteristics in common. In addition to the overlap between these areas, many of these characteristics are not unique to auditory processing disorders or phonological awareness difficulties. Some characteristics may also be noted in individuals with attention deficits, hearing loss, behavioral problems, and learning difficulties.

In general, auditory processing disorders tend to have broader effects than do phonological disorders, particularly related to distinguishing words and creating a clear link with meaning. They generally affect overall comprehension of orally delivered communication. In contrast, phonological awareness skills relate to the ability to manipulate the sound elements: understanding and producing rhymes and segmenting and blending sounds or sound units. For example, an early phonological awareness skill is the ability to recognize each separate word within a sentence or syllables within a word, while a more advanced skill is identification of the individual sounds within a word. The latter of these skills is most directly related to reading and spelling.

The following table lists characteristics of auditory processing and phonological awareness disorders that teachers should watch out for. The table indicates whether the effects of the characteristics might be moderate (M) or strong (S).

Characteristics	Auditory Processing Disorders	Phonological Awareness Disorders
Acts as if a hearing loss is present, despite normal hearing	S	
Has difficulty hearing in noisy situations	S	
Seems to perceive speech differently; for example, the student cannot distinguish word, phrase, or sentence boundaries; is unable to tell where one ends and the next begins	S	S
Has difficulty following speech spoken at a normal or fast rate	S	
Has difficulty remembering spoken information	S	
May mispronounce words and repeat them as they are perceived	S	S
Has difficulty learning sound-symbol associations	M	S
Has difficulty with sound blending	M	S
Has difficulty with word discrimination	M	S
Has difficulty learning to read or spell	M	S

Characteristics	Auditory Processing Disorders	Phonological Awareness Disorders
Has difficulty following long conversations	S	
Has difficulty hearing conversations on the telephone	S	
Has difficulty learning a foreign language or challenging vocabulary words	S	S
Has a history of chronic otitis (infection or inflammation of the ear) or other otologic or neurologic sequelae	S	S
Has significant differences between subtest scores within domains assessed by the speech and language pathologist and psychologist, with identified weaknesses in auditory-dependent areas	S	S
Has a verbal IQ that is often lower than his or her nonverbal IQ	S	M

In general, there is no single cause for the presence of auditory processing disorders. They may be related to differences in brain development or documented neurological problems, disease, or brain trauma. Prevalence of auditory processing disorders in American children is estimated to be between 2 and 3 percent, with the prevalence twice as high for males as for females (Chermak & Musiek, 1997). Auditory processing disorders often coexist with other disabilities, including speech and language disorders and delays, learning disabilities, reading disabilities, ADHD, and social and emotional problems.

Assessment

A problem-solving team met halfway through Maya's second-grade year to review her situation and determine the next steps. Maya's mother wondered why she struggled so with reading and if she had some type of memory problem. Maya's teachers also expressed concern about her ongoing problems with reading. The teachers noted that, despite her poor vision, Maya tired much more quickly when she was asked to perform auditory tasks that were not accompanied by visuals.

The first step was to refer Maya to the speech-language pathologist for assessment of her articulation and language skills. Based on the testing and a classroom observation, the speech-language pathologist noticed that Maya reacted to language-based information more slowly than her peers, appearing to process language at a very slow rate. The speech-language pathologist also determined that Maya was eligible for services to improve her articulation, overall intelligibility, and phonological processing. Maya performed poorly on a screening for auditory processing disorder. The speech-language pathologist wondered, given Maya's history of recurrent ear infections and failed hearing screenings, if she might have a hearing loss or an auditory processing disorder that might account for her slower-than-average speed for comprehending and processing language. Maya was consequently referred to an audiologist.

By this time Maya was 8 years old. Her educational team decided that a psychoeducational battery of tests was also indicated due to Maya's slow language-processing speed and the questions about her memory. Maya's poor reading skills were becoming a greater concern since she would soon be entering third grade, when the curriculum typically relies increasingly on reading to learn content. It was decided that testing by the learning disabilities specialist would establish a reference point between her skill levels and those of typically developing peers. The team knew that Maya scored below grade level on criterion-referenced measures but sought to document the degree of her difficulty through standardized measures. The psychologist and learning disabilities specialist consulted with the teacher of students with visual impairments regarding visual displays to ensure that Maya would demonstrate her best performance on the test instruments.

The psychologist noted that during many verbal tests Maya stated that she was "tired" or "bored," whereas she was highly animated and engaged during visual tasks. The psychologist was able to document low-average cognitive ability overall (with modified test materials), with a marked disorder of auditory processing speed and auditory memory. In contrast, Maya's visual memory (when materials accommodated her visual impairment) was average. Maya performed best on auditory tasks that were embedded in context and with accompanying visuals, in contrast to rote auditory memory (unrelated lists of information).

Testing by the speech-language pathologist and audiologist demonstrated a scattered pattern of performance in auditory-dependent areas, despite documentation that Maya's hearing acuity was within normal limits. Maya understood the content of listening passages and had a fairly well-developed vocabulary. However, she had not yet mastered basic sound-symbol relationships (phonemic awareness) necessary for reading and spelling. In addition, she failed a screening in auditory processing that involved listening in a noisy environment, listening to degraded speech (like listening to someone with a cold), and listening to competing auditory messages. It was determined that Maya had an auditory processing disorder, which had resulted in the phonological processing weakness and consequent difficulty in learning phonics. The additional effects of the auditory processing disorder for Maya were a slowed processing speed for interpreting auditory messages and weak auditory memory.

The learning disabilities specialist documented that Maya's reading skills were significantly below average for use of phonics skills and word identification. In contrast, her sight-word vocabulary was low average, indicating a relative strength for visual memory of high-frequency words.

Maya's auditory processing difficulties made both words and sounds unclear and confusing to her against an interfering background. This, in turn, led to indistinct mental representations of auditory patterns for words and individual sounds. When she was expected to link sounds with letter representations (phonics skills), her difficulty in distinguishing between similarly sounding phonemes made learning the corresponding letter very confusing and difficult.

The result of the multidisciplinary assessment—interviews with Maya's parents, teachers, and specialists; observation in the classroom, during small-group instruction, and on the playground; and formal and informal testing—confirmed Maya's diagnosis of auditory processing disorder, which was judged to be the basis for a language-based reading disability. Despite her visual impairment, visual processing was her strongest modality.

The IEP team decided to classify Maya with the additional handicapping condition of speech-language impaired and to provide special education services from the speech-language pathologist and the learning disabilities specialist, in close collaboration with the teacher of students with visual impairments. Upon recommendation by the audiologist, Maya's parents decided to consult with an ear, nose, and throat specialist to determine if removal of her tonsils or adenoids might improve her hearing acuity and the quality of her sleep, which was negatively affected by her snoring.

When the teacher of students with visual impairments and educational team suspect a problem with auditory processing, the student needs to be referred to a multidisciplinary team, as Maya was in the vignette just presented. Consistent with the approach described by ASHA (2005a) and Bellis (2003), the speech-language pathologist needs to take the lead to ensure that screenings are multidisciplinary. Assessment needs to begin with evaluation of the student's cognitive, psychoeducational, and language skills. Since symptoms of auditory processing disorders can also be attributed to other disabilities, other potential causes need to be ruled out, including but not limited to hearing loss, a more generalized language disorder, or ADHD.

An initial standard battery of tests, generally consisting of an intelligence test, an achievement test, and a broad language test, may not be sufficient to determine the diagnosis. The psychologist, educational diagnostician, or special educator may need to perform additional assessment to investigate areas of concern indicated by the initial battery. By starting the process with these more global measures, school personnel can focus on the area or areas that are contributing to the student's classroom difficulties. They can then perform additional assessments in these targeted areas to pinpoint the nature, breadth, and depth of the difficulty.

When the speech-language pathologist has evidence of auditory-based deficits, referral to an audiologist for additional testing specific to auditory processing disorders is warranted (DeBonis & Moncrieff, 2008). A definitive diagnosis of auditory processing disorders requires specialized testing completed by an audiologist, in conjunction with a multidisciplinary team (ASHA, 2005a). This needs to include testing to rule out any peripheral hearing loss. Additionally, a referral to an ear, nose, and throat specialist may be appropriate to rule out organic causes for listening and hearing problems.

Key Strategies for Students with Auditory Processing Difficulties

Maya was provided with phonemic awareness activities orally as a portion of her speech and language therapy. The speech-language pathologist also worked on goals for improved speech intelligibility and self-advocacy skills for asking questions when Maya did not comprehend oral directions or discussion points. Maya was also educated about the conditions that best supported effective listening for her. Trial use of an FM system was begun. The speech-language pathologist arranged for preferential seating in the classroom; that is, choice of her desk location based on the best listening conditions according to the results of her audiological exam.

Work with the learning disabilities specialist focused on connecting her developing phonemic awareness with print for reading and spelling, working in a small-group setting. The learning disabilities specialist trained Maya's parents in read-aloud techniques and joint book-reading activities to support comprehension when reading to and with Maya. Within the general education classroom, the teacher was coached to provide ample wait time when asking

Maya questions and given ways to deliver directions and lectures that would support language comprehension.

The concentrated and coordinated efforts of Maya's teachers and special education team were effective in helping her make progress in both literacy skills and overall language comprehension. Although Maya remained at the low-average range for her academic skills, by sixth grade she was able to handle general education instruction when appropriate accommodations were in place.

Maya will require ongoing direct and consultative services from a teacher of students with visual impairments throughout her schooling to ensure proper provision of large-print materials in a timely manner, instruction in the use of a video magnifier (closed-circuit television system) and other technology, and ongoing consultation to her family, teachers, and the other specialists who work with her. Once the optimal conditions to support Maya's learning are determined and her self-advocacy skills develop, the teacher of students with visual impairments may be able to delegate some modifications and adaptations to other school staff, but ongoing assessment of additional areas within the expanded core curriculum is appropriate for continuation throughout Maya's school career. Intensified services are needed at transition points, to provide consultative services as new teaching staff begin to work with Maya.

In the listening and learning environments, a number of adjustments are likely to be helpful. These include providing optimal listening conditions; providing comprehensible input, including from electronic media; and providing support for responses, performance, and learning.

Providing Optimal Listening Conditions

The first step in supporting a student with auditory processing difficulties such as Maya is to evaluate the listening environment. Auditory processing deficits can be exacerbated in unfavorable acoustic settings (Jerger & Musiek, 2000). The classroom environment needs to be examined to look for ways to eliminate competing noise and to improve the quality of the auditory signals received by the student. An audiologist can be consulted to identify influences that negatively impact the sound quality, such as sound reverberation off the walls. Some speech-language pathologists also may be able to provide recommendations. Simple solutions include insulation, such as carpeting or hanging cloth banners from the ceiling to decrease reverberation and absorb sound. In some cases, the student's physical location within the room can make a difference. For example, seating close to the teacher or away from competing noise may be beneficial. (See Chapter 8 for a more detailed discussion of the listening environment.)

If an auditory processing disorder is identified, the audiologist needs to evaluate the benefit of using a frequency-modulation (FM) system in the classroom (discussed in Chapter 8), which increases the volume of the desired signal through the use of an amplification device and enhances the spoken word over the background noise, creating an optimal auditory environment for listening.

There are two types of FM systems:

▸ Wireless system: The teacher wears a lapel microphone. The child wears a headset and receiver. Only the student wearing the receiver and headset receives the modified signal. It is important for the teacher to turn off the microphone when speaking to other individuals because any message spoken while the microphone is on will be delivered straight to the ears of the child with the headset.

▸ Sound-field system: The teacher wears a microphone. The message is broadcast through speakers that have been carefully placed around the classroom. In this case, the entire room receives the modified signal.

If such a system is recommended, there needs to be a period of diagnostic trials during which data are gathered on the student's responses to different conditions and settings to identify effective sound levels and adjustments for the student. It is important to solicit the student's opinion, as well that of the instructor. Information the student provides may indicate adjustments that are needed and which system is preferred.

Providing Comprehensible Input

The guiding principle when working with students who have auditory processing disorders is to ensure that comprehensible input is being provided. The speaker needs to make any necessary adjustments to augment the clarity of the auditory input and to ensure that information is being transmitted in ways that support comprehension. These adjustments include the following:

▸ ensuring that the student's attention is gained

▸ using accessible language and delivery

▸ using techniques for verifying comprehension and clarifying, as needed

▸ making sure that audio recordings, if used, or synthetic speech is appropriate for the student

To ensure that the student has the best opportunity to process the orally presented information or questions, it is important to gain the student's attention before giving assignments and before beginning classroom lectures, discussions, or question-and-answer sessions. The teacher can use such attention-getting techniques as calling the child's name; saying "Listen"; or asking "Are you ready?" It is important to check for comprehension of verbal directions and information frequently. A classroom routine that requires students to repeat the instructions or explain them to a buddy helps to ensure that students understand the information while avoiding confrontational questioning on the part of teachers.

The teacher's rate of speech and length of utterance and quantity of verbal information can have a substantial influence on the student's ability to listen effectively. Directions need to be given in a logical, time-ordered sequence using words that make the directions clear, such as *first*, *next*, and *finally*. Speech needs to be delivered slowly and clearly, but not in an overexaggerated way. Variations in loudness and pauses to emphasize phrasing can increase attention (Paul-Brown, 2003).

Redundancy of information and the organization of the presentation are important features to monitor. When information is rephrased and restated, the ensuing redundancy supports comprehension. When information is presented with explicitly stated connections (such as the use of time-sequence labeling—*first*, *then*; *first*, *second*; *earlier*, *later*—and causal connectors—*because*, *so*, *since*, *due to*), this results in a more concise and organized message, which is more easily understood. It is important to make the transition from one topic to another clear.

Teachers are often not aware of their presentation style, so recommendations based on classroom observation can facilitate comprehensible input for students. It is often helpful to supply examples when providing recommendations based on observation; it can be hard to translate general descriptions into change. For Maya, the coaching provided to her general education teacher by the speech-language pathologist played an important role in improving her listening comprehension.

Pre-teaching of concepts and vocabulary for new learning topics can significantly raise a student's ability to comprehend a lecture or discussion. This can be provided in introductory lessons or small group instruction; sometimes it is provided by a special educator (usually the learning disabilities teacher, speech-language pathologist, or a paraprofessional assistant) to prepare students to participate in the whole class lesson. When students have vocabulary lessons of key words or have the opportunity to develop background information on upcoming topics, comprehension is facilitated. For additional information about vocabulary and comprehension of the meaning of an auditory message, see also the section on semantics, later in this chapter.

Listening to Audio Recordings or Synthetic Speech

As discussed in Chapter 5, listening to books as audio recordings or as text read aloud through synthetic speech using text-to-speech features on a computer or other device is an important method of gaining access to books. Listening to books in a digital format that can be speeded up to increase the student's reading speed has many advantages for students with visual impairments and unimpaired language processing and comprehension.

For students with auditory processing disorders or language-based learning disabilities, however, speed is not always an advantage and audiobooks may not always be beneficial. The majority of students with auditory processing disorders have difficulty with the temporal aspect of speech processing; that is, they process speech at a much slower rate than the average listener. They often have difficulty deciphering where one word ends and the next one begins. They may perceive accelerated or synthesized speech as "degraded" and find it even more challenging to process accurately. The teacher of students with visual impairments needs to work closely with the speech-language pathologist, the learning disability specialist, and the students' classroom teachers to determine the utility of accelerated or synthesized speech for students in this unique population.

Providing Support for Responses, Performance, and Learning

Students with visual impairments and auditory processing disorders will likely need additional response time in the classroom for both asking and answering questions. Conversations and classroom discussions can move very rapidly from one speaker to the next and from topic to topic. This interaction style can be frustrating for a student with a visual impairment and concomitant auditory processing difficulty, because by the time the student has processed the information, organized his or her thoughts, and formulated a response, the conversation may have moved on or changed topic.

Teachers can support the student's full participation and inclusion by making sure that the student has enough time to respond during discussions before others jump in, or before the topic changes. If the student falters in his or her response, the adult can say, "I'll get back to you in a minute," or some other simple, respectful phrase that allows the student additional time in a way that does not call attention to his or her difficulties. When this kind of exchange becomes an accepted pattern in the classroom discussion for all the students, it becomes the group norm; either the student raises a hand when ready to respond, or, in a more teacher-directed discussion, the teacher calls on the student a second time a few minutes later if he or she is not ready to respond when first called on. Techniques such as these supported Maya's listening in the classroom and were passed along as effective accommodations to new teachers as she progressed from grade to grade.

The ability to review information and check that homework assignments have been recorded accurately, or at all, is a problem area for many students and their caregivers. Students can audio-record lectures and homework assignments to give them a reminder or review system for any notations they may have made. Some teachers have found e-mail or postings on websites to be effective in giving a student a place to check on assignments or review lecture outlines and key points. Such information can be posted as an audio file; alternatively, students can use braille, or text-to-speech software can "read" the information to them.

A buddy system can also be set up to provide students with a partner to check in with for homework assignments or other instructions, including clarification of what the teacher really meant. Such a system helps create a community of learners and encourages communication outside of class and school hours; additionally, it eliminates potential excuses such as "I didn't know" or "I didn't get it." It is best to assign buddies in triplets or quartets to reduce the chance that a buddy is not available.

The suggestions offered in the sections of this chapter on attention and semantics can also be used as strategies to support students with auditory processing disorders. Many characteristics of these three conditions overlap, and the strategies are often effective for more than one specific source of difficulty.

LISTENING DISORDERS RELATED TO PHONOLOGICAL AWARENESS

Explicit awareness of the sound structure of a spoken word is referred to as phonological awareness (McCauley & Fey, 2006). In its purest sense, phonological awareness does not involve interaction with print media of any kind. Phonological awareness disorder can be considered a subset or type of auditory processing disorder; it is directly related to how the mind interprets sounds, such as identifying sounds to learn sound-letter correspondence for reading. Characteristics of phonological disorders are compared with those of auditory processing in Sidebar 9.2. As presented in the vignette for this section, Maya's difficulties were related to both phonological awareness and auditory processing. The phonological component created difficulty hearing sounds clearly in order to differentiate them to learn sound-symbol associations and also caused her imprecise articulation.

Tasks involving phonological awareness require a student to listen, analyze, make judgments about, and manipulate sounds in spoken words. For example, a student may be asked if *mat* rhymes with *bat*; he or she may be asked to tell the number of syllables in *baseball bat*. Phonological awareness is the foundation for the literacy skills of both reading and spelling and is critical to the formation of connections between sounds and letters. Anthony and Lonigan (2004) listed three levels of commonly identified phonological awareness:

- ▸ awareness that words have a syllabic structure (syllable awareness)
- ▸ awareness that a syllable has a beginning part (onset) and a rime unit, for example, *b-at* (onset-rime awareness; *onset* is the part of the word

before the vowel; *rime* is the vowel and the remaining consonants in the final part of the word)

▸ awareness that words are formed from individual speech sounds, or phonemes, such as *b-a-t* (phoneme awareness)

Phonemic awareness, a subtype of phonological awareness, refers to the degree of understanding about the separateness of individual sounds (phonemes) and the ability to use them as building blocks for the construction of words. In particular, it is the awareness that the sounds can be separately identified, broken apart from a word, and recombined to form different words (see the discussion of phonemic awareness in Chapter 4). The ability to manipulate phonemes strongly correlates with decoding for reading and understanding, as well as spelling (Blischak, Shah, Lombardino, & Chiarella, 2004).

Research indicates that in general there is no difference between the phonological skills of sighted students and those of students who are blind (Dodd & Conn, 2000; Gillon & Young, 2002). Beginning readers of braille can be expected to develop phonological awareness skills in the same manner as readers of print (Gillon & Young, 2002). The phonological skills of braille readers may be strong because they rely heavily on auditory input as a primary mode of sensory input (Clark & Stoner, 2008).

Despite these research findings, teachers of students with visual impairments encounter children with poor phonological awareness skills and difficulty with processing and holding phonological information in memory. Visually impaired children who are diagnosed with an additional disability of speech and language impairment frequently have difficulty in this area. These students are more likely to experience early literacy difficulties and are at risk of developing persistent failure in the areas of reading and spelling (Gillon, 2004). Indeed, difficulty in processing phonological information is considered a causative factor in reading disorders (Catts & Kamhi, 2005).

Assessment

When a student has difficulty with early literacy activities involving awareness of syllables, rhyming, or awareness of phonemes, the teacher of students with visual impairments, along with the educational team, may engage in more intense and explicit training for these skills to track the student's response to intervention. (A further discussion of Response to Intervention appears in Appendix 9B.) He or she may also collaborate with the speech-language pathologist or reading specialist for screening, assessment, and teaching strategies in this area. Numerous tools for phonological and phonemic awareness skills are available, as both skill surveys and standardized assessments. Two tests in this category are the Phonological Awareness Test–2 (Robertson & Salter, 2007) and the Test of Phonological Awareness–2+ (Torgesen & Bryant, 2004). Skill surveys are recommended because they facilitate planning for intervention; they make it easy to tell which areas are developing and which need work, because skills are generally listed within a learning hierarchy. Coordinated phonological awareness goals and activities may be implemented in a variety of learning environments simultaneously, such as in different classes or during designated instructional services.

Key Strategies for Phonological and Phonemic Awareness Difficulties

Phonemes are the smallest units of sounds that can differentiate meaning. For example, the vowel phonemes in the words *mat* and *met* help listeners determine the meaning of each word. Phonemic awareness is a subset of phonological awareness and is taught and practiced only via oral exercises since the goal is to develop the student's ability to manipulate sounds. A primary focus of initial teaching for literacy, however, is to promote the student's awareness and understanding of the relationship between alphabet letters and the sounds they represent, or sound-letter correspondence, one of the building blocks for literacy development. For students, such as Maya, who experience difficulty with the correspondence between sounds and letters, practitioners often use concrete strategies such as finger tapping, counting, or moving objects from one location to another as sounds are identified.

Phonemic awareness may begin by focusing on sounds only, but later sound-symbol correspondence develops in concert with early braille or visual reading skills. It is important to be aware of the interactive nature of this learning; as students learn about letters and learn to read easy phonetic words, their knowledge of phonemic awareness expands. More advanced phonemic awareness, such as separating one sound from a two- or three-sound consonant blend (for example, saying *brand* without /r/ produces *band*), develops later and is not essential for beginning reading. Practitioners need to coordinate phonemic awareness and early reading instruction to the extent possible.

Several authors have mapped out a sequence of phonological awareness instruction (Gillon, 2004; McCauley & Fey, 2006; Schuele & Boudreau, 2008). In general, five characteristics make a task of phonological recognition easier or harder (Kame'enui, 1996):

▶ The size of the phonological unit: It is easier to break sentences into words and words into syllables than to break syllables into phonemes.

▶ The number of phonemes in the word: It is easier to break up phonemically short words such as *no, see,* and *cap* than it is to break up longer words such as *snort, sleep,* and *scrap.*

▶ Phoneme position in words: Initial consonants are easier to hear than final consonants, and middle consonants are most difficult.

▶ Phonological properties of words: Continuant, or drawn-out, lengthy consonants such as /s/ and /m/ are easier to recognize than very brief sounds such as /t/.

▶ Phonological awareness challenges: Rhyming and initial phoneme identification are easier to perform than blending and segmenting. (*Blending* involves merging individual sounds together—for example, *m-a-p* equals *map*—whereas *segmenting* involves breaking the word *map* up into its components).

A recommended sequence of instruction (Schuele & Boudreau, 2008) begins with the syllable unit and progresses through onset-rime (*br-and, tr-ack*) to sound blending. Table 9.2 illustrates this sequence and provides examples.

A supportive structure and visual representation for discriminating sounds within words and eventually representing sounds as letters is provided by word boxes, also known as Elkonin boxes after their originator, D. B. Elkonin, a Russian psychologist. A word is represented by a row of boxes, each box representing one sound unit (phoneme). Initially, a student moves chips or small blocks into each box to segment and sequence the individual sounds in a dictated word. Students may also be asked to listen for a target sound and place a marker in the box that represents the position of the sound within the dictated word. The same types of activities can be used with letter blocks or magnetic letters to practice sound-letter correspondence and spelling and can be adapted for braille learners (Blachman, Ball, Black, & Tangel, 2000).

For students with visual impairments who have difficulty with phonological awareness, it is advantageous to teach within natural contexts using familiar words that can be represented in concrete forms (such as objects or pictures). This supports generalization of teaching across different learning settings. Words that represent personal life and interests are highly motivating and relevant, for example, words from familiar books that are accompanied by story objects; words from movement activities in adaptive physical education, physical therapy, and orientation and mobility; and words from classroom thematic units.

TABLE 9.2
Building Phonological Awareness: Sequence of Instruction

Skill	Examples
Syllable Awareness	
Segment sentences into words	*Bob likes his bike*: Repeat with pauses between words or clap for each word while repeating the sentence.
Segment compound words into their component words	*Cupcake, hotdog*: Repeat with pauses between parts (*cup/cake*).
Segment words into syllables	*Alphabet, tomato*: Repeat with pauses between syllables (*al/pha/bet*) or clap for each syllable while repeating the word.
Onset-Rime Awareness	
Determine what doesn't fit	Which one does not rhyme? *ball, boy, fall*?
Rhyme matching/recognition	Which one rhymes with *hat*? *cat, ball, cup*?
	Do *pan* and *pack* rhyme? Do *shoe* and *blue* rhyme?
Rhyme production	Tell me a word that rhymes with *house*.
Phoneme Awareness	
Judge initial sounds	Do *cat* and *ball* start with the same sound?
Determine what doesn't fit	What word starts with a different sound: *cap, key, can, mat*?
Match initial sounds	What begins the same as *man*? *can, boy, map*
Identify initial sounds	What is the first sound in *lunch*?
	Tell me a word that begins the same as *pencil*.
Judge final sounds	What doesn't fit? What word ends with a different sound: *cat, cap, tap, pop*?
Match final sounds	What word ends the same as *bat*? *ball, light, car*
Identify final sounds	What is the last sound in *dog*?
	Tell me a word that ends the same as *red*.
Phoneme deletion	Say *cup*. Now say it again without the /c/.
Sound Blending	
Build from shorter, simpler to longer, more complex constructions.	
Consonant (C) with vowel (V): CV, VC	*no, up*
Short vowel words: CVC	*cup, bag, log*
Initial consonant blends: CCVC	*small, black*
Final consonant blends: CVCC	*jump, nest*

Source: Adapted with permission from C. M. Schuele & D. Boudreau, "Phonological Awareness Intervention: Beyond the Basics," *Language, Speech, and Hearing Services in Schools, 39* (2008), 3–20.

Reading Disability

Phonological awareness is a highly specialized area of listening. Difficulties in this area may not be recognized until a student attempts to learn to read. Students like Maya, who fail to understand the sound pattern of their language and how sounds within a language function to signify meaning, are at risk for difficulty learning to read. Figuring out a word based on its letters and letter patterns requires the ability to identify and associate the letters and letter patterns with sounds, remember them while maintaining their sequence, and blend them into a recognizable word. Students who experience difficulty learning to decode or spell words need to receive both a hearing screening and an assessment of phonological awareness skills to rule out problems in these areas, as discussed in earlier sections of this chapter. A student who is struggling to learn sound-letter correspondence may require additional instruction and practice in segmenting sounds and differentiating similar-sounding, frequently confused sounds, such as b/v, d/t, and b/p.

When a student experiences persistent difficulty with the correspondence of phonemes to graphemes (the written or tactile symbols for a spoken sound) in braille or print, whether in processing, remembering, or reading them, collaboration (including assessment) with the reading specialist or learning disability specialist may be warranted. It is always important to separate braille-reading errors due to a student's difficulty with tactile discrimination from errors that may be related to a lack of auditory skills involved in reading. When remedial reading intervention is warranted, instruction needs to be frequent, explicit, systematic, cumulative, and multisensory to the highest degree possible.

No matter what media is used for reading (braille or print), students with visual impairments will be negatively affected by a weakness in the area of phonological awareness. Early literacy learners with underdeveloped phonological awareness need to rely on visual memory, or, in the case of a student with visual impairments, on the memory of tactile patterns transmitted via braille. This leaves them without strategies for figuring out unknown words; that is, they can read only the words they have previously learned. Consequently, in such cases it is critical to intervene in a timely manner. Teachers and caregivers need to closely monitor progress in phonological awareness and learning sound-letter correspondence in order to provide additional instruction and practice as early as possible for those who are struggling.

LISTENING DISORDERS RELATED TO SEMANTICS AND LANGUAGE COMPREHENSION

David's mother was concerned about his listening comprehension for text read aloud, his reading comprehension, and his difficulty putting his ideas into writing. As a 10-year-old, David attended a home-school program in which he received special education support from his local county office of education, including services from a resource specialist, occupational therapist, teacher of students with visual impairments, and orientation and mobility specialist.

David's visual diagnosis was widespread rod-cone degeneration. He used his vision well for orientation to avoid obstacles while traveling and to read large print. David had mastered the fundamentals of reading and spelling and had diverse interests including trains, videos, sports statistics, and his family.

David's story retellings, an informal measure of comprehension, were a string of details with little reference to the sequence of the story. He had difficulty identifying the main idea or the problem in a narrative. His understanding seemed literal; he was unable to make inferences or understand the implications of actions or events.

Although David had many creative ideas to express, he spoke in very simple, short sentences and struggled to get them into writing. David could handle structured tasks much better than open-ended ones that lacked a clear completion point or well-defined product.

Learning the Meaning of Language

Semantics is the aspect of communication that deals with word meanings and vocabulary. Semantics refers to the labeling of objects, actions, and relationships in the world. In general, an individual's knowledge of objects and actions and the relationships between them is learned through exposure, experience, and personal interests. A typically developing student learns the labels for concrete objects and for actions by a combination of visual, auditory, and kinesthetic input. For a student with a visual impairment, language labels are learned through these same channels, but the importance of the auditory and kinesthetic channels increases with the severity of the student's visual impairment. Children with low vision can use vision for learning with appropriate modifications for their individual vision needs. Some students, such as David, may fail to use language successfully to compensate for their visual impairments. In such cases, impediments to listening for meaning become a major stumbling block on the road to learning. The impact of listening comprehension varies widely depending on the magnitude and pervasiveness of the student's language weaknesses. At the extreme end of the continuum, students may appear to be hearing impaired or deaf because they do not respond in any observable fashion to verbal input due to lack of understanding on their part.

Students with visual impairments may be vulnerable to gaps in the acquisition of semantics or word meanings, as David was in the vignette just presented, unless they receive deliberate and repeated hands-on exposure to a variety of experiences and concepts. It is difficult, for example, to understand the essence of animal fur or snake skin from a verbal description only. Therefore, providing constant opportunities for direct experience is a sound technique for building semantics. Chapters 2 and 3 provide detailed descriptions of methods for promoting the development of language concepts, but for some students these will not be sufficient. It is of paramount importance to identify students with visual impairments for whom the acquisition of the meaning of language is deficient despite careful instruction and exposure. These students, like David, have language comprehension difficulties that are unexpected based on their cognitive ability and the accommodations that have been provided to compensate for their visual impairments. It is important to recognize that students who have difficulties with receptive language (language comprehension) often have accompanying expressive language difficulties. Although expressive language difficulties are beyond the focus of this book, sometimes a student's difficulty in expressing his or her ideas is more easily recognized and may alert a teacher or parent to the possibility that the student is also having difficulty with comprehension.

Generally speaking, research on the acquisition of language has revealed relatively small quantitative differences between the size of vocabulary of children who are blind and that of children who are sighted (Bigelow, 2005; Brambring, 2003, 2005). Fraiberg (1977) was the first researcher to document that, overall, children with visual impairments attain milestones such as uttering the first word at the same ages as their peers who are sighted. Other research has indicated that although children who are blind experience a slight delay in the acquisition of their first meaningful words, they overcome this delay rapidly, so that generally no qualitative differences can be found when 10- or 50-word vocabularies are compared (Bigelow, 2005).

However, Bigelow and Brambring have found qualitative or characteristic differences between the *types* of words used by children who are blind and the types used by children who are sighted. Children who are blind tend to use more specific nouns; that is, they may use *high chair* to refer a specific chair but may have difficulty generalizing that differently shaped chairs all belong to the category of *chair*. Children who are blind also find it difficult to acquire spatial prepositions (Brambring, 2007). They are less able than their sighted peers to perceive their surroundings and the objects or persons located within them. Difficulties with comprehension and use of personal and possessive pronouns have also been documented in the literature. Without cues from facial expressions and gestures that frequently accompany the roles of speaker and listener, for example, it is apparently more difficult to learn to correctly classify personal pronouns such as *I* and *you* (Brambring, 2007). On the other hand, children who are blind appear to learn to name objects spontaneously and can give their own first names, along with their addresses, at an earlier age than can sighted children.

The teacher of students with visual impairments, the teaching team, and parents may notice that a student is slow in development of vocabulary and has a poor understanding of language concepts and verbal directions. Many students with extended periods of echolalia (immediate or delayed repetition of words or phrases) have great difficulty attaching meaning to new words, phrases, and sentences that they hear. Sidebar 9.3 lists characteristics that are likely to indicate problems with semantics and language comprehension.

Before coming to any conclusions about the listening skills of a student who is visually impaired or blind, it is important to consider the environmental support, or lack thereof, for listening to language. In the preschool and early elementary school years, visual materials predominate. The presence of visual information in the surrounding environment provides many supports for students with unimpaired vision for maintaining attention and obtaining clues about the topic of discussion and details being referred to verbally. However, when students with visual impairment are not sufficiently prompted or supported by being provided with routine "calls to attention" cues, tactile materials, and hands-on opportunities for exploration, they may appear distracted, inattentive, or unengaged, that is, judged as poor listeners with poor comprehension.

The signs of language comprehension difficulties sometimes coincide with symptoms of other difficulties, including attention deficit/hyperactivity disorder (ADHD), an auditory processing disorder, slow processing speed, autism spectrum disorders and intellectual disability, potentially masking the source of the problem. Conversely, some behaviors that frequently accompany visual impairment, such as echolalia and atypical hand movements, may be misinterpreted as signs of difficulties with language comprehension. These circumstances make it possible to overlook comprehension problems and disabilities in the area of receptive language in students with visual impairments and attribute these delays to poor visual skills. When a student's classroom performance is negatively affected by poor listening skills, the IEP team should consider a language assessment and implementation of accommodations discussed thoughout this chapter.

((SIDEBAR 9.3
Red Flags for Disorders Related to Semantics and Language Comprehension

When the difficulties in listening comprehension relate to semantics, or understanding the meaning of language, the characteristics in the following list are likely to be present. Although these characteristics *may* indicate the presence a receptive language disorder, for students with visual impairments it is also important to consider how their development of language skills compares with that of other students who have visual impairments.

Children with disorders related to semantics and language comprehension may display the following characteristics:

- history of delayed language acquisition
- longer than average response time for questions and for conversational turn taking
- limited receptive vocabulary
- difficulty following directions
- periods of confusion or "checking out"
- off-topic responses or responses related to an earlier topic
- poor comprehension for story details, main idea, or inferences
- extended periods of echolalia

These characteristics also *may* be accompanied by expressive language problems, such as the following:

- simple or limited vocabulary
- short sentence length
- simple sentence structure
- use of memorized words and phrases without the underlying knowledge of their meaning

---

Assessment

Based on the concerns about David's understanding and expression of language, his IEP team decided to have him evaluated for a language disorder by the speech-language pathologist, in consultation with other team members. On formal and informal measures, David demonstrated strengths in abstract visual reasoning and spatial orientation, compared to his speech and language abilities. Assessment tools included tests of intellectual functioning and cognitive processing. comprehensive language tests and language samples, as well as puzzles and games that require problem solving skills. His nonverbal reasoning fell in the low-average range when compared to that of his sighted peers, as indicated by standard scores. David's ability to remember and follow verbal directions was poor.

The IEP team determined that David had a receptive and expressive language disorder, which made attaching meaning to the words he heard very challenging for him. He had trouble with language structure and the grammar for more than the simplest of sentences. This affected his ability to understand what he heard and to express his ideas.

If educational team members are seeing evidence indicating that a student is having difficulty with language comprehension, further assessment may be warranted. The speech and language pathologist, in collaboration with the teacher of students with visual impairments, the orientation and mobility specialist, the psychologist, the family, and the teaching team, needs to contribute to the diagnosis of a receptive language disorder. The teacher of students with visual impairments can provide essential information to the speech pathologist and psychologist regarding the appropriateness of visual materials used in assessment and how to adapt test materials, such as enlarging text or pictures, using a video magnifier or other assistive technology, or creating greater visual contrast when a student uses vision. For those who do not use vision, braille, objects, or both will be needed. Both the teacher of students with visual impairments and the orientation and mobility specialist have critical information to share concerning the student's concept knowledge. Because formal speech and language tests are not normed on students with visual impairments, the speech and language pathologist needs to use other means of assessing the students, such as informal measures, observations, interviews, and review of records including psychological testing, in addition to well-chosen formal tests, in order to determine whether the student's behavior is the result of a receptive language disorder. Frequently used speech-language assessment tools are listed in the Resources section.

Children who speak a language other than English (or the dominant language of their society) at home need to be tested in that language if possible. It is necessary to distinguish whether the child's ability to understand and communicate in English is the source of difficulties in understanding language, not his or her competence with spoken language in general. (See Chapter 10 for additional information about English language learners.)

Strategies for Promoting Language Comprehension

Once it was determined that David had a receptive and expressive language disorder, his IEP team added the services of a speech and language pathologist to his program. Goals were set to build vocabulary and receptive language (comprehension) and to increase the length and complexity of his sentences expressively.

In concert with his language goals, the resource specialist added instruction in plot and story structure, using graphic organizers (visual or tactile representations of text, concepts, or ideas) to record information and represent the relationship of the ideas to each other. Building from the models of stories read and studied, David was guided to write his own stories using parallel structures. Graphic organizers helped him record his ideas using a note-taking technique. These notes were then expanded into sentences and paragraphs.

For reading comprehension, the amount of time spent previewing the story was increased to help David learn new vocabulary and to build and activate his background knowledge. Pauses during story reading were structured into a review of details, as well as queries designed to encourage summarizing, predicting, and inference. This same process was used by the teacher of students with visual impairments during work with David to teach him how to use recorded literature and curriculum materials.

David's teacher of students with visual impairments is an active member of his instructional team. In addition to making certain that David's learning materials were visually accessible, the teacher of students with visual impairments helped choose and develop forms of the graphic organizers for note taking that were accessible for David. These diagrams rely on physical layout and visual information to represent the interrelationships between ideas. Some experimentation was needed to determine the best means for David to record notes in preparation for writing. These activities were carried out in conjunction with the resource specialist and speech and language pathologist.

The purpose of language is as a vehicle for conveying meaning, that is, communicating ideas. Unless that purpose is achieved, language is merely a random string of sounds. The goal of any communicative partner in conversation is to provide language in a way that can be understood in the moment it is presented; in other words, there needs to be comprehensible input combined with the student's ability to comprehend the information. Only when the language that is expressed can be understood is the child able to learn (Krashen, 2003).

When assessment has determined that a student has difficulty with comprehension, those who work with the student need to investigate the source of the student's difficulties and make plans to implement supports and compensatory strategies. Initially, the IEP team analyzes how to improve the comprehensibility of the input provided to the student and develops appropriate support strategies. (See also the discussion of comprehensible input related to an auditory processing disorder earlier in this chapter). These beginning steps are discussed in this section, followed by recommended strategies tailored for both preschool and primary-grade students and for middle elementary and beyond. Strategies to promote listening and language comprehension are covered extensively here because they are so critical for all students with visual impairments, including those with additional listening difficulties. (See also the discussions of listening comprehension in Chapters 3, 4, and 5.) Strategies and techniques in this section may also be helpful for students with attention or auditory processing difficulties.

Providing Comprehensible Input

A critical first step for language comprehension is to ensure that the delivery of the material presented to the student is clear. Clear input is affected by a variety of factors, particular to both the student and the environment. The student's educational team needs to consider the acoustic environment, as well as the language load (the length and complexity of the material) for the content that the student is expected to understand. Difficulties may arise from the medium (delivery mode, such as lecture versus audio recordings) or the message (language content/ideas) or both. Although it is not always possible to determine precisely the source of the problem, trying out different intervention strategies and techniques can help determine which ones have a positive effect to promote optimal listening comprehension. In addition to factors related to language, attention and auditory processing, discussed earlier in this chapter, may affect a student's reception of the auditory information.

Teachers and parents need to strive to present information in a form that is most likely to be received by the listener, that is, to provide comprehensible input. Language adjustments may involve

- simpler vocabulary
- simpler or shorter sentence structure, or both
- repetition
- paraphrasing
- segmenting or chunking information by dividing its delivery with pauses and gestures
- stopping frequently to check for understanding and clarifying as needed

Providing Environmental and Multisensory Supports

Because they may miss verbal information, students with visual impairments and listening difficulties benefit from increased emphasis on the naturally occurring environment. Helping these students to become oriented in time and space, in a developmentally appropriate manner, can support them in learning concepts, anticipating what will happen next, and making appropriate generalization to new tasks, as in the following examples. Large-print, braille, or audio-recorded directions can provide the student with multiple sources for obtaining information.

▸ The *time of day, based on the sequence of the classroom schedule,* can cue the student that it is time for group circle, and he or she can anticipate counting the number of classmates present.

▸ The student's *position in the room* can cue the student that it is time for art, and he or she can anticipate discovering new materials and textures.

▸ A *routine sequence in a series of steps* can cue the student that he or she needs to throw away the napkin after lunch.

▸ Presenting the student with two *objects* can cue the student to make a choice between the two items.

Language Comprehension Strategies for Preschool and Primary Grades

An overall strategy for supporting language comprehension in beginning language learners with visual impairments in preschool and primary grades is to tap into their own interests and comment upon them. Taking these interests and expanding upon them helps engage and maintain a young learner's attention. This section addresses strategies and techniques to assist a student's language learning, including the following:

▸ functional routines

▸ calendar systems

▸ use of objects to support language growth

▸ vocabulary development

▸ development of higher-level comprehension through guided listening

Using Functional Routines throughout the Day

Functional routines—recurrent events that provide a predictable structure to a child's life—create a meaningful and repetitive structure that is essential for learning language for students with visual impairments and comprehension difficulties. These ordered sequences allow the student to anticipate events, promoting active participation and creating a sense of security and control over events. Routines, such as activities within a student's school day or the steps for making a snack, provide a natural way for learning vocabulary, concepts, and sequences. For example, a snack routine includes steps for washing and drying hands, steps for collecting ingredients, steps for eating, and steps for cleaning up, all conducted in the natural environment. The inherent repetition and context provided by routines introduces and reinforces the information the student is learning, which supports the student in understanding and beginning to use the new knowledge.

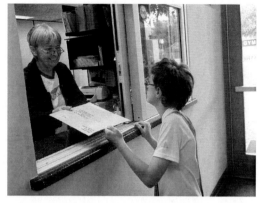

Routines, such as a school job, provide a natural way for learning vocabulary, concepts, and sequences. This student has learned the steps for delivering the school mail.

Lizbeth A. Barclay

Auditory (recorded), brailled, picture, object, icon, or written cues can be used to outline and organize work expectations, daily schedules, and activity sequences, such as steps to preparing lunch or a snack. For those times when a routine needs to change, it is important to provide an explicit explanation. In addition, use of a written or physical symbol to represent change needs to be considered for such situations, depending on the student's visual needs. The symbol would be inserted into the calendar box, written or placed on an activity chart, or other system—for example, the universal *no* sign (a circle with a slash running through it) for a cancellation, or a plus sign for an addition (+). These can be embossed paper icons placed within the chart or large print icons. For the student who is blind, an object or tactile symbol can be used for this same purpose. This serves as a reminder when referring to the schedule, activity list, or calendar box later.

The following is an example of the steps in a routine for watering plants, an appropriate routine for a primary school–age student that can be used to reinforce vocabulary and concepts:

▸ Locate the plants in the classroom.
▸ Check the soil to see if it is wet or dry.
▸ Bring the plant to the sink to water it, or water it in its location in the class.
▸ Locate the watering can.
▸ Fill the can with water.

▸ Water the plant.

▸ Feel the soil and the tray to determine when the plant is wet.

▸ Return everything to its place and clean up.

This routine supports the understanding of individual descriptive vocabulary items, such as *wet* or *dry*; directional vocabulary, such as "Find the plant *next* to the refrigerator"; and time sequences with words, such as *first* and *last*. It provides a predictable sequence from which to anticipate next steps and to participate more actively.

Establishing a Calendar System

In curricula for students with visual impairments and multiple disabilities, a calendar system refers to a method for representing activities or events within a sequence. The sequence may refer to the morning activities, such as arrival routines, or a sequence of steps in a prevocational job. A divided calendar box or a strip can be designed with real objects or parts of objects attached to some type of backing used to represent the steps in the sequence. For young students, the calendar would consist of two distinct containers with objects representing *now* and *done*. (Additional information about calendar systems appears in Chapter 7.)

The details of the system for a particular student are a collaborative decision by the student's IEP team and may require some trial and error with respect to what icons to use, how frequently to present the calendar, and where to place the calendar. Once the system is designed, the student could then look at the activity icon (for example, a juice glass), perform the snack preparation activity, return to the calendar, and then put the object into a "done" box. Once established, the system needs to remain consistent, accompanied by a consistent language script that occurs across activities. Examples of language for the snack activity are: "Time for snack and "Put the juice glass in the 'done' box." (For further information on how to set up a calendar system and use it effectively, see *Calendars*, by Blaha [2001], and *Tangible Symbol Systems Manual*, by Rowland and Schweigert [2000].)

Supplementing Language Input with Relevant Objects

In order to maximize opportunities for comprehension, the educational team can decide upon a standardized language repertoire to accompany regularly occurring activities and routines. This labels the activity and sets it apart from other classroom events. The goal is to match language with its referent in the clearest manner possible. For the young student, handing the student a tambourine while saying "Time for music" makes the words very clear and salient. The tambourine helps define "music" and supports the message that music is the next activity. Consistent use of an object paired with a phrase helps the student form the association more quickly and avoids confusion.

Larson and McKinley (2003) used the phrase *narrow listening opportunities* to refer to situations in which key vocabulary is purposefully controlled and frequently repeated. For the student with visual impairments, teachers often use this technique during routine daily jobs such as taking attendance to the office. The student hears words and sentences in a real context, such as "Keep going straight," "Put it in the box," or "Good morning," and associates them with particular actions and the environmental context. The teacher may repeat words that represent spatial concepts, for instance, *over* and *under*, in many situations, such as in gross-motor activities, desktop activities, or adaptive physical education, without using a lot of additional language before or after these key words. For the language learner, isolating words or phrases in this way separates the most important information from the less important and allows the student to focus on learning in a less verbally cluttered environment.

The selected vocabulary and concepts to be taught through real experience and daily routines can also be represented through enlarged or high-contrast pictures, line drawings, or objects in a scrapbook, with the word or concept label written near it. The scrapbook can be revisited numerous times, "reading" the images by labeling them orally. Some students can learn language structure and vocabulary more readily through reading and writing than through listening and conversation.

Objects provide a natural and concrete way to augment a student's understanding of language. Objects can be used multiple times within a classroom routine, circle time, or curriculum to provide the student with the consistency and exposure necessary to fully understand the language and specific vocabulary. Team members need to jointly agree on words and phrases to label objects and actions consistently while communicating with the student. When different teachers refer to the same item or activity with different labels, it can be potentially confusing. Objects can make concepts in a story more concrete and understandable, and an object can serve as a symbol to represent an activity, either during conversation about an activity that has taken place or to represent part of an activity sequence.

Real objects, or parts of objects, are always preferable to representative objects such as plastic models or miniatures, because the sensory features of such models frequently do not provide meaningful information to students with little or no vision. Please see the Resources section at the back of this book for sources of information about using real objects for language and comprehension support.

Organizing Instruction with a Unifying Topic

An integrated, thematic approach is a practical way to expand a student's vocabulary for understanding and expression; this type of approach provides multiple opportunities for the student to hear and use the targeted words frequently within a short period of time. Lessons and units of study need to be planned to incorporate all areas of language arts—listening, speaking, reading, and writing—combined with experiential learning, that is, the use of real objects with hands-on activities.

Thematic teaching is a technique for organizing instruction across different subject areas, domains of the expanded core curriculum, and designated instructional services (different teachers or service providers). Instruction can be organized into thematic units (broad topics, such as transportation), around a specific concept (such as climate), around a specific piece of literature (such as *Corduroy* [Freeman, 1968]) or around a specific vocabulary item (such as latitude) which is taught in a variety of activities throughout the student's day. Thematic teaching is a highly effective and appropriate technique for students who have receptive language disorders because it explicitly links categories of information, highlighting vocabulary and concepts in a multisensory and repetitive fashion. Although this method is more commonly employed during preschool and the primary grades, it can be extended to children at any age and developmental level by choosing appropriate topics and activities. For example, some middle and high schools coordinate their history and language arts courses so that students read or listen to the literature of the same time period, country, or region that they are studying in history.

Themes such as "All about Me," the senses, foods, clothing, nature, and the community are appropriate for many younger students. Other examples include family, work/job awareness, and "Transportation in My Neighborhood." An example of a unit-based curriculum, designed around the theme of water, is presented in Sidebar 9.4.

((SIDEBAR 9.4
Thematic Unit: Water

Thematic units are planned around a topic that has many related categories. They provide a way to help students learn about commonalities and differences. A thematic unit, such as water, allows teachers to connect information that students may have originally learned separately into a unified category.

Categories of Ways We Use Water

Recreation and Leisure	At Home	Vocational
Swimming	Brushing your teeth	Watering plants
Sink and float games	Washing	Washing cars
Playing in the sprinkler	Making a snack	Selling lemonade
Painting with watercolors	Making ice	Mopping the floor

Source: Adapted from L. Hagood, *Communication: A Guide for Teaching Students with Visual and Multiple Impairments* (Austin: Texas School for the Blind and Visually Impaired, 1997).

Many vocabulary items and concepts can be emphasized through this type of teaching, such as *heavy/light, dry/wet, cold/hot*. For more information about thematic units, see Hagood (1997), O'Sail et al. (2001), and Lybolt (2007).

Monitoring and Supporting Vocabulary Development

Vocabulary development runs as an undercurrent throughout this discussion of language comprehension; however, vocabulary also needs to be an important focus in its own right throughout the school years and, indeed, beyond. Fully sighted typical learners maintain a vocabulary growth rate of about 3,500 words per year until age 30, for a total vocabulary of close to 100,000 words (Gleitman & Newport, 1995). Supporting the learning of all this vocabulary for students with visual impairments with objects and hands-on experiences is a time-consuming challenge that needs to be addressed proactively.

Vocabulary learning takes place both incidentally—through observation—and through direct instruction. Effective instruction makes use of lessons and activities that ensure that students encounter the words they need to learn both embedded in context and explicitly discussed and demonstrated. For example, carving pumpkins and roasting pumpkin seeds in conjunction with reading books about Halloween and the harvest provide a context in which vocabulary instruction can take place while learning subject material and enjoying literature.

Text Talk (Beck & McKeown, 2001; McKeown & Beck, 2003) is a research-based method of vocabulary instruction that coordinates well with an organized program in which the teacher reads stories aloud to students to incorporate background knowledge and vocabulary development along with the enjoyment of story. Key features of Text Talk include active involvement, asking open-ended questions, and a gradual increase in the expectations for students to take on more responsibility for their own vocabulary learning (Graves, 2006).

Books chosen for the Text Talk method need to have a plot structure that will capture students' interest, motivate them to participate in the discussion, and promote higher-level thinking. Two to four vocabulary words from the book are selected to focus on. The read-aloud starts with a discussion of the students' prior knowledge related to the topic of the book. As the book is read aloud, the teacher pauses periodically to encourage discussion that will guide comprehension; students may be encouraged to predict what will happen next. Vocabulary words essential to understanding the plot need to be explained briefly.

After the story is read, directed vocabulary work takes place with activities designed to enhance student participation, motivate students to make the word "their own," and clarify and enrich word knowledge. Each focus vocabulary word is highlighted within the context of the story and the sentence or sentences in which it occurs. The students are asked to repeat the word ("Say it with me") to create a phonological representation and allow them to hear the cadence and feel the movements of their mouths as they say it. The teacher explains the meaning and then provides a second example of how the word is used. Discussion aims to extend understanding of the word from the context in the story to other suitable contexts. Students are asked to give an example of another way they might use the word, and sentences are adjusted and rehearsed to ensure that the usage is accurate. For example, if the story character was desperately looking for a lost item, the teacher would be working to extend the concept of *desperation* to other contexts beyond *lost* and *looking for,* such as desperately wishing for a certain toy as a birthday gift or desperately waiting for a ride to a friend's house.

The guidelines for Text Talk suggest working with one to two books per week (Beck, McKeown, & Kucan, 2002). Words that are most useful for instructional focus for primary-level students are frequently occurring, high-utility words that are essential for comprehension and concept learning and create the opportunity to build deeper understanding and form connections with other words and concepts. Such words build conceptual understanding through their precision and specificity. For example, when using the Text Talk approach with *A Pocket for Corduroy* (Freeman, 1978), the teacher might introduce the word *reluctant* in the context of the girl being reluctant to leave the laundromat when she couldn't find Corduroy, her toy bear.

In preschool and for primary-level students with weak vocabulary skills, it may be necessary to concentrate on more basic words (such as *clock, baby, happy, walk*) and other concrete nouns, actions, or feelings that need explicit representation for the struggling language learner who is blind or visually impaired. (Further discussion of vocabulary development at the higher level appears in "Strategies for the Middle Elementary Level and Beyond" later in this chapter.)

Supporting Higher-Level Comprehension

An active process of constructing meaning and the explicit teaching of comprehension strategies are essential for struggling learners (Fielding & Pearson, 1994). Higher-level comprehension, beyond literal recall, requires prioritizing, summarizing, and connecting. Literature and research on comprehension strategies within the field of reading apply equally to the process of comprehension when listening, particularly the auditory comprehension of texts. Such strategies may be implemented before, during, or after reading—or, in this case, listening (Carlisle & Rice, 2002). Strategies such as activating background knowledge with students by discussing what they may already know about a topic, and previewing the topic take place prior to listening to the material. During listening, strategies such as stopping to summarize, making connections, and predicting are appropriate. Strategies that take place after listening are ones that involve synthesizing and interpreting. Many highly effective comprehension instructional practices support the listener throughout all three portions of the experience. For example, K-W-L (Know-Want to Know-Learned) and Predict-Support-Adjust strategies, discussed later in this chapter, begin before the listening experience but are revisited during and after the listening event.

Guided Listening

Guided reading of a text by a teacher is a process of modeling the noticing, thinking, and questioning that a person needs to do as he or she makes sense of the text. The goal is to provide a window into the thinking behind good comprehension; that understanding is constructed of connecting and extending information. The teacher explicitly states what a reader or listener might think and how the reader would combine information, think about related information or situations, and seek information from somewhere else in order to make sense of the passage. In this way, comprehension is presented as an active process of constructing meaning. Guided listening is one purpose for teacher read-alouds. It is designed to bridge the gap between teacher lessons and discussions, on the one hand, and students' independent application of the comprehension skills they have learned and practiced, on the other.

For example, a teacher reading *Corduroy* (Freeman, 1968) might pause to say, "Oh, this makes me remember a time when I was little and I wanted something, but my mother tried to tell me that it wasn't worth having," or "One time when I was about six, I saved up my money for a month to buy something, and it was *so* hard to not spend my allowance on little things so I could get it."

During guided listening, the teacher guides the student to use comprehension strategies appropriate for the passage and purpose of the reading. The teacher might ask for predictions or pose open-ended questions, such as, "What do you think Norman was feeling?" or "What is a good ending for the story?" The teacher might also ask questions that allow students to take more of a lead, such as "What are you wondering?" or "What does Brian's situation remind you of?" The purpose of such questioning is to encourage students to think beyond a literal understanding of the text, to connect ideas within the story or with their background knowledge, and to consider the various story elements, including setting, plot, and point of view, at a deeper level. The role of the teacher is to provide support (scaffolding) to help students get to the next stage or level of thinking. These types of strategies were very effective for David in the vignette at the beginning of this section, and were among those taught to Maya's mother discussed in an earlier section.

Depending on the lesson focus, a fiction or nonfiction text might be chosen for the guided listening activity. Literature selections support discussions of story elements (characters, setting, and so on) and plot structure for narratives. Biographical and history selections assist with an emphasis on sequence or cause and effect. Nonfiction selections (on topics such as animals, natural phenomena, and the like) can provide a backdrop for other methods of examining logical connections between ideas, such as compare and contrast, cause and effect, or main idea and supporting details. Buehl (2001) recommended that for this purpose teachers choose selections with a clear structure—those that constitute an organized, coherent whole with interrelated ideas rather than those that consist of a series of descriptions, such as a picture book of animals.

Predict-Support-Adjust. The Predict-Support-Adjust strategy is highly effective for promoting engagement and teaching students that predictions need to be derived from solid evidence that can be described or explained. It promotes active listening by guiding the student to make logical predictions based on prior knowledge and information from the text. This helps students develop logical connections and discourages students from making wild, unsubstantiated guesses. Students are asked to predict what will happen, or what will happen next, in a book being read to them, and need to explain how they arrived at the idea; that is, what information supports the prediction. Students' predictions and supporting information are recorded in the first two columns of a three-column chart: "Predict" and "Support." After a portion of the text is read or listened to, the discussion returns to the original predictions. Some will be confirmed; some will be modified. This information is recorded in the final column, "Adjust." A quality prediction is grounded in evidence, whether it is accurate or not in terms of the outcome in the story. Although it may not always be feasible to create a group chart that can be read, this valuable monitoring strategy can be adopted in teacher read-alouds and guided listening activities if the instructor takes notes and returns to the ideas to adjust the predictions and allow for revisions.

K-W-L Strategy. For nonfiction text, use of the K-W-L strategy (Ogle, 1986) is appropriate in the primary grades and can be continued for older students. The strategy of K-W-L focuses on setting a purpose for reading or listening. The information can be recorded in a chart with three columns. First, students are guided to focus on what they already know (K) about a topic. Once this background knowledge has been elicited, students are encouraged to state information they want to know or wonder (W). Finally, students are asked what they have learned (L) from what they have read or heard as a summarizing activity. The K-W-L model provides a structure for the important comprehension strategies of activating background knowledge, setting a purpose (that is, searching for new information about predetermined topics), and summarizing learning. The format can also be used to guide information gathering, a research unit, or a nonfiction book read-aloud. It provides a way to keep track of information in order to return to it later to continue the discussion.

Strategies for the Middle Elementary Level and Beyond

As students gain more listening experience and grapple with more complex topics, instructional focus necessarily changes. As students mature, they are learning to handle more abstract concepts and topics with an increasing number of details. They may also need to begin to prioritize the relative importance of information. Thus, as students move into late elementary school and beyond, they require a different style of instruction and support.

Many of the techniques and instructional strategies discussed here for older students apply to both reading and listening comprehension and concept learning in subject areas such as science and social studies. Whether instruction is provided by listening to audio versions of text or by structured lessons and discussions, students with visual impairments who have concomitant language comprehension difficulties require active systems to support their language and content comprehension.

Strategies for older students include methods for the following:

- ▶ teaching of active listening
- ▶ comprehension strategies to teach and use prior to listening
- ▶ comprehension strategies to support review and learning after the listening experience
- ▶ explicit vocabulary instruction
- ▶ teaching strategies for note taking

Teaching Strategies and Techniques That Support Good Listening

For students who are at the stage in their educational career when subject content learning predominates, it is essential for instructors to recognize that the skills of listening for details and remembering, as well as study techniques, do not necessarily develop naturally and automatically. Strategies and techniques to use prior to listening to the material involve both the presenter and the listener. Instructors need to revisit the concept of making input comprehensible, discussed previously in this chapter, that is, methods of presenting information so that it is organized and more easily understood. Readers may also want to revisit the sections on active listening in Chapters 4 and 5.

Many of the strategies listed in the sections on pre- and post-listening strategies need to be explicitly taught to students and practiced. Class time may need to be specifically scheduled for some of these steps until students have internalized the study cycle.

Pre-listening Strategies

In contrast to casual conversation, lectures and teacher's classroom instruction are packed with information that the student needs to comprehend, connect with other information, and learn. Knowing strategies for being a competent and attentive listener is a start, but students also need to understand that review and study of the information is usually necessary to comprehend and remember it. The following pre-listening strategies prepare students for listening to learn:

▶ Help students become aware of the difference between good and bad listening habits. For example, good listeners get ready to listen when cued by the teacher that a new topic or activity is about to begin (Larson & McKinley, 2003). Poor listeners are still shuffling through their backpacks while the teacher has begun instruction.

▶ Help students be mentally prepared to listen. Explicitly review the previous day's materials and then relate them to the current day's topic.

▶ Teach students to listen for organizing cues. Guide them to listen for verbal cues that signal key points or introductory statements, for example, "Today we will discuss," "In summary," "First of all," "Then," and so on.

▶ Demonstrate and discuss the use of emphasis that can cue students to key ideas. These cues may be verbal, for example, "You need to know," "This is key," "Listen carefully," or they may be nonverbal, for example, a slowed speaking pace, louder volume, repetition of key words or phrases, and asking questions that the speaker answers him- or herself (Deshler, Ellis, & Lenz, 1996).

▶ Guide students to listen for main ideas and supporting ideas. Students can practice by listening to a short lecture and then suggesting a title, summarizing a story, or picking out the main ideas and supporting details. When presented in advance, graphic organizers or guided notes can assist students to focus on essential ideas.

▶ Teach students to ask questions for clarification. Students can be taught how and when to ask questions during a lecture. Provide scripts for the students to use until they have become more expert at the technique. Possible phrases include "Can you explain . . . ?" and "What did you mean when you said . . . ?"

Post-listening Strategies

Following a lecture or class discussion, students need to be responsible for ensuring that they have understood the information and have the notes or study guides to review in order to prepare for any tests or culminating activity. To reinforce listening after the lecture, Larson & McKinley (2003) suggested that students do the following:

- ▸ review materials and key ideas
- ▸ add missed information and correct or modify notes
- ▸ ask questions about the lecture
- ▸ write a set of summary statements and conclusions; rewrite the ideas in their own words
- ▸ review their notes before the next lecture
- ▸ employ pre-listening strategies to prepare for the next lecture

These techniques rely in part on students' ability to take notes that they will understand later, notes that accurately record the information that they are expected to learn. Note taking is an art in and of itself and is discussed in more detail later in this chapter.

Explicitly Teach Vocabulary

Vocabulary knowledge has long been established as highly correlated with reading comprehension (Carlisle & Rice, 2002; Tabors, Snow, & Dickinson, 2001). Likewise, it is expected that it would strongly affect listening comprehension, both for understanding classroom instruction and discussion and for listening to audio versions of literature and content-area text.

The techniques for vocabulary development used in the Text Talk method (Beck & McKeown, 2001; McKeown & Beck, 2003), discussed earlier in this chapter for students in the preschool and primary grades, can be extended into the higher grades with judicious choices of age- and developmentally appropriate texts. In the older grades, the use of nonfiction texts needs to increase to support content-area learning and essential vocabulary development for those topics. Decisions for vocabulary to study can be made for the book as a whole; there may not be a suitable word in each chapter. A word lesson would take place following any chapter in which one or more words are introduced.

Explicit and direct vocabulary instruction is expected to increase for older students. Students at upper elementary school age and beyond have typically developed a broad word base. By this time, students are ready to refine and expand, clarify and enrich, their word knowledge. Graves (2006) described a variety of activities for working with known and new words that are associated with either known or new concepts, including the use of examples of words that both fit and do not fit the category, as well as explanations of similarities to other words in order to avoid false associations.

Graves (2006) described three methods for clarifying and extending meanings that can be adapted to meet the needs of students with visual impairments because they create a physical representation of the relationships between words and ideas as a chart or graphic organizer. Semantic maps, feature analysis, and Venn diagrams all record information about words and word relationships in ways that allow for an uncluttered spatial representation.

Semantic Maps

Semantic maps are laid out in a grid form around a central concept or topic. Their purpose is similar to that of semantic webs, a diagram of circles and lines that looks like a spider and its web. Semantic webs are often used with younger students; however, the chaotic and subordinate diagramming of word and concept relationships is likely to be confusing for students with visual impairments who may be able to see only one portion of the chart at a time and fail to grasp the gestalt.

Each category in a semantic map is given a physical area, which can be enclosed by a dark or textured line, so that the grouping and separation physically represent the relationships. Graves (2006) provided an example in which telecommunication is the central topic, with separate boxes for costs, types, potential problems, potential benefits, places used, and users. Another example is presented in Figure 9.1. Use of semantic maps also promotes the development of categorization skills.

Semantic Feature Analysis

Semantic feature analysis is a technique for refining students' understanding of word meanings, in which similarities and differences between related words or characteristics that distinguish them are recorded on a grid. The words are listed in a vertical row on the left side, while the features are listed across the top. At the intersection of each word and feature, a plus or minus sign, or both, is inserted to denote whether the characteristic applies to a word. This type of chart can be adapted by enlargement, with braille, or with the use of color or textured symbols. Graves (2006) presented an example comparing different types of roads and walkways (path, road, freeway, and so on) with characteristics such as paved, unpaved, narrow, wide, walking, driving. Sidebar 9.5 gives an example comparing the uses of different rooms in a house.

Venn Diagram

The visual and spatial layout used in a Venn diagram is appropriate for investigating meanings of similar words or terminology—words or labels that have some attributes

((‹ FIGURE 9.1   **Semantic Mapping: An Example**

For a semantic map, information is classified with each category listed in a separate box. It is recommended that the main topic be enclosed in a different shape, such as a circle or an oval, for easier identification. Many adaptations are possible for students with visual impairments based on individual need: Labels might be enlarged or made in braille; pictures may be added; or each category could be a separate card or piece of paper.

Mammals
- Warm-blooded
- Have hair or fur
- Have 4 legs (or 2 legs & 2 arms)
- Have lungs, breathe air
- Have external ears
- Give birth to young
- Most live on land, but some live in water

Examples: human, bear, elephant, mouse, whale

Birds
- Warm-blooded
- Have feathers
- Have 2 legs
- Have wings
- Have ear holes
- Lay eggs

Examples: robin, eagle, chicken, ostrich

Reptiles
- Cold-blooded
- Have scales
- Have dry skin
- Have ear holes
- Usually lay eggs, but some give birth

Examples: turtle, snake, crocodile, lizard

Fish
- Cold-blooded
- Have scales & fins
- Live in water
- Breathe underwater with gills
- Lay many eggs

Examples: trout, salmon, goldfish, guppy, shark

Vertebrates

Animals with a Backbone

Amphibians
- Cold-blooded
- Moist, smooth skin, no hair or fur
- Usually have 4 legs
- Webbed feet
- Breathe with lungs & gills
- Live on land & in water
- Lay many eggs

Examples: frog, toad, salamander, newt

((SIDEBAR 9.5
Semantic Feature Analysis: An Example

A semantic feature analysis is designed to record similarities and differences between vocabulary words to aid in the development of vocabulary precision. This type of charting can be individualized in a variety of ways, based on a student's visual needs and essential features that need to be represented.

Areas of a House

Room	Function						Location	
	Wash	**Cook**	**Sleep**	**Sit**	**Eat**	**Storage**	**Inside**	**Outside**
Kitchen	+	+	–	+	+/–	+	+	–
Bedroom	–	–	+	+	+/–	+	+	–
Living room	–	–	+/–	+	+/–	+	+	–
Bathroom	+	–	–	+/–	–	+	+	–
Dining room	–	–	–	+	+	+	+	–
Patio/deck	–	+/–	+/–	+	+	–	–	+
Garage	+/–	–	–	–	–	+	+/–	+/–
Laundry room	+	–	–	–	–	+	+/–	+/–

\+ The function or location applies to this room
– The function or location does not apply to this room
+/– The function or location may apply, and may not. It is not an essential element.

in common yet cannot be considered synonyms due to a few distinct differences in meaning. A Venn diagram is constructed with two overlapping circles, with their intersection representing the commonalities between two words or concepts; the differences are represented by the sections that do not overlap; terms describing similarities and differences can be listed in the appropriate sections of the diagram. Graves (2006) provided an example that compares features of short stories as fiction and essays as nonfiction. They both are prose, have paragraphs, and vary in difficulty. Short stories are typically read for pleasure and written in first or third person, while essays are often read to learn something and usually written in third person. In the photograph of an adapted Venn diagram, the categories *food* and *plants* are represented.

Teaching Strategies for Text Comprehension

Listening and reading can be considered parallel language functions because they are both forms of receptive language, one based on oral input and the other on written.

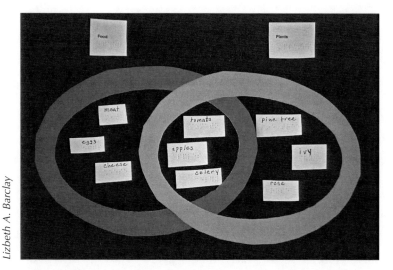

Lizbeth A. Barclay

Venn diagrams are easily adapted to accommodate a range of visual needs, in this case by enlarging the diagram, using texture and contrasting colors, and adding braille to the labels.

Both have an ultimate goal of language comprehension; that is, the language input in either form needs to be processed by the receiving mind before it can have value. For students with visual impairments, listening and reading are doubly intertwined, as students listen not just to lectures and discussions, but also to audio recordings of text or digitized (synthesized) speech. These recordings may be locally recorded, or they may come from Learning Ally (formerly Recordings for the Blind and Dyslexic) or from publishers or a variety of other commercial sources in the form of electronic textbooks. Because of this increased reliance on the auditory mode, students who are visually impaired and have language and learning disabilities require especially strong support. (See also the previous discussion of listening to audio recordings and digital versions of text in the section of this chapter on auditory processing.)

High school and middle school teachers rely on a combination of lecture and text. Listening to expository, nonfiction text to learn new information creates a substantial challenge for students. It is recommended that text comprehension—methods of analyzing text to improve comprehension—be explicitly taught to all students, and particularly to students with language disabilities (Carlisle & Rice, 2002). Many methods for developing comprehension in students base their curricula on Bloom's taxonomy of education objectives (Bloom, 1956), which presents the increasingly complex levels of comprehension and interpretation. These are represented variously as steps, levels in a pyramid, or rungs in a ladder (Wiig & Wilson, 2002), with suggested types of questions at each level for teachers to ask students to elicit increasingly complex levels of understanding. Conscious lesson planning, based on an understanding of how to use these levels of questioning to signal depth of comprehension, can assist teachers and curriculum developers in promoting increased comprehension and higher-order thinking skills.

Reciprocal teaching (Oczkus, 2003) is a technique designed to improve text comprehension for students by teaching the four comprehension strategies of predicting, questioning, clarifying, and summarizing. Although originally developed for reading, these strategies translate well to listening comprehension. Based on the work of Palincsar and Brown (1984), Oczkus's method expands the concepts into lessons suitable for both fiction and nonfiction texts and for a variety of instructional group sizes. All strategies are used with each text, but each receives specific emphasis during a series of lessons designed to deepen students' understanding of the strategies. Texts can be read to, or by, the student, in whatever modified format is necessary. Follow-up activities can be done singly or in cooperative groups, in written form such as a graphic organizer, or through oral discussion and questioning. For students with visual impairments, these lessons may be suitable for inclusionary settings or small-group or individual instruction.

Teaching Note Taking

For older, more academically inclined students, the complexity and density of lecture and text content continue to increase. It is critical that students with language-related learning difficulties have explicit instruction and practice in determining the logical relationships between facts and ideas, as well as their relative importance. Older students are also expected to learn increasingly from text—in print, large print, braille, or audio recordings. Students may listen to recorded text in conjunction with braille or enlarged text. Language and auditory processing difficulties strongly impact students' listening comprehension and consequently their comprehension of the content of the text and/or lecture. (See also information about listening to audio recordings and digital versions of text in the auditory processing section of this chapter and Sidebar 4.9, "Instructional Strategies for Audio-Assisted Reading.")

Note-taking strategies need to be taught to help students become more efficient in outlining key concepts and to provide them with study guides. This relates to both listening to audio versions of text and lectures in the classroom. Some key formats are bulleted lists and charts. Bulleted lists function as a hierarchical form, a modified outline. Charts and graphic organizers are often used to reorganize, prioritize, and integrate ideas; they may be used separately or in conjunction with outline or bulleted systems. For David, the student discussed earlier in this section, graphic organizers used for note taking represented sequence, main idea with supporting detail, and to represent similarities and differences, such as comparing and contrasting.

Materials in content areas such as science and history are often organized with headings and subheadings that may be conducive to outlining. Instructors likewise can adopt a standard format for lectures or reading of texts aloud in the classroom to refer to an idea's place within the hierarchy of ideas; for example, "There are X [number] of results from the Cuban embargo—Y positive ones and Z negative ones. We'll cover the positive ones first. These are . . . ," and so on. Some instructors choose to label the levels explicitly: "The level 1 idea is that the Cuban embargo had both positive and negative effects." Level 2 would be elucidation of the positive versus negative effects: "The positive effects are . . . ; the negative effects are . . ." These lists would be followed by detailed explanations and descriptions of each effect. When presenting each detailed section, the instructor needs to refer back to the broader category: "The second positive effect was . . ."; "Of the negative effects, B had the strongest impact." Regardless of the structures and specific organizers that the team chooses to teach, it is essential that such key linguistic signals for the relationships between ideas be explicitly taught and discussed with students. These include signal words such as *one*, *another*, *yet another*, *first*, *then*, *finally*, *similarly*, *on the other hand*, *however*, and so on. It is important to recognize that work on listening comprehension also has a strongly positive effect on a student's ability to express ideas in spoken and written language. Students with language impairments benefit from explicit instruction in the specific vocabulary needed to express the relationships between ideas. Well-written texts, whether read or listened to, and translation of key ideas into outlines or organizers provide models for students' future writing.

Keeping track of the increasingly complex ideas and their relationships is supported by visual or tactile representation or both, such as graphic organizers. Oral messages are transient; their physical representation in charts or notes allows the student to refer back to the information to understand and learn it. Listening again to a recording of a book or lecture is time-consuming and often inefficient. Students may have difficulty locating the material they need to review. The notes in charts and organizers may be written in phrases that assist the learner to reconstruct the original content without needing to reread an entire sentence or paragraph. Teachers may want to consider graphic organizers that emphasize key relationships between the ideas being studied. The most prevalent are ones that stress comparing and contrasting, main idea with supporting details, and sequence (such as a timeline for history or a biography).

Learning to be an effective note taker requires instruction and practice. Guidance provided to students needs to be carefully planned to support the student in taking increasing responsibility for note taking. It should begin with demonstrations and teacher think-alouds, then proceed with guided note taking, until the student can function independently. It is helpful for the student's instructional team to collaborate on which note-taking formats they can all adopt; it is much more effective for the student to learn to use a few formats very well than to be exposed superficially to many. (See Chapter 5 for additional information on note taking and electronic note taking).

In the guided note-taking phase, the instructor provides the format for the notes, either a graphic organizer or an outline. The instructor fills out portions of the chart or outline in advance to keep the student on track and to demonstrate the use of key phrases, abbreviations, and so on. As the student has more exposure, the instructor can gradually decrease the amount of information entered in advance.

Although graphic organizers and outlines can serve as notes and study guides, these at first are more likely to be the end product of a discussion or activity subsequent to reading or listening. However, students need to be able to take notes during a lecture or discussion. On a practical level, students need to be taught standard abbreviations that allow them to take notes more quickly. Students can be shown simple ways to create their own abbreviations. These can be adapted from techniques discussed in Deshler et al. (1996), such as omitting vowels (*abt* for *about*), using standard abbreviations or symbols (*st* for *street*, > for *greater than*), using initial letters (*IT* for *information technology*), or using the first several letters (*freq* for *frequent*, *bec* for *because*). Students also need to be made aware that the same abbreviation may mean something different depending on its context; for example, *NA* might mean *North America*, *not applicable*, or *not available* depending on the subject or context.

CONCLUSION

Although the specific source of difficulty in listening cannot always be definitively identified, it is critical that all teaching staff and caregivers be alert to the characteristics of language and learning disabilities within the learning environment, so that they can develop appropriate strategies to meet students' needs. This is true for all students, not just students with visual impairments. After appropriate assessment, the IEP team is encouraged to maintain a practical, goal-oriented focus characterized by diagnostic teaching and periodic adjustments devised to improve learning outcomes. As discussed throughout this chapter, the teacher of students with visual impairments is a critical member of the educational team, in the decision-making process and in the implementation of the interventions chosen.

Early investigation into the reasons for listening difficulties that are beyond those related to visual impairment is critical. When caregivers and a team of professionals understand the student's additional learning challenges, then educational modifications, supports, and interventions can be implemented so the world can be made accessible and comprehensible to each and every student. It is only when we understand what we have heard that true listening can take place.

REFERENCES

American Psychiatric Association. (2000). *Diagnostic and statistical manual of mental disorders* (4th ed., Text Revision) *(DSM-IV-TR).* Washington, DC: American Psychiatric Association.

American Psychiatric Association. (2010). Attention deficit/hyperactivity disorder. Retrieved September 10, 2010, from www.dsm5.org/ProposedRevisions/Pages/proposedrevision .aspx?rid=383.

American Speech-Language-Hearing Association (ASHA). (2005a). (Central) Auditory processing disorders—The role of the audiologist [position statement]. Retrieved July 10, 2010, from www.asha.org/docs/html/PS2005-00114.html.

ASHA. (2005b). (Central) Auditory processing disorders. Washington, DC: American Speech-Language-Hearing Association, Working Group on Auditory Processing Disorders. Retrieved August 8, 2011, from www.asha.org/docs/html/TR2005-00043.html.

ASHA. (2011). Speech language disorders and diseases. Retrieved July 27, 2011, from www.asha.org/public/speech/disorders.

Anthony, J. L., & Lonigan, C. J. (2004). The nature of phonological awareness: Converging evidence from four studies of preschool and early grade school children. *Journal of Educational Psychology, 96*(1), 43–55.

Barkley, R. A. (2000). *Taking charge of ADHD: The complete, authoritative guide for parents.* New York: Guilford Press.

Barkley, R. A. (2005). *ADHD and the nature of self-control.* New York: Guilford Press.

Barnes, A. C., & Harlacher, J. E. (2008). Clearing the confusion: Response-to-intervention as a set of principles. *Education and Treatment of Children, 31*(3), 417–431.

Barraga, N. C., & Erin, J. N. (2001). *Visual impairments and learning* (4th ed.). Austin, TX: Pro-Ed.

Bauwens, J., & Hourcade, J. J. (1989). Hey, would you just L.I.S.T.E.N.? *Teaching Exceptional Children, 21*(4), 61.

Beck, I. L., & McKeown, M. G. (2001). Text talk: Capturing the benefits of read-aloud experiences for young children. *The Reading Teacher, 55,* 10–20.

Beck, I. L., McKeown, M. G., & Kucan, L. (2002). *Bringing words to life: Robust vocabulary instruction.* New York: Guilford Press.

Bellis, T. J. (2003). *Assessment and management of central auditory processing disorders in the educational setting: From science to practice.* Delmar, NY: Thompson Learning.

Bigelow, A. (2005). Blindness. In B. Hopkins (Ed.), *The Cambridge encyclopedia of child development.* New York: Cambridge University Press.

Blachman, B. A., Ball, E. W., Black, R., & Tangel, D. M. (2000). *Road to the code: A phonological awareness program for young children.* Baltimore, MD: Paul H. Brookes Publishing.

Blaha, R. (2001). *Calendars: For students with multiple impairments including deafblindness.* Austin: Texas School for the Blind and Visually Impaired.

Blischak, D. M., Shah, S. D., Lombardino, L. J., & Chiarella, K. (2004). Effects of phonemic awareness instruction on the encoding skills of children with severe speech impairment. *Disability and Rehabilitation, 26*(21–22), 1295–1304.

Bloom, B. S. (1956). *Taxonomy of educational objectives: The classification of educational goals. Handbook I: Cognitive domain.* New York: McKay.

Brambring, M. (2003). Sprachentwicklung blinder Kinder [Language development in children who are blind]. In G. Rickheit, T. Herrrmann, & W. Deutsch (Eds.), *Psycholinguistik: Ein internationals Handbuch* (pp. 730–753). Berlin: de Gruyter.

Brambring, M. (2005). Divergente Entwicklung blinder und sehender Kinder in vier Entwicklungsbereichen [Divergent development in children who are blind or sighted: Four developmental domains]. *Zeitschrift fur Enwicklungspsychologie und Padagogische Psychologie, 37,* 173–183.

Brambring, M. (2007). Divergent development of verbal skills in children who are blind or sighted. *Journal of Visual Impairment & Blindness, 101,* 749–762.

Buehl, D. (2001). *Classroom strategies for interactive learning* (2nd ed.). Newark, DE: International Reading Association.

Carlisle, J. F., & Rice, M. S. (2002). *Improving reading comprehension: Research-based principles and practices.* Baltimore: York Press.

Catts, H., & Kamhi, A. (2005). *Language and reading disabilities* (3rd ed.). Boston: Allyn and Bacon.

Chermak, G. D., & Musiek, F. E. (1997). *Central auditory processing disorders: New perspectives.* San Diego, CA: Singular.

Clark, C., & Stoner, J. B. (2008). An investigation of the spelling skills of braille readers. *Journal of Visual Impairment & Blindness, 102*(9), 553–563.

Conners, C. K. (2008). *Conners* (3rd ed.). San Antonio, TX: Pearson Education.

Council for Exceptional Children. (2007a). Position on Response to Intervention (RTI). Retrieved July 6, 2010, from www.cec.sped.org/AM/Template.cfm?Section=Home& CONTENTID=9640&TEMPLATE=/CM/ContentDisplay.cfm.

Council for Exceptional Children. (2007b). RTI summit delves into implementation, current and future issues. Retrieved July 6, 2010, from www.cec.sped.org/AM/Template.cfm ?Section=Home&CONTENTID=9639&TEMPLATE=/CM/ContentDisplay.cfm.

DeBonis, D. A., Moncrieff, D. (2008). Auditory processing disorders: An update for speech-language pathologists. *American Journal of Speech-Language Pathology, 17,* 4–18.

Deshler, D., Ellis, E., & Lenz, B. (1996). *Teaching adolescents with learning disabilities* (2nd ed.). Denver, CO: Love Publishing Company.

Dodd, B., & Conn, L. (2000). The effect of braille orthography on blind children's phonological awareness. *Journal of Research in Reading, 23,* 1–11.

Dote-Kwan, J., Chen, D., & Hughes, M. (2001). A national survey of service providers who work with young children with visual impairments. *Journal of Visual Impairment & Blindness, 95,* 325–337.

Erin, J. N., & Koenig, A. J. (1997). The student with a visual disability and a learning disability. *Journal of Learning Disabilities, 30*(3), 309–320.

Ferrell, K. A., with Shaw, A. R., & Dietz, S. J. (1998). *Project PRISM: A longitudinal study of developmental patterns of children who are visually impaired.* Greeley: University of Northern Colorado.

Fielding, L. G., & Pearson, P. D. (1994). Reading comprehension: What works. *Educational Leadership, 51*(5), 62–68.

Fraiberg, S. (1977). *Insights from the blind: Comparative studies of blind and sighted infants.* New York: New American Library.

Freeman, D. (1968). *Corduroy.* New York: Viking Press.

Freeman, D. (1978). *A pocket for Corduroy.* New York: Viking Press.

Fuchs, D., & Fuchs, L., (2006). Introduction to response to intervention: What, why, and how valid is it? *Reading Research Quarterly, 41*(1), 93–99.

Fuchs, D., Mock, D., Morgan, P. L., & Young, C. L., (2003). Responsiveness-to-intervention: Definitions, evidence, and implications for the learning disabilities construct. *Learning Disabilities and Practice, 18*(3), 157–171.

Gillon, G. T. (2004). *Phonological awareness: From research to practice.* New York: Guilford Press.

Gillon, G. T., & Young, A. A. (2002). The phonological awareness skills of children who are blind. *Journal of Visual Impairment & Blindness, 96,* 38–49.

Gleitman, L. R., & Newport, E. L. (1995). The invention of language by children: Environmental and biological influences on the acquisition of language. In L. R. Gleitman & M. Liberman (Eds.), *An invitation to cognitive science,* Vol. 1, *Language.* Boston: MIT Press.

Goodman, S., & Wittenstein, S. (2003). *Collaborative assessment working with students who are blind or visually impaired, including those with additional disabilities.* New York: AFB Press.

Graves, M. F. (2006). *The vocabulary book: Learning and instruction.* New York: Teachers College Press.

Haager, D., Klingner, J. K., & Vaughn, S. (Eds.). (2007). *Evidence-based reading practices for response to intervention.* Baltimore, MD: Paul H. Brookes Publishing.

Hagood, L. (1997). *Communication: A guide for teaching students with visual and multiple impairments.* Austin: Texas School for the Blind and Visually Impaired.

Hatton, D. D. (2001). Model registry of early childhood visual impairment: First-year results. *Journal of Visual Impairment & Blindness, 95,* 418–433.

Hunt, R. D. (2006). Functional roles of norepinephrine and dopamine in ADHD: NE function. *Medscape Psychiatry & Mental Health, 11*(1). Available from www.medscape.org/viewarticle/523887.

Individuals with Disabilities Education Improvement Act of 2004 (IDEA), Pub. L. No. 108-446 (2004).

Jerger, J., & Musiek, F. (2000). Report of the consensus conference on the diagnosis of auditory processing disorders in school-aged children. *Journal of the American Academy of Audiology, 11*, 467–474.

Kame'enui, E. J. (1996). Shakespeare and beginning reading: "The readiness is all." *Teaching Exceptional Children, 28*(2), 77–81.

Kovaleski, J. F. (2007). Response to intervention: Considerations for research and systems change. *School Psychology Review, 36*(4), 638–646.

Krashen, S. (2003). *Explorations in language acquisition and use.* Portsmouth, NH: Heinemann.

Larson, V. L., & McKinley, N. (2003). *Communications solutions for older students assessment and intervention strategies.* Eau Claire, WI: Thinking Publications.

Loftin, M. (2005). *Making evaluation meaningful: Determining additional eligibilities and appropriate instructional strategies for blind and visually impaired students.* Austin: Texas School for the Blind and Visually Impaired.

Lybolt, J. (2007). *Building language throughout the year.* Baltimore, MD: Paul H. Brookes Publishing.

McCauley, R. H., & Fey, M. E. (2006). *Treatment of language disorders in children.* Baltimore, MD: Paul H. Brookes Publishing.

McKeown, M. G., & Beck, I. L. (2003). Taking advantage of read alongs to help children make sense of decontextualized language. In A. van Kleeck, S. A. Stahl, & E. B. Bauer (Eds.), *On reading books to children: Parents and teachers* (pp. 159–176). Mahwah, NJ: Erlbaum.

National Institute of Neurological Disorders and Stroke. (2010). *NINDS learning disability information page.* Retrieved June 27, 2010, from www.ninds.nih.gov/disorders/learningdisabilities/learningdisabilities.htm.

Oczkus, L. D. (2003). *Reciprocal teaching at work: Strategies for improving reading comprehension.* Newark, DE: International Reading Association.

Ogle, D. (1986). K-W-L: A teaching model that develops active reading of expository text. *Reading Teacher, 39*, 564–570.

O'Sail, B., Levack, N., Donovan, L., & Sewell, D. (2001). *Elementary concepts.* Austin: Texas School for the Blind and Visually Impaired.

Palincsar, A. S., & Brown, A. L. (1984). Reciprocal teaching of comprehension-fostering and comprehension-monitoring activities. *Cognition and Instruction, 2*, 117–175.

Paul-Brown, D. (2003). What are auditory processing problems in children? *Lets Talk.* Retrieved June 28, 2010, from www.asha.org/uploadedFiles/aud/LetsTalkAuditory Processing.pdf#search=%22let%22.

Reynolds, C. R., & Kamphaus, R. W. (2004). *Behavior assessment system for children* (2nd ed.) (BASC-2). San Antonio, TX: Pearson Education.

Robertson, C., & Salter, W. (2007). *The phonological awareness test* (2nd ed.) *(PAT-2).* East Moline, IL: LinguiSystems, Inc.

Rotz, R., & Wright, S. D. (Fall 2008). *When ADHD kids fidget: Better focus through multitasking.* Retrieved September 30, 2010, from www.additudemag.com/adhd/article/3967.html.

Rowland, C., & Schweigert, P. (2000). *Tangible symbol systems manual.* Portland, OR: Design to Learn.

Scahill, L., & Schwab-Stone, M. (2000). Epidemiology of ADHD in school-age children. *Child and Adolescent Psychiatric Clinics of North America, 9*(3), 541–555. Retrieved September 30, 2010, from www.ncbi.nlm.nih.gov/pubmed/10944656.

Schuele, C. M., & Boudreau, D. (2008). Phonological awareness intervention: Beyond the basics. *Language, Speech, and Hearing Services in Schools, 39,* 3–20.

Tabors, P. O., Snow, C. E., & Dickinson, D. K. (2001). Homes and school together: Supporting language and literacy development. In D. K. Dickinson & P. O. Tabors (Eds.), *Beginning literacy with language* (pp. 313–334). Baltimore: Paul H. Brookes Publishing.

Tadic, V., Pring, L., & Dale, N. (2009). Attentional processes in young children with congenital visual impairment. *British Journal of Developmental Psychology, 27,* 311–330.

Torgesen, J. K., & Bryant, B. R. (2004). *Test of phonological awareness* (2nd ed., plus) *(TOPA-2+).* Austin, TX: Pro-Ed.

U.S. Office of Special Education Programs. (2004, February). Teaching children with attention deficit hyperactivity disorder: Instructional strategies and practices. Retrieved August 28, 2011, from www2.ed.gov/rschstat/research/pubs/adhd/adhd -teaching.html.

Weiss, B., & Landrigan, P. J. (June 2000). The developing brain and the environment: An introduction. *Environmental Health Perspectives, 108*(Suppl. 3), 373–374. Retrieved September 30, 2010, from www.ncbi.nlm.nih.gov/pmc/articles/PMC1637828.

Wiig, E. H., & Wilson, C. C. (2002). *The learning ladder: Assessing and teaching text comprehension.* Eau Claire, WI: Thinking Publications.

⟨⟨ Appendix 9A
Avenues for Intervention for Students with Concomitant Language and Learning Disabilities

In the United States, the Individuals with Disabilities Education Act (IDEA) is the federal legislation that governs the provision of special education services to children with disabilities. Students with demonstrated visual impairments are typically eligible to receive special education services by virtue of their visual condition. When a student with a visual impairment has additional language or learning disabilities that may also require special services, these conditions may often be overlooked or may be attributed to the effects of the student's visual impairments on learning or the use of language. To ensure that students receive all the services to which they are entitled to address their learning needs, it is important for teachers of students with visual impairments and other professionals to be aware of the various avenues through which intervention can be provided. These vary by state, and by district within a state, and relate to ways in which students become eligible for additional special education services and how they may be served under the Response to Intervention (RTI) process (discussed in more detail in Appendix 9B).

SPECIAL EDUCATION

IDEA requires that students receive a comprehensive assessment and that a structured process of planning for students' educational goals and services (known as an Individualized Education Program, or IEP) be carried out by educational teams, whose members represent different disciplines and expertise. The IEP team, of which the teacher of students with visual impairments is a member, determines how a student is categorized within the special education system; therefore, knowledge of the eligibility categories that may coincide with visual impairment is essential to active participation in team meetings and to advocacy for meeting the student's unique learning needs.

IDEA defines 13 "handicapping conditions" that may qualify a child for special education services, and it sets the criteria for eligibility for special education services under each designation. Three of these are most relevant to students with average cognition who experience difficulty with listening: Specific Learning Disability, Speech or Language Impairment, and Other Health Impairment. Eligibility criteria for each of these categories is summarized below.

Although it is important to be familiar with the eligibility categories under which students may receive special education services, it is also important to understand that the relationship of these categories to the actual learning characteristics observed in a student is not straightforward. In addition, the categorization of language and learning disabilities can vary greatly from one location to another. Moreover, despite the specificity of the definitions of the federal handicapping conditions for special education eligibility, it is important to keep in mind that recommendations for intervention need to be based on students' needs, rather than determined by any label or category that might be applied to them.

Specific Learning Disability

A combination of federal and state mandates (including IDEA) determines how eligibility for special education services under the category of Specific Learning Disability is determined. Specific Learning Disability has a two-part definition; first, "a disorder in one or more basic psychological processes" and, second, that the result is "imperfect ability to listen, think, speak, read, write, spell, or do mathematical calculations" (34 CFR300.8(c)(10)). The psychological or cognitive processing areas that may be identified as a likely cause for the student's difficulty include attention, visual processing, auditory processing, sensory motor, or cognition.

The definition of Specific Learning Disability also lists the following exclusionary factors: difficulties primarily attributed to "visual, hearing, or motor disability; mental retardation; emotional disturbance; cultural factors; environmental or economic disadvantage; or limited English proficiency" (34 CFR300.8(c)(10)). The exclusionary factors clause ensures that learning difficulties are not attributed to a Specific Learning Disability when the source of the difficulty would, theoretically, lead to a different type of intervention.

These exclusionary factors often lead IEP teams to assume that a student with a visual impairment cannot have a coexisting learning disability. In such a situation, the student's IEP team needs to address the phrase in the legal description "primarily attributed to." The role of teachers of students with visual impairments, then, is to provide evidence that the extent of the student's learning difficulties is above and beyond what would be expected due to his or her visual impairment.

Prior to the 2004 reauthorization of IDEA, one of the key criteria for including a student in the category of Specific Learning Disability was a significant discrepancy between cognitive ability and academic performance. With reauthorization in 2004, however, use of this criterion is no longer required. For additional information regarding alternatives to the discrepancy criteria, see the discussion of Response to Intervention in Appendix 9B.

Speech or Language Impairment

The category of Speech or Language Impairment covers "a communication disorder, such as stuttering, impaired articulation; a language impairment; or a voice impairment" (IDEA, 2004, 34 CFR300.8(c)(11)) that adversely affects the student's educational performance.

Other Health Impairment

The special education eligibility category of Other Health Impairment is defined as "having limited strength, vitality, or alertness . . . that results in limited alertness with respect to the educational environment, that . . . is due to chronic or acute health problems such as . . . attention deficit disorder or attention deficit hyperactivity disorder" (CFR300.8(c)(9)). Attention is the primary concern related to listening, although other health concerns that affect a student's educational progress may fall under this category.

RESPONSE TO INTERVENTION

In 2004, under the periodic reauthorization of IDEA (the Individuals with Disabilities Education Improvement Act), a new option was established to address the needs of struggling students with learning difficulties within the framework of general education, prior to a student's referral for special education services. This program, known as Response to Intervention (often referred to as RTI), has been implemented in many states and districts and has become the initial avenue in many localities through which students' learning problems are addressed. Only if the student makes what is deemed insufficient progress within the RTI instruction will he or she be referred for special education services to evaluate potential eligibility based on the 13 federal handicapping conditions discussed previously. With its focus on intense reinforcement and structured intervention, the RTI model can be effective in promoting students' learning, including addressing students' listening skills. A more detailed discussion of the program and how a student with a visual impairment may fit into this model appears in Appendix 9B.

Although a student with a visual impairment is likely to be already receiving special education services based on the presence of a visual impairment or some other identified need, the student may also be entitled to Response to Intervention services if he or she is experiencing learning difficulties that are not attributable to the visual impairment. Teachers of students with visual impairments and others who work with students who are visually impaired who appear to be struggling with a language-related or other learning disability need to be prepared to advocate for their inclusion in an RTI program and, should RTI services not adequately address the student's learning needs, for a concomitant diagnosis that will make them eligible for special education services related to other nonvisual issues. Teachers of students with visual impairments need to be prepared to help the IEP team determine which areas of difficulty may be related to the student's visual impairment and which are above and beyond what would be expected due to his or her visual condition.

The RTI Process
Cheryl Kamei-Hannan

Alicia is a second-grade student who is visually impaired, fully included in her neighborhood elementary school, and receiving services from an itinerant teacher of students with visual impairments. According to a report from her most recent eye exam, Alicia has myopia, amblyopia, and congenital cataracts. She has had numerous surgeries to remove the cataracts and correct the inward eye turn. Her visual acuity is 20/80 in one eye and 20/100 in the other. Alicia also participates in a school-wide Response to Intervention (RTI) program as a result of her difficulties in reading, particularly in the areas of basic decoding and phonological skills, which were identified early in her educational career. The RTI program, implemented by a collaborative multidisciplinary team, consists of core academic content and benchmark assessments or periodic probes (checkpoints that are designed to monitor performance and which are aligned with the scope and sequence of the curriculum). A teacher of students with visual impairments has been working with Alicia since kindergarten on a consultative basis to ensure that her classroom teachers understand her vision needs and to provide adapted materials.

When she started kindergarten, Alicia's teacher identified her significant difficulty with letter-sound correspondence and basic phonological skills early in the year. Alicia participated in an alternate full-day kindergarten program specially designed for children who struggled to meet the criteria for adequate progress and received additional literacy instruction. Alicia's teacher of students with visual impairments continued consultation services and added 30 minutes of weekly direct instruction to provide real-life experiences for Alicia, pre-teach concepts from the general education curriculum, and adapt materials. Typical adaptations for Alicia included reducing visual clutter, using bold dark line outlines for some pictures, and increasing contrast between the print and the background. The assessments within the RTI program were modified to reduce the number of words per line and to use a font without serifs.

Despite the increased duration and frequency of instruction, Alicia continued to struggle in reading, particularly in the areas of basic decoding and phonological skills. Alicia's teacher of students with visual impairments previewed first-grade classrooms prior to the start of the school year. Following her recommendation, Alicia was placed in an instructional group that focused on phonological awareness and sound-letter correspondence. In addition to the regular curriculum, a reading specialist provided small-group literacy instruction with a supplemental curriculum.

RESPONSE TO INTERVENTION

Response to Intervention was established by the 2004 reauthorization of the Individuals with Disabilities Education Act (IDEA) as an option for providing more intense instruction in a timely fashion outside of special education for students who are struggling and for identifying whether such students have a specific learning disability. RTI is designed to provide appropriate, high-quality instruction using evidence-based interventions to meet the needs of all students in core academic subject areas (Council for Exceptional Children, 2007a). Through RTI, a struggling student may be provided with a combination of more targeted instruction, reduced instructional group size, and increased instructional time for the area of concern within the general education framework. It is up to each state to create its own RTI model to be implemented at the district level.

In the IDEA reauthorization, RTI was established as an acceptable method of identifying students with a specific learning disability. Prior to 2004, eligibility for special education services under the category of mild/moderate disability was determined by a discrepancy between a student's expected performance based on his or her intellectual ability (as measured by IQ) and the student's actual performance in reading, language, or mathematics. In practice, this method requires a child to show "no progress" or "very little progress" for a significant time period before he or she can receive access to remediation, more intensive instruction, or proper interventions. In contrast, RTI uses the provision of research-based intervention as a method of distinguishing students with an actual learning disability from those whose learning difficulties can be resolved with more intense and targeted general education interventions.

RTI involves an inclusive collaborative approach among general and special education educators, specialists, and families. Sugai (2007, as quoted in paragraph 5, Council for Exceptional Children, 2007b) identified six critical elements to effective RTI programs:

- implementing interventions with fidelity, as specified by the intervention's developers
- a continuum of evidence-based interventions

- student performance, which demonstrates the effectiveness of instruction and determines placement
- continuous progress monitoring
- universal screening for all students and a school-wide approach
- multiple tiers of support or levels of intervention that increase in frequency, duration, or intensity, or that adjust the type of intervention, instructional methods, or specialists who provide support, as a student moves into the next level

Although RTI models differ in how they are conceptualized and implemented, their unifying purpose is to use a problem-solving, data-driven method in a system-wide approach to ensure quality instructional programs and a continuum of options to all children (Fuchs & Fuchs, 2006). Students who are at risk are identified early on and provided with access to needed interventions. Assessments, progress monitoring, and data collected about how students respond to evidence-based interventions are designed to identify students with actual learning disabilities (Council for Exceptional Children, 2007b). Collaboration among educational specialists, special education teachers, and administrators is fundamental to the multitiered framework of the model.

The RTI model is conceptualized as a school-wide systematic approach with multiple tiers of instruction (Barnes & Harlacher, 2008; Council for Exceptional Children, 2007a, b; Fuchs & Fuchs, 2006; Haager, Klingner, & Vaughn, 2007; Kovaleski, 2007). All children who attend schools with RTI models participate in school-wide assessment and ongoing progress monitoring. Scores from these assessments are used to identify children who are underperforming, and these students are provided with additional supports, at varying levels, so that they have the opportunity to demonstrate progress (Fuchs & Fuchs, 2006). Assessment data are supposed to drive the use of evidence-based practices and ensure that best practices are used to develop students' skills and eliminate the chance that slow progress is the result of inadequate or inappropriate instruction (Kovaleski, 2007). A decision-making process, based on the use of data collected on students, together with a multitiered model, is designed to identify students who are struggling and ensure that their individual needs are addressed (Fuchs & Fuchs, 2006).

A Multitiered Approach

Although three levels of intensity are standard in the RTI approach, the specific models vary among states and localities (Fuchs, Mock, Morgan, & Young, 2003). The following example is based on a position paper from the Council for Exceptional Children

(2007a). In the first tier, children receive a "universal core program." Typically, this is the general education curriculum and is at the heart of the RTI process. Children who are not making adequate progress receive additional academic supports such as increased frequency or duration of instruction, instruction by a specialist in the area of academic need (such as a reading or mathematics specialist), or provision of a more intensive intervention to target the area of academic need. For children who are visually impaired, input from a teacher of students with visual impairments must be included. Children who do not show response to the additional supports may be moved to the second tier of the RTI model.

Second-tier interventions are more intensive than and supplement the universal core program. They may be designed in a variety of ways, including small-group instruction, direct instruction, tutoring, extended-day programs, increased frequency or duration of instruction, use of a specific intervention program, or support provided by a specialist (Fuchs & Fuchs, 2006).

If a child does not show adequate progress within the second-tier intervention, he or she may be referred to special education services under the eligibility category of Specific Learning Disability. A team of educational experts assesses the student to determine whether a specific learning disability exists. The assessment team should include, at minimum, a special educator and a school psychologist or educational diagnostician trained in academic and cognitive assessment, as well as other specialists determined by the individual student's needs (for example, speech, language, visual impairments, motor skills). If a student is determined to be eligible for services under the category of Specific Learning Disability, he or she begins third-tier intervention. This may be a pull-out service or the student may be placed in a self-contained special education classroom for intensive instruction with a special educator. In some programs, tier three is special education. In others, special education is beyond, or after, tier three. (For addition information, the reader is referred to the National Center on RTI website, www.rti4success.org.)

RTI AND CHILDREN WHO ARE VISUALLY IMPAIRED

Alicia began her first-grade school year in a general education classroom specifically designed for children who were struggling readers. She continued to receive services from a teacher of students with visual impairments who worked with her weekly and provided consultative services to her classroom teacher. Despite whole-class and small-group intensive instruction with a scripted reading intervention by a certified reading specialist, Alicia still showed minimal progress. After two months, Alicia's teacher of students with visual impairments updated her functional vision and learning media assessments. The recommended adaptations of high-contrast materials, reduced visual clutter, and large print were continued. The learning media assessment data reported that Alicia's listening comprehension was at grade level, despite her reading ability being below a pre-primer level.

By the second half of first grade, Alicia was referred for additional special education eligibility areas. Her teachers had documented her minimal response to intervention programs designed specifically for struggling readers. Assessment results determined that vocabulary and oral language were strengths for Alicia. Using an informal reading inventory, she scored at a pre-primer level at oral reading; particular difficulty was noted with phonemic awareness and phonics. Alicia's IEP team determined that she qualified for services as a student with a specific learning disability, with a disorder in auditory processing, which interfered with learning to identify sounds and directly affected the development of phonemic awareness and phonics skills. At her IEP meeting, the services of a specialist in learning disabilities were added. Because the team directly addressed the auditory processing deficit through targeted instruction (isolating phonemes, segmenting and blending them for word recognition) and provided Alicia with additional practice, Alicia progressed to a second-grade reading level by the end of third grade. Alicia was now able to participate in her school's program of leveled reading groups within general education. (Alicia's school grouped children for reading instruction based on their reading levels across all classrooms within an entire grade.) Alicia's IEP team continued to monitor her reading progress to ensure that she was able to maintain her progress during fourth grade, knowing that students who have needed intense intervention may continue to require support to continue their progress.

A key aspect of RTI is that it is a school-wide approach. Therefore, students who are visually impaired and who are in general education classes participate in RTI with nondisabled classmates. If a child is fully participating in on-grade-level general education instruction with services of a teacher of students with visual impairments, as Alicia was, he or she is included in tier one with others, regardless of the fact that he or she is receiving special education services. Movement from one RTI tier to another is dependent on data documenting responsiveness to interventions. Students who are blind or visually impaired have the same array of supports available as do all children who do not respond to the initial interventions and may have the additional option of increased frequency and duration of services by a teacher of students with visual impairments and interventions designed specifically to meet their individual needs.

When an RTI model is in place, one important role of a teacher of students with visual impairments is to evaluate assessment tools and data for individuals with visual impairments. In particular, teachers of students with visual impairments should consult with school personnel to determine the appropriateness of assessment tools, adapting them when necessary. Another role of the teacher of students with visual impairments is explaining the impact of a student's visual impairment on test taking, performance, and results. A teacher of students with visual impairments should determine the impact of an individual's visual functioning and provide consultation on proper assessment, adaptations to testing materials, and interpretation of results. Some measurements may be inappropriate for students with visual impairments for a variety of reasons. Input from a teacher of students with visual impairments may include a discussion of whether vision is stable, if the student maximizes his or her vision, if the student needs visual efficiency training, if alternate learning media are appropriate, or if scores are valid for a student with visual impairments. Additional assessment and triangulation of data (using multiple data points) should take place to verify the student's ability and skill levels. While data from school-wide assessment may be used to identify areas of weakness, they should not be used to adjust placement and level of service without further evaluation and input from a teacher of students with visual impairments.

RTI IN SPECIALIZED SCHOOLS FOR STUDENTS WHO ARE BLIND AND VISUALLY IMPAIRED

Although RTI was conceptualized as a general education function to be implemented in local education agencies, its fundamental principles can be applied at specialized schools for students who are blind and visually impaired. Key aspects of RTI include providing a range of instructional programs, each of which is comprised of evidence-based interventions implemented with fidelity, and using benchmark assessment and continuous progress monitoring (Council for Exceptional Children, 2007b). Each of these concepts is applicable to specialized schools for students with visual impairment and blindness.

First, the concept of providing a range of instructional programs is not new to special educators, especially in the field of visual impairment and blindness. However, RTI reminds teachers to maintain the instructional programs provided to students who are blind and visually impaired and to offer a range of services and placement options. RTI provides an avenue to use a problem-solving approach to determine instructional programming. Data collected from progress monitoring presents the evidence required to support specific levels of intervention, including adjusting the frequency, duration, and intensity of services. In certain instances, an adjustment of placement may need to occur to provide the necessary level of support. Short-term programs and long-term programs offered at specialized schools are options that ought to be made available to students who are in need of these types of instructional supports.

Second, the use of evidence-based interventions that are implemented with fidelity is the biggest challenge for the field of visual impairment and blindness. Data to evaluate curriculum effectiveness is typically from sighted, non-disabled students and may not necessarily be relevant to the requirements for success with the select population of students with visual impairments. Researchers are now responding to the need to evaluate effectiveness for other populations. Despite the lack of literature in evidence-based interventions at present, the instructional programs that are being used can be implemented with fidelity and measurements can be taken to gauge the outcomes. (For additional information regarding evidence-based interventions, see the U.S. Department of Education Institute of Education Sciences website, What Works Clearinghouse at http://ies.ed.gov/ncee/wwc/.)

Finally, evidence from progress monitoring should be used to determine the effectiveness of a program for any individual. For example, routine reviews of skills can determine if students who are at specialized schools for the blind are progressing at expected rates. Together with information about a student's individual level of performance, aptitude for achievement, and rate of skill acquisition, this data can help determine if progress toward goals is being made at levels appropriate for each individual. If a student is not responding to a particular intervention, a change should take place. The change can be in the intensity, frequency, or duration of instruction or in the use of a different instructional program. One caution is that a student's ability and the academic demands on him or her must be taken into consideration before a change in intervention occurs. It may be possible that a student responds slowly and monitoring needs to take place many times before growth can be seen.

Chapter 10

Listening Guidelines for English Language Learners

Madeline Milian

How am I to understand anything the teacher says? English sounds like popcorn popping fast and hard on the stove.

—A. Veciana-Suarez, *Flight to Freedom,* 2002

My first day at school I sat quietly at my desk while the teacher talked about CAT. She wrote CAT on the chalkboard. She read a story about CAT. I did not know what the words meant, but I knew what the pictures said. She sang a song about CAT. It was a pretty song, and I tried to sing the words, too.

—H. Recorvits, *My Name Is Yoon,* 2003

CHAPTER PREVIEW

- ▶ Who Are English Language Learners?
- ▶ Principles of Second Language Listening and Learning
- ▶ Listening to a New Language
- ▶ Proficiency Levels and Standards
- ▶ State Language Development Standards for English Language Learners
- ▶ Listening Skills: Bottom-Up and Top-Down Processes

▸ Designing Listening Activities for English Language Learners
▸ Attentive Listening Skills

Entering a new school is both an exciting and a frightening experience for most students, as there are multiple unfamiliar situations to encounter, with challenges such as learning about a different physical environment, establishing social relationships, and learning the academic expectations of the new setting. For students who are absorbing the details of a new school in a new language and may have recently moved from their native country, this situation offers additional challenges such as the inability to communicate with teachers and peers, learning new cultural norms and behavior expectations, exposure to unfamiliar foods, and navigating a new educational system that may function very differently from previous educational settings they have experienced. For students who are visually impaired—those who have low vision or are blind—other factors, such as exposure to new environmental sounds, fragrances, technologies, and physical settings, are also part of the adjustment process.

For students who cannot rely on vision or have limited use of it, touch and hearing become the primary interpretative senses. When students with visual impairments enter school with little or no understanding of the language of instruction, however, their reliance on listening skills as a vehicle to understand the world and to communicate suffers a significant setback. Learning the new language of instruction that will facilitate understanding and making use of new environmental sounds provide students with visual impairments with a sense of belonging, orientation, and comfort; all of which they need to learn academic subjects, daily living skills, and orientation and mobility.

Teaching students who are blind or visually impaired requires that educators use language often and effectively to communicate visual concepts that students may not have access to because of the nature or degree of their visual impairment. Consequently, language is one of the primary vehicles students who are blind or visually impaired use to access new learning; this emphasizes the importance for educators to become aware of the language needs of English language learners and to be able to support the English language development of students who are English language learners who are visually impaired.

WHO ARE ENGLISH LANGUAGE LEARNERS?

Students who enter classrooms in the United States without having a proficiency level in the English language that allows them to access the regular curriculum are classified as English language learners (often known as ELLs); that is, they are still in the process of developing their English skills and require special language programs. These students may have been born in other countries or in the United States in homes where English is not the primary language. As of the 2008–9 school year, 5.3 million students attending school in the United States were identified as English language learners (National Clearinghouse for English Language Acquisition, 2011). According to a 2006 report published by the American Federation of Teachers, 60 percent of all pre-K–12 educators nationwide have at least one English language learner in their classroom. Enrollment of English language learners accounts for 46 percent of the students in grades pre-K–3; 35 percent in grades 4–8; and 19 percent in grades 9–12. Eighty percent of English language learners in the United States are Latinos; 13 percent are Asian; and 4.5 percent come from Africa, the Caribbean, Europe, the Middle East, New Zealand, India, or Australia. Additionally, 2.5 percent of English language learners are Native Americans, Alaska Natives, or Hawaiian Natives. The 10 most common languages spoken by English language learners in the United States, ranging from most to least common, are Spanish, Vietnamese, Hmong, Cantonese, Korean, Haitian Creole, Arabic, Russian, Tagalog, and Navajo.

Although there is extensive information on the number and the countries of origin of English language learners in the general school population, the information available on students who are both learning English and have visual impairments is much more limited. In 1998, Milian and Ferrell conducted a study with a sample of 4,640 students with visual impairments in Arizona, California, Colorado, Florida, New Mexico, New York, and Texas. Of these students, 27.3 percent lived in homes where a language other than English was spoken, and 8.2 percent were identified as having limited English proficiency. Of the students who lived in homes where a language other than English was spoken, 30.1 percent were still in the process of learning English. Of the teachers who participated in the study, 80.2 percent reported working with students whose families spoke a language other than English at home, and 43.8 percent reported working with students who were still classified as English language learners.

One can conclude that given the increase in the number of English language learners attending school in the United States, it is likely that many teachers of students with visual impairments will have the experience of teaching English language learners during their teaching careers, particularly if they work in states with large numbers of immigrant students or multilingual communities. Listening skills, fundamental to the learning of a new language, are an area on which teachers need to focus when working with English language learners with visual impairments. Sidebar 10.1 suggests some strategies that will be helpful for teachers as they get to know these students.

(((SIDEBAR 10.1
Getting to Know Your English Language Learners

The following suggestions will help teachers to know their students who speak a language other than English and better understand their learning needs.

- Read and ask questions about the students' culture and country of origin.
- Find out about students' educational experiences prior to entering the new educational setting.
- Find out basic differences about students' native language and the English language.
- Find out differences in the braille system the student uses and the English braille system (such as whether they use contracted or uncontracted braille).
- Find out about students' literacy levels in their native language, as literacy levels in the native language can predict academic progress in English.
- Meet students' relatives and develop an open and respectful relationship with them.
- Observe students in different school settings to get an idea of how they are adapting to the new school and to their classmates.

PRINCIPLES OF SECOND LANGUAGE LISTENING AND LEARNING

When teaching English language learners how to listen, educators need to understand the skills and knowledge that are required in order to master the skills of listening in a new language. Following are important questions to consider:

▶ What is the role of listening in language acquisition?

▶ How does the listener process and recognize incoming speech?

▶ How does prior knowledge facilitate listening in a new language?

▶ How can already acquired learning strategies assist in the listening process?

Vandergrift (2003) summarized significant research findings on the importance of listening when learning a new language:

▶ Listening is an important component in the process of acquiring a second language, particularly in the early stages of language learning.

▶ Listening comprehension relies on the process of matching incoming speech with what listeners already know about a topic. Thus, prior knowledge of the topic under discussion is essential for listening comprehension.

▸ Listening comprehension is an interactive and interpretive process in which listeners use both prior knowledge and linguistic knowledge to understand a message. Listeners' knowledge of the language, their familiarity with the topic under discussion, and the purpose for listening determine the degree to which listeners use prior knowledge or linguistic knowledge.

▸ Instead of paying attention to every detail, listeners listen selectively according to the demands of the task.

▸ Listening is helped by listeners' use of metacognitive, cognitive, and socio-affective strategies.

- *Metacognitive* strategies require that students think about the learning process to plan, monitor, and evaluate their learning.

- *Cognitive strategies* consist of specific learning tasks such as repetition, translation, concentrating on key words, practice, and memorization.

- *Socio-affective strategies* refer to the interactions between learners and those around them, such as cooperation and clarification.

▸ Skilled listeners use more metacognitive strategies than less skilled listeners do. In order to develop independent listening skills outside the classroom, English language learners need to:

- analyze the requirements of a listening task
- use prior knowledge and linguistic knowledge
- make appropriate predictions
- monitor their comprehension
- problem solve to guess the meaning of what they do not understand
- evaluate their approach to listening to determine if it is successful

From these findings, one can conclude that instruction designed to develop or improve listening skills needs to include attention to prior knowledge, linguistic knowledge, and the teaching of metacognitive, cognitive, and socio-affective strategies. The guidelines for listening instruction presented in Sidebar 10.2 are intended to ensure that English language learners with visual impairments receive the extra support they require.

((‹ SIDEBAR 10.2

Guidelines for Listening Instruction with English Language Learners

The following guidelines will help educators provide extra support to English language learners during listening instruction:

- Match the listening activity to the English language level of the students.
- Begin instruction with activities that include functional vocabulary, such as body parts, school supplies, names of foods, and areas around the school.
- Learn basic differences between the language spoken by the students and English, as these differences can influence some of the sounds students may have difficulties learning in English.
- Teach key phrases that will help students ask for listening assistance, such as "Please repeat"; "Slower, please"; "I don't understand"; and "Sorry, I did not hear that."
- Teach key questions that will allow students to obtain or verify information, such as "What is that?" "How do you say . . . ?" "Did you say . . . ?"
- Reinforce listening activities through literacy activities, as the written or brailled representation of sounds is helpful to students.
- Include opportunities in listening activities for students to demonstrate the skills being learned. For example, when teaching rules for telephone conversation, first have students listen to a few examples of telephone conversations, provide sufficient practice opportunities, and then have students engage in a real telephone conversation.

LISTENING TO A NEW LANGUAGE

Many students who are learning English as a new language have already developed appropriate listening skills in their native language that assist them in learning academic content in school. This is particularly true for students who have attended schools in their native countries and have been academically successful. Other students who enter school already fluent in their native language may experience difficulties with listening skills in their native language as a result of hearing or auditory processing difficulties (see Chapters 8 and 9), making the learning of the second language an even more complex process than it would be ordinarily. Younger children whose home language is not English and who are receiving educational services from English-speaking educators are learning two languages at the same time, as well as developing their listening skills. Thus, English language learners may have different learning needs, depending on where they are in the process of acquiring both listening and English language skills. As a result, teachers need to individualize listening

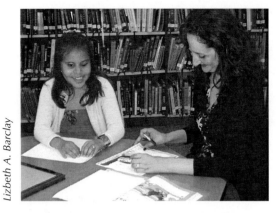

This student is learning to read English braille. She is continuing to learn concepts, pairing her native language, Spanish, to her second language, English.

instruction for English language learners based on their English proficiency levels, prior academic experiences, and native language skills.

Taylor (1981) proposed a developmental sequence that describes the process students experience as they refine their listening skills in a new language. Taylor proposed five stages:

▶ stream of sound
▶ isolated word recognition within the stream
▶ phrase and formula recognition
▶ clause and sentence recognition
▶ extended speech recognition

The stages explained in Taylor's (1981) work are instructive in helping teachers understand the process students go through when learning to listen in a new language.

Stream of Sound

When they begin to hear a new language, listeners at first perceive what can be compared to a "stream of sounds." Subsequently they begin to distinguish certain sounds. Learners concentrate on the sounds of the new language and begin to distinguish the target language from other languages. While they may not understand what they are listening to, they begin to distinguish the new language from other languages. They are, at this stage, learning the distinct sounds of English and may begin imitating sounds to practice, pretending to be speaking the language. Teachers can demonstrate intonation patterns, speed, pitch, and basic differences in language patterns either through direct instruction or through the use of recorded materials. For example, teachers can begin using simple sentences such as "This is your cane" and "This is your braillewriter" and then turn these sentences into questions to reinforce both vocabulary and intonation: "Is this your cane?" "Is this your braillewriter?" These examples introduce differences in language patterns as well as basic important vocabulary.

At this stage, sighted students who are learning a new language focus on pictures and gestures to make sense of a language they do not understand. Educators can make substitutions for pictures for students who are visually impaired, for example, by using objects and the student's native language to facilitate understanding, when possible.

Educators can provide many listening activities through music, basic poetry, and learning the names of the students' peers in the classroom and the names of teachers and other service providers. For students with very low vision or those who are blind, this is an excellent time to explain new environmental sounds students may be encountering. For example, if a student came from a rural environment and is now living in a city, the sounds of airplanes, cars, trains, motorcycles, and other common city sounds will necessitate explanation. Sounds as common to educators as a flushing toilet may be foreign to a child who has spent his or her life in a rural area in another part of the world. These sounds are important to learn, not only for orientation and mobility, but also to alleviate students' anxiety created by unfamiliar sounds. For students with visual impairments who are learning a new language, developing listening skills at this stage is not limited to the sounds of the language, but also involves the sounds of the new neighborhood and school setting. Sidebar 10.3 presents strategies that help develop students' understanding of environmental sounds.

Isolated Word Recognition within the Stream

In the next stage of learning a new language, what were once sounds without meaning now begin to become recognizable words, although in isolation. Students may recognize one or two words in a sentence at the beginning of this stage and progress to recognizing many words in a passage, but meaning is still limited to words in isolation.

Educators can design activities that provide repetition and predictable vocabulary, which offer the opportunity to reinforce functional vocabulary needed for the school setting. Books with repetitive phrases and those that involve actions, such as Eric Carle's *From Head to Toe* (1997), with its focus on teaching body parts and simple body movements, can be very helpful in assisting students who are functioning at this stage of listening.

Other helpful activities at this stage are those used in the language teaching methodology known as Total Physical Response. When using this method, developed by Asher (1977), students are engaged in body movements to demonstrate understanding of oral language. For example, when the student is becoming familiar with a classroom, the teacher first uses commands and modeling of physical actions and then asks the student to demonstrate the action. Possible actions can include walking to the door, opening the window, or finding the first seat. Total Physical Response has been used successfully in the teaching of new languages in the United States and around the world. Because of its emphasis on body movements, Total Physical Response is appropriate and easy to use in orientation and mobility lessons with students who have visual impairments (Conroy, 1999). For example, when teaching the

---

((Sidebar 10.3
Strategies for Introducing Environmental Sounds

For students with visual impairments who are new to a country and language of instruction, developing listening skills includes not just the sounds of the language, but also the environmental sounds of the new neighborhood and school setting. The following suggestions will help students learn about the sounds in their new environment:

- Take a walk around the school and listen to the sounds found in different areas, such as the cafeteria, main office, playground, gym, and so on. Identify each room or area for the student.
- Make a recording of the sounds around the school, and then play the sounds for the student, to reinforce both the sounds and the names of the rooms where those sounds were found. This activity can be repeated around the school neighborhood or student's neighborhood.
- Record the voices of school personnel who work with the student, and then play the recording to match the name of the person with the voice.
- Take the student to the music room and introduce him or her to the different sounds of the instruments. This provides an opportunity to match the names of the instruments to the sounds they create.
- Play guessing games using school objects that create sounds and are typically assumed to be known by all children, such as scissors, staplers, computer keyboards, keys, and so on. Match the names of the objects to the sounds, and then have the student identify the objects.
- Use commercially available materials to illustrate animal sounds, city sounds, and other relevant sounds in the student's life.

---

student to get around the classroom, important verbs and nouns such as *walk, stop, turn,* and *touch; table, chairs, bookcase,* and *wall* can be introduced as part of the activity. Unlike a traditional O&M lesson for students who are visually impaired that aims at facilitating movement and orienting students to the environment, the Total Physical Response lesson for English Language Learners aims at introducing new vocabulary that will then facilitate not only movement, but also communication skills.

Taylor (1981) emphasized that at this stage of listening it is important for students to develop a positive attitude about learning a new language and concentrate on the words and sounds that they can recognize to avoid the frustration that often crops up about not understanding other parts of the language. Educators can provide positive reinforcement when they see students showing evidence of understanding and avoid presenting materials or activities that are not appropriate for the student's language level. During the first two listening stages, students need to be given the opportunity to concentrate on developing their receptive language skills and so need to not be required to produce language.

Phrase and Formula Recognition

In the next stage of learning a new language, phrase and formula recognition, students begin to recognize phrases and language patterns that are frequently used in the classroom or school setting that will assist them in grasping the general idea or request that is being discussed. Understanding frequent comments such as "It is time for lunch"; "Let's get ready to go home"; and "Do you like this game?" begins to provide students with a sense of familiarity that, although limited, will help them with the process of adapting to their new educational setting. With knowledge of typical phrases and language patterns, students begin to have a functional understanding of the language to succeed in the English-speaking setting. For example, at this stage students may be able to understand greetings such as "How are you?"; basic instructions such as "Open your book"; and simple questions such as "What is your name?" One important aspect of this stage is that students begin to attach meaning to syntactic groupings of words instead of to individual words.

At this stage, educators may be able to engage students in simple functional dialogues that require oral expression from the students. For example "telephone conversations" can serve both as a way to develop listening skills and as a daily living skill. The teacher and the student can practice making telephone calls to learn appropriate telephone phrases, such as "May I speak to . . ."; "This is . . ."; and "You have the wrong number." Other activities appropriate at this stage include listening to recorded stories that provide repetitive language patterns and appropriate vocabulary; use of computer programs that engage students in listening to dialogues; and more advanced Total Physical Response activities that require students to remember longer phrases such as "Stand up, walk to the door, and turn right." At this stage students may be also able to start singing simple songs and remembering basic poetry. For younger children, learning songs such as "If You're Happy and You Know It" and "Ten Little Monkeys" offers opportunities to support the learning of developmentally appropriate phrases and concepts that are often used in the learning setting. For older students, using popular songs with simple lyrics often provides the motivation to speak (or sing) the language, while also developing listening skills.

Clause and Sentence Recognition

In the next phase of language learning, students begin to attach meanings to clauses and sentences even when they have not previously heard these clauses and sentences. These students can be considered to be minimally functional in their understanding of spoken language and still have great vocabulary deficits in content areas. However, at this stage students typically have enough knowledge of English syntax to combine many word groups and be able to function in situations in which the vocabulary is familiar to them. It is possible for students at this stage to understand common classroom routines that they are exposed to on a daily basis within the school environment; students at this stage may also be able to contribute basic sentences and commands needed to communicate with teachers and peers.

While it may be unrealistic to expect rapid oral expression at this stage, students can be exposed to discussions and conversations about topics that they are unfamiliar with and can expect a general understanding of the topic under discussion. For example, at this stage, students may be able to participate in a science or social studies class and get a basic understanding of the topic. Thus, additional support, such as the use of tangible materials, pairing a student with a bilingual peer, and paraphrasing the information in more understandable terms, assists the student to make more connections with the content, since at this stage the student's listening ability still misses many important details that facilitate true content comprehension.

Extended Speech Recognition

True listening comprehension can be considered to have been achieved when students begin to follow the meaning of a new passage, even though they may not understand every word or phrase. However, if students encounter much unfamiliar vocabulary or extremely complex content, they may function at a lower level of comprehension. Although at this level students demonstrate general comprehension of conversations and discussions, their listening functioning in the new language is not as advanced as it is in their native language. Therefore, additional support is needed in order to facilitate understanding. This is particularly the case when students are exposed to new content that contains unfamiliar vocabulary or new situations in which students cannot use their background knowledge to navigate meaning. The strategies presented in Sidebar 10.4 include ways to support English language learners with visual impairments in the classroom while they are learning other subject matter.

As Taylor (1981) noted, native speakers who typically function at the stage of extended speech recognition in some areas may function at a lower level of listening comprehension depending on the complexity of the conversation. This is an important idea for educators to remember when exposing students who are still learning a second language to new content or situations.

The stages explained by Taylor's (1981) work are instructive in helping teachers understand the process students go through when learning to listening in a new language.

((SIDEBAR 10.4

Supporting the Educational Needs of English Language Learners

The following strategies will help English language learners to better follow teachers' oral instruction in the classroom:

- Pair English language learners with bilingual classmates who can serve as good English role models and also assist with students' native language if needed.
- Teach vocabulary that is essential to understanding content before presenting the lesson.
- Encourage English language learners to paraphrase information in their own words so that the teacher can verify that they have truly understood.
- Repeat instruction or directions more than once to facilitate understanding.
- Increase the wait time given to English language learners to respond to questions. Typically 15 to 20 seconds should be provided to allow learners to process a question in the new language.
- Gear questions to the student's English language proficiency level. Students at the beginning levels of language proficiency are typically able to respond only to "yes/no" or "either/or" questions. Allow nonverbal responses.
- Limit the use of slang and idioms, which are very confusing to English language learners at the beginning stages. As students progress in their English language development, idioms can be introduced through direct or indirect instruction.
- Pay attention to the rate of speech used to present information, as following fast speech is more challenging for English language learners.
- Use tangible and tactile materials as often as possible, as some items that are common to teachers may be unknown to English language learners because of cultural differences. For example, common items in U.S. homes such as blenders, toasters, and mixers, may be unknown to students who have moved from rural communities in developing countries or refugee camps in Africa or Southeast Asia.
- Provide support for the native language as much as possible, as students can continue to learn content while they are in the process of learning English.

PROFICIENCY LEVELS AND STANDARDS

Another way to understand the development of listening skills for English language learners is to become familiar with the proficiency levels that have been developed by various state departments of education and local school districts in order to follow the language progress of English language learners. For example, the Office of Bilingual Education and Foreign Language Studies of the New York State Education Department (2004) has developed a clear and sequential list of listening behaviors as part of its English language development standards' handbook, which is available online (see Sidebar 10.5). Educators can use the proficiency levels to design activities that facilitate progress to more advanced listening levels.

Another example of proficiency-level indicators has been created by the World-Class Instructional Design and Assessment (WIDA) Consortium (2007), which has developed an extensive system of assessment and materials to support its English language proficiency standards. Twenty-four states are currently members of the consortium, and many other states use the WIDA English language proficiency standards as well.

The standards are organized using the following categories or levels to reflect students' ability to process, understand, express, or use the English language:

1. entering
2. beginning
3. developing
4. expanding
5. bridging
6. reaching

Examples of selected indicators of listening proficiency for the different levels of language proficiency as described by the WIDA Consortium are provided in Table 10.1. Examples are not provided for level 6 (reaching), as students at that level can demonstrate communication skills that are comparable to those of proficient English-speaking students. Additionally, since all of the activities were developed for English language learners without visual impairments, teachers who work with English language learners with visual impairments may have to provide modifications depending on the visual functioning of the students in their caseload.

STATE LANGUAGE DEVELOPMENT STANDARDS FOR ENGLISH LANGUAGE LEARNERS

State and federal requirements, such as the No Child Left Behind Act of 2001, have influenced the development of content and subject standards and the use of standardized tests to measure those standards. Similarly, states have also been required to develop language standards for English language learners and corresponding tests to measure the language growth of students who are still identified as needing language support because they have not yet reached the language proficiency level required to be classified as fluent English speakers. Excerpts of listening skills or goals from California's English Language Development Standards (California State Department of Education, 1999) are presented in Sidebar 10.6 as examples of some of the standards

Listening Proficiency Levels and Indicators

The following descriptions of listening proficiency levels provide the typical skills that are often achieved at different levels when learning a new language. Teachers and administrators who work with English learners in New York State developed the descriptors based on previously published proficiency level descriptions.

BEGINNING-LEVEL LISTENING

Low Beginning

1. Students at this low beginning level of ESL [English as a second language] can recognize a very limited number of common individual words and learned phrases, even in a predictable context and on everyday personal topics.
2. They can understand greetings and some simple instructions, and depend on gestures and other contextual clues.
3. They require extensive assistance to make language comprehensible.

Mid Beginning

1. Students at this mid-beginning stage can understand a number of individual words, common social phrases, and simple short sentences on topics of immediate personal relevance or related to the immediate physical environment.
2. They can understand simple personal information questions and simple commands or directions related to the immediate context.
3. They continue to struggle to understand simple instructions without clear contextual clues.
4. Students at this stage continue to rely on visual support and other assistance.
5. They frequently understand some short, previously learned words or phrases, particularly through use of cognates (such as accident/*accidente*, captain/*capitán*, or list/*lista*) or when the situation strongly supports understanding, although they can rarely understand an ongoing message. (Cognates are words in two languages that are related in origin, have the same meaning, and have similar spelling such as in the word "brother" in English and "*Bruder*" in German. For a list of English/Spanish cognates, educators can visit the following website: http://www.colorincolorado.org/pdfs/articles/cognates.pdf.)
6. They usually require repetition, rephrasing, or modified speech.

High Beginning

1. Students can understand key words, formulaic phrases, and most short sentences in simple, predictable conversations on topics of immediate personal relevance.

Source: Adapted from Office of Bilingual Education and Foreign Language Studies, "The Teaching of Langauge Arts to Limited English Proficient/English Language Learners: Learning Standards for English as a Second Language. Introduction." Albany: New York State Education Department, 2004.

(Continued)

2. They understand questions related to personal experience and requests related to the immediate context.

3. They frequently need assistance to comprehend meaning and sometimes may understand the main idea of short simple speech on familiar topics.

4. They can sometimes understand an ongoing message but still often require repetition, rephrasing (repeating the idea in different ways), or modified speech (either slower or simplified sentences).

INTERMEDIATE-LEVEL LISTENING

Low Intermediate

1. Students can recognize many topics by familiar words and phrases.

2. They understand simple, short, direct questions related to personal experience and general knowledge and can understand many common everyday instructions and directions related to the immediate context.

3. With strong support and clear context, students often understand new information.

4. They can sometimes identify the main idea and details when listening to extended speech on a familiar topic.

5. They benefit from repetition or rephrasing.

Mid Intermediate

1. Students can understand with some effort the overall message of oral discourse in moderately demanding contexts, including media broadcasts, and personally relevant topics.

2. They may require repetition, rephrasing, or some modifications of speech for unfamiliar topics.

3. They can understand a range of common vocabulary and a very limited number of idioms.

4. They can understand simple, short, predictable phone messages, but have limited ability to understand extended speech on the phone and sometimes in person.

5. They sometimes understand new information in brief personal interactions.

6. They can often identify details when listening to extended speech and usually understand natural speech when the situation is familiar or fulfills immediate needs.

High Intermediate

1. Students can usually understand main ideas and identify key words and important details in oral discourse in sustained personal interactions.

2. Students understand language in moderately demanding contexts, such as audio-tapes and media broadcasts on everyday topics.

3. They can understand a range of common vocabulary and a limited number of idioms.

4. They comprehend contextualized, short sets of instructions and directions, but may still need repetition.

5. They can understand simple, short, predictable phone messages.

6. They sometimes understand speech on abstract or academic topics, although this understanding is often affected by length, topic familiarity, and cultural knowledge.

7. They show evidence of understanding inferences.

ADVANCED-LEVEL LISTENING

Low Advanced

1. Students can usually comprehend main points and most important details in oral discourse in moderately demanding language contexts, including media broadcasts.

2. They often cannot sustain understanding of conceptually or linguistically complex speech and require slower speech, repetitions, and rewording.

3. They often understand implications beyond surface meaning.

4. They recognize but do not always understand an expanded inventory of concrete and idiomatic language.

5. They can understand more complex indirect questions about personal experience, familiar topics, and general knowledge.

6. They can understand short, predictable phone messages on familiar matters, but have problems understanding unknown details on unfamiliar matters.

7. They have some difficulty following a faster conversation between native speakers.

8. Their understanding of speech continues to be affected by length, topic familiarity, and cultural knowledge.

High Advanced

1. Students can comprehend many important aspects of oral language on social and academic topics, such as main points, most details, speaker's purpose, attitudes, levels of formality, and inferences.

2. They can comprehend an expanded range of concrete, abstract, and conceptual language and can sustain understanding of conceptually or linguistically complex speech.

3. They can understand sufficient vocabulary, idioms, colloquial expressions, and cultural references to understand detailed stories of general popular interest.

4. They often have difficulty following rapid, colloquial, or idiomatic speech between native English speakers.

5. Their understanding of English is much less frequently affected by length, topic familiarity, and cultural knowledge.

TABLE 10.1

Selected Examples of Listening Indicators Based on the WIDA Proficiency Levels

Examples and Topics	Level 1: Entering	Level 2: Beginning	Level 3: Developing	Level 4: Expanding	Level 5: Bridging
Music and movement	Mimic musical beats or movements modeled by teachers (for example, hop, hop-jump; one clap, two claps)	Respond to chants using gestures, movement, or instruments modeled by the teacher	Respond to songs using gestures, movement, or instruments modeled by the teacher	Interpret songs (for example, melodies from diverse cultures) through movement or playing of instruments	Follow lyrics of songs and respond accordingly in small groups or in the whole class (for example, "Put your right foot in . . .")
Recreational objects and activities	Identify recreational objects (for example, balls, swings) and locate recreational settings (for example, playground, gym)	Follow one-step oral directions using recreational object (for example, "Pick up the ball.")	Follow two-step oral directions using recreational object (for example, "Pick up the ball. Then give it to a friend.")	Indicate use of recreational objects from complex oral directions (for example, "Show me how to pass the ball from person to person.")	Simulate playing according to sequential oral descriptions (for example, "Make two rows. Choose a friend. Have the friend go between the rows.")
Concepts about print (or braille)	Point to features of books (for example, cover, title, illustrator) according to oral commands	Show directionality of print or braille in various sources (for example, left to right, beginning, ending, top, bottom) according to oral commands	Identify features of text in context with a partner (for example, spaces between words, sentences) according to oral directions	Sort features of text with a partner (for example, lower- and uppercase letters, period, question mark) according to oral directions	Match illustrations or graphic representations to oral reading of related sentences or short stories

Patterns	Imitate pattern sounds with physical movement from modeling (for example, clap, snap, stomp)	Select "What comes first, next, or last?" in illustrations or tactile models according to oral directions	Sort patterns from nonpatterns in pictures or tactile models according to oral directions	Identify patterns from pictures, graphics, or tactile models (for example, "girl, boy, girl, boy") according to oral directions	Form patterns from pictures, graphics, or tactile models (for example, "the tall girl, the short girl, the tall boy, the short boy") according to detailed oral directions
Transportation	Associate sounds of different modes of transportation with pictures, graphics, or tactile models (for example, "Which goes choo choo?")	Identify modes of transportation from visually or tactilely supported rhymes or chants (for example, "The Wheels on the Bus")	Match pictures or tactile modes of transportation with descriptive statements (for example, "Airplanes go fast.")	Pair models of transportation with their environment (for example, "Jets fly in the air.") based on pictures, tactile models, and oral directions	Differentiate modes of transportation from the past or present based on visual or tactile models and oral descriptions

Source: Excerpted and adapted from WIDA Consortium, *English Language Proficiency Standards and Resource Guide, 2007 Edition, Pre-Kindergarten through Grade 12* (Madison: Board of Regents of the University of Wisconsin System, 2007).

Note: Minor adaptations were included to make activities more appropriate for students with visual impairments.

that are guiding listening instruction for English language learners throughout the country. These selected examples can facilitate ideas as to how educators can structure activities around the standards. It is recommended that educators locate and use the standards that have been developed for their own state by contacting the administrator in charge of services for English language learners in their district or by consulting their state department of education.

An additional source of information related to language standards for English language learners can be found through professional organizations. For example, Teachers of English to Speakers of Other Languages (TESOL) has developed standards for pre-K–12 English language learner students that have been published in print and are available through its website. The TESOL pre-K–12 standards are organized by grade level and take into consideration both social and academic language. The following proficiency standards (TESOL, 2006) are the foundation of TESOL's English language learner standards:

> **Standard 1:** English language learners *communicate* for *social, intercultural, and instructional* purposes within the school setting.
>
> **Standard 2:** English language learners *communicate* information, ideas, and concepts necessary for academic success in the area of *language arts.*
>
> **Standard 3:** English language learners *communicate* information, ideas, and concepts necessary for academic success in the area of *mathematics.*
>
> **Standard 4:** English language learners *communicate* information, ideas, and concepts necessary for academic success in the area of *science.*
>
> **Standard 5:** English language learners *communicate* information, ideas, and concepts necessary for academic success in the area of *social studies.*

Educators who work in states where English development standards have not been designed to guide instruction for English language learners can use the TESOL standards as a framework for understanding the educational needs of students who are learning English as a new language.

It is important that all teachers who work with English language learners become familiar with the English-language proficiency levels and standards that are used in their states so that they can appropriately align their instruction to the language expectations and requirements for English language learners. When educators who work with English language learners who have visual impairments understand the natural

((• SIDEBAR 10.6

Excerpts of Listening Skills from California's English Language Development Standards

STANDARD: COMPREHENSION OF ORAL COMMUNICATION

Beginning Level

1. Answer simple questions with one to two word responses.

2. Respond to simple directions and questions using physical actions and other means of non-verbal communication (e.g., matching objects, pointing to an answer, drawing pictures).

3. Begin to speak with a few words or sentences, using a few Standard English grammatical forms and sounds (e.g., single words or phrases).

4. Independently use common social greetings and simple repetitive phrases (e.g., "Thank you." "You're welcome.").

5. Ask and answer questions using phrases or simple sentences.

6. Retell stories by using appropriate gestures, expressions and illustrative objects.

STANDARD: ORGANIZATION AND DELIVERY OF ORAL COMMUNICATION

Beginning Level

1. Begin to be understood when speaking, but with inconsistent use of Standard English grammatical forms and sounds (e.g., plurals, simple past tense, pronouns, and appropriate pronunciation of simple English words).

2. Orally communicate basic personal needs and desires (e.g., "May I go to the bathroom?").

STANDARD: COMPREHENSION OF ORAL COMMUNICATION

Intermediate Level

1. Ask and answer instructional questions using simple sentences.

2. Listen attentively to stories/information and identify key details and concepts, using both verbal and non-verbal responses.

3. Ask and answer instructional questions with more extensive supporting elements (e.g., "What part of the story was the most important?").

STANDARD: COMPREHENSION, ORGANIZATION AND DELIVERY OF ORAL COMMUNICATION

Intermediate Level

1. Actively participate in social conversations with peers and adults on familiar topics by asking and answering questions and soliciting information.

(Continued)

(⚬ SIDEBAR 10.6 *(Continued)*

STANDARD: ORGANIZATION AND DELIVERY OF ORAL COMMUNICATION
Intermediate Level

1. Be understood when speaking, using consistent Standard English grammatical forms and sounds; however, some rules are not in evidence (e.g., third person singular, male and female pronouns).

_____

Source: Excerpted from California State Department of Education, *English Language Development Standards* (Sacramento: California State Department of Education, 1999).

---

process students follow in their journey to learning a new language and develop activities that support this natural process, they are able to create an effective educational environment where both students and teachers achieve their desired academic goals.

LISTENING SKILLS: BOTTOM-UP AND TOP-DOWN PROCESSES

Two types of listening skills are needed to develop effective listening: linguistic knowledge, or bottom-up processing, and prior knowledge, or top-down processing. Teachers working with English language learners need to work on both types of language processing or listening skills with their students.

Bottom-up processing involves turning the sounds of the language into meaning. It requires that students know the sounds of the language they are learning and how these sounds can be connected together to create meaning. It also requires students to distinguish how meaning can change when similar sounds are connected (for example, "You are going to the park" has a different meaning than "You are going to the park?"). A telephone conversation in which directions to a certain location are given requires bottom-up listening.

Top-down processing requires students to use the cultural, academic, and social knowledge they already have to find meaning in what they hear in the new language they are learning. Predicting how a story will end requires top-down processing.

Morley (2001) described these processes as follows: Bottom-up processing involves the attention to every detail of language input. It refers to the decoding process of language into meaningful units. The listener processes the language he or she heard from sounds, to words, to grammatical relationships, and to meaning. Top-down skills, on the other hand, require the listener's ability to bring prior information or knowledge to what is heard in order to understand the message. The basic distinction between these two processes is that the bottom-up process occurs externally as the sounds come from an external speaker to the listener, and the top-down process occurs internally as the listener interprets the message according to prior experiences.

Peterson (2001) provided the following examples to illustrate bottom-up skills:

1. discrimination between intonation in sentences, as when students listen to rising and falling intonation and use appropriate punctuation for statements, questions, surprise, or excitement
2. discrimination between sounds, as when students can identify difference in sounds between pairs of words
3. listening for ending sounds, as when students can tell the difference between verbs ending in -s or -es
4. recognizing syllable patterns, number of syllables, and word stress, as when students can listen to sentences and count the number of syllables in words and identify or underline the stressed syllable
5. awareness of sentence fillers in informal speech, such as when students can identify fillers such as "well," "like," or "you know" in sentences
6. selecting detail from a conversation, as when students are able to listen to a recorded message and write down essential information, such as the times a movie is playing or when a store is open or closed

Some examples provided by Peterson (2001) to describe top-down skills include:

1. discrimination between emotional reactions, as when students can listen to a conversation about a trip and determine if the speaker enjoyed the experience
2. understanding of the gist or main idea of a passage, as when students listen to a short conversation and can write a title that describes the theme of the conversation
3. recognition of the topic of conversation, as when students can predict appropriate topics that two people who do not know each other can discuss
4. employment of features of speech to decide if a statement is formal or informal, as when students can predict if the conversation between two teenagers or the conversation between a patient and a doctor will be formal or informal
5. making of inferences after listening to a conversation, as when students listen to the weather report and then decide if sandals, snow boots, or rain boots are appropriate to wear given what they heard

6. identification of the speaker of a topic, as when students listen to a recorded conversation and can identify the speaker, for example, teacher,
priest, president, or principal

Understanding bottom-up and top-down processes guides teachers to examine
the complexities and prerequisites involved in the typical listening activities students encounter in the classroom and in the school setting. The examples provided
can assist teachers to develop their own appropriate activities for the students in their
caseload. Devoting time to work on specific listening skills helps second language
learners to navigate the often confusing new environment they confront and promotes academic learning.

DESIGNING LISTENING ACTIVITIES FOR ENGLISH LANGUAGE LEARNERS

Listening activities for students with visual impairments are provided in many of the
chapters in this text according to age level. The suggestions included in this section
offer additional considerations that can be helpful when implementing listening activities with students who, in addition to having a visual impairment, are also going
through the process of learning English as a new language.

The recommendations included here have been adapted from the work of Horwitz
(2008) and Van Duzer (1997), as they also apply to the population of students with
visual impairments:

▶ Listening needs to be relevant: Connect listening activities to content,
knowledge, rules, and regulations that students need to know in order
to succeed in their environment. Listening activities disconnected
from the realities of students' lives will not generate the purpose and
interest that is required for students to engage in listening activities.

▶ Materials need to be authentic: The use of materials that have a real
connection to students' lives is required for both students who are visually impaired and students who are not familiar with U.S. culture.
Authentic materials for listening activities can include materials available through the Internet or on CD-ROMs, television, or DVDs that illustrate real-life situations. For example, conversations at a work-site
environment such as a doctor's office, grocery store, train station, or department store can be used to learn target vocabulary or other structures
of language that are appropriate to those situations. Later, educators can
conduct additional activities in the classroom or on a field trip to enhance
and support the content and language learned through the activity.

▶ Listening activities need to provide opportunities to develop both top-down and bottom-up processing skills: Activities need to allow students to practice the learning of sounds, words, intonation, and grammatical structures as needed according to their language proficiency levels; they also need to encourage students to relate their previous knowledge to what is being learned.

▶ Listening strategies need to be taught: Strategies such as predicting, asking for clarification, using attentive listening behaviors, verifying understanding, and other cognitive, metacognitive, and socio-affective strategies need to be included as part of listening activities.

▶ Listening activities need to teach, not test: Listening activities need to teach the process of listening, not simply test memory. Activities need to assist the student to focus attention on the task, assess the accuracy of what they do, and transfer the listening skill they are learning to other situations outside of the school setting.

▶ Expectations need to match students' language proficiency levels: When designing activities, educators need to have realistic expectations of students' listening abilities. Students' proficiency levels in the new language can range from beginning to advanced; their listening abilities will therefore also range from basic activities that will discriminate

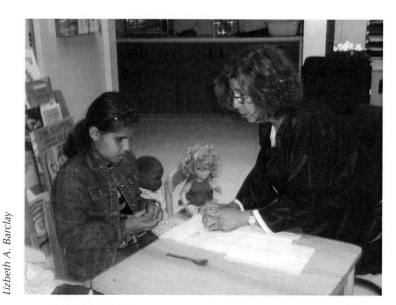

Lizbeth A. Barclay

Vocabulary practice with use of authentic materials—objects with meaning in the student's life—provides an engaging and purposeful listening activity.

sounds or words, to more sophisticated activities that will involve students in explanations, clarifications, and other discussions that require advanced levels of language proficiency.

▸ Activities need to facilitate cultural understanding: Often English language learners may not understand the true meaning of a passage because it may be based on cultural knowledge that they do not yet have, for example, passages making references to certain holidays, historical events or historical figures, specific places, or important people in the community. To prevent unnecessary difficulties, educators need to anticipate how the content of the passage may interfere with listening skills.

▸ Listening activities need to encourage sharing of experiences with other English language learners: When English language learners share their experiences related to listening skills, they understand that learning to listen to a new language is a process that everyone experiences and begin to view the process as a shared experience with others.

Additionally, when designing activities for English language learners, educators for students with visual impairments may want to request the assistance of a teacher of English as a second language assigned to the student's school or the assistance of the district English language learner coordinator. These professionals can provide ideas, materials, and recommendations for listening activities and can also clarify questions concerning language proficiency levels and expectations for students at different proficiency levels.

ATTENTIVE LISTENING SKILLS

An area of importance that should not be overlooked for students with visual impairments is that of listening behaviors and the social dimension of listening. When students are visually impaired, how do they know when a person is listening to them? How do they demonstrate that they are listening to others? Although some attentive listening behaviors involve visual cues, such as eye contact, head nods, or leaning forward, other behaviors such as attentive silence, encouraging sounds, and relevant questions do not rely on visual skills. Educators who work with English language learners with visual impairments are encouraged to concentrate on attentive listening skills as part of their social skills curriculum since social norms such as eye contact, head nods, and physical proximity are different and have different uses across cultures. When a student who is visually impaired comes from another culture and is an English language learner, certain behaviors may have different meanings and may be interpreted differently from those used in this country. For example, while in the United States eye contact is understood as a sign of respect and attention, in many Latin American countries if children have eye contact with an older person or an authority figure when they are being reprimanded, it is perceived to be lack of respect. It is important to teach English language learners with visual impairments how attentive listening behaviors are used in the United States so that they can both practice these behaviors to demonstrate when they are listening to others, and understand when others are listening to them. While these skills are important for all learners, they are essential for students with visual impairments, who may not be able to simply model some of these behaviors through the use of vision.

CONCLUSION

As is stressed throughout this book, listening skills for students with visual impairments are essential not only because of their connection to the learning of academic content, but also because of their role in other primary areas in students' lives, such as orientation and mobility, daily living skills, leisure activities, relationships with friends and family members, and, eventually, job training. When students with visual impairments are English language learners, it is essential for educators to understand and utilize strategies that support the development of listening skills, which are fundamental to learning a new language. Learning the new language of instruction that will facilitate understanding and making use of new environmental sounds provides students with visual impairments with a sense of belonging, orientation, and comfort, which students need for learning both academic subjects and the areas of the expanded core curriculum.

The time spent working with students on developing effective listening skills therefore has the potential to create long-lasting changes in students' lives. Students can become not only better learners, but possibly also better employees, supervisors, friends, spouses, or parents. Listening skills are critical tools for all students with visual impairments for engaging in learning and in life. By providing effective instruction in these skills, teachers can make a major contribution to the well-being and success of their students.

REFERENCES

American Federation of Teachers. (2006). *Where we stand: English language learners.* Washington, DC: American Federation of Teachers.

Asher, J. J. (1977). *Learning another language through actions. The complete teacher's guide book.* Los Gatos, CA: Sky Oaks Productions, Inc.

California State Department of Education. (1999). *English language development standards.* Sacramento: California State Department of Education.

Carle, E. (1997). *From head to toe*. New York: Harper Collins.

Conroy, P. (1999). Total physical response: An instructional strategy for second-language learners who are visually impaired. *Journal of Visual Impairment & Blindness, 93*(5), 315–318.

Horwitz, E. K. (2008). What should I know about teaching listening? In E. K. Horwitz, *Becoming a language teacher: A practical guide to second language learning and teaching* (pp. 67–90). Boston: Pearson Education.

Milian, M., & Ferrell, K. A. (1998). *Preparing special educators to meet the needs of students who are learning English as a second language and are visually impaired: A monograph*. Retrieved from ERIC database (ED 426545).

Morley, J. (2001). Aural comprehension instruction: Principles and practices. In M. Celce-Murcia (Ed.), *Teaching English as a second or foreign language* (pp. 69–85). Boston: Heinle and Heinle.

National Clearinghouse for English Language Acquisition. (2011). *The growing numbers of English learner students 1998/99–2008/2009*. Washington, DC: National Clearinghouse for English Language Acquisition.

No Child Left Behind (NCLB) Act of 2001, Pub. L. No. 107-110, § 115, Stat. 1425 (2002).

Office of Bilingual Education and Foreign Language Studies. (2004). The teaching of language arts to limited English proficient/English language learners: Learning standards for English as a second language. Albany: New York State Education Department. Retrieved September 7, 2011, from www.p12.nysed.gov/biling/resource/ESL/standards.html.

Peterson, P. W. (2001). Skills and strategies for proficient listening. In M. Celce-Murcia (Ed.), *Teaching English as a second or foreign language* (pp. 87–100). Boston: Heinle and Heinle.

Recorvits, H. (2003). *My name is Yoon*. New York: Frances Foster Books.

Taylor, H. M. (1981). Learning to listen to English. *TESOL Quarterly, 15*(1), 41–50.

Teachers of English to Speakers of Other Languages. (2006). PreK–12 English language proficiency standards framework. Retrieved September 9, 2011, from www.tesol.org /s_tesol/sec_document.asp?CID=281&DID=13323.

Vandergrift, L. (2003). From prediction through reflection: Guiding students through the process of L2 listening. *Canadian Modern Language Review, 59*(3), 425–440.

Van Duzer, C. (1997). Improving ESL learners' listening skills: At the workplace and beyond. Center for Applied Linguistics, Washington, DC. Retrieved September 9, 2011, from www.cal.org/caela/esl_resources/digests/LISTENQA.html.

Veciana-Suarez, A. (2002). *Flight to freedom*. New York: Orchard Books.

World-Class Instructional Design and Assessment (WIDA) Consortium. (2007). *English language proficiency standards and resource guide, 2007 edition, pre-kindergarten through grade 12*. Madison: Board of Regents of the University of Wisconsin System.

Epilogue: A Personal and Professional Perspective

As a life-long learner who is visually impaired, if my fingers replace my eyes to take in the world, I can see only what I can reach. My ears give definition and dimensionality to the larger environment beyond my range of touch. *Learning to Listen/Listening to Learn* provides a framework with examples of strategies that will guide parents and educators in helping individuals with visual impairment understand what we are hearing, how that information affects our awareness of what is around us, and how to use that information and resulting awareness to fully engage in life's offerings.

It is critical to learn how to use one's hearing to acquire information and process it. I cannot stress enough the importance of verbally labeling sounds—the source, direction, and value—for a blind child or even an adult. The lexicon of labeled sounds becomes a means of assessing and interpreting one's surroundings and safety. Learning to listen requires continual labeling, verification, and feedback.

As a child with low vision, I was constantly trying to identify whether the sound I heard required additional attention. I asked, and now, as a blind adult, continue to ask, "What was that? What is that?" Sighted people often turn toward the source of a noise and visually decipher its nature or origin. Does the reception of a sound require a response? Should I be afraid, defensive, entertained, pleased, or excited? The mere fact of hearing a sound without ability to interpret how to respond can make the difference in one's enjoyment, comfort, safety, or survival. It is not only important to learn to label sounds; it is also very important to learn to interpret the nature and source of sounds so as to identify their implications for future occurrences.

Learning to listen provides enjoyment, safety and satisfaction. If a child is not physically introduced to the shape and sound of an instrument in a band or orchestra, how can he or she learn what instruments make what sounds? Likewise, if one never learns to distinguish between the sound of a happy or hostile dog, one cannot make a valid decision about whether it is approachable. The sound of a smile can bring as much satisfaction to the listener as seeing it.

The subtle skill of interpreting sounds is acquired over time and requires nurturing. I hope those of you who read this incredible book expand your ability to help people who are blind or visually impaired learn to listen so we can engage more fully in life.

Jerry Kuns
Technology Specialist
California School for the Blind
Fremont, California

Appendix A

The Listening Skills Continuum

The Listening Skills Continuum provides a compilation of the many listening skills that students with visual impairments may acquire over time, depending on their individual differences in development, starting in infancy and continuing from preschool through high school. The skills are presented for parents, teachers, and other professionals to use as a guide to help promote the development of these skills as children progress from infancy and throughout their school years. The continuum includes listening skill development that requires deliberate instruction for students to maximize their ability to interpret auditory input and use it as a basis for learning and growth.

The structure of the Listening Skills Continuum was inspired by the work of Lueck, Chen, Kekelis, and Hartmann in *Developmental Guidelines for Infants with Visual Impairments: A Guidebook for Early Intervention.*[1] A similar format is used in Anthony's "Typical Developmental Timeline of Auditory Skills."[2]

Although the continuum specifies ages and grade levels in relation to the skills it includes in order to provide a general guide to the progression of skill development, it should be regarded as an outline of the sequence in which students with visual impairments typically acquire these skills, rather than a blueprint for when during early development a child will acquire a given skill. True comparisons based on developmental level and age cannot be made due to the tremendous variation within the population of students who are visually impaired. Moreover, although the skills

---

1. A. H. Lueck, D. Chen, L. S. Kekelis, & E. S. Hartmann, *Developmental Guidelines for Infants with Visual Impairments: A Guidebook for Early Intervention*, 2nd ed. (Louisville, KY: American Printing House for the Blind, 2008).
2. T. Anthony & S. S. Lowry, "Sensory Development," in T. Anthony, S. S. Lowry, C. Brown, & D. Hatton (Eds.), *Developmentally Appropriate Orientation and Mobility* (pp. 125–240) (Chapel Hill: Early Intervention Training Center for Infants and Toddlers with Visual Impairments, University of North Carolina at Chapel Hill, 2004).

are listed in the developmental and grade-level order presented in the individual sources used, a student's acquisition of the skills needed to learn to listen will take place according to the progress of his or her individual development, and in fact may differ from the sequence presented.

The continuum is a guide to the skills that will optimize learning at home, in school, and in community settings. Progress in attaining listening skills can be monitored using the Informal Checklist for Listening Skills Development, which follows the continuum in Appendix B.

The sources for the items used in the Listening Skills Continuum were chosen to reflect a broad developmental range and variety of listening skills within assessment tools that are used with children with and without visual impairments. They were selected because of their relevance to listening skill development, a topic of importance for students with visual impairments about which little has been published. Consequently, some of the sources are older, such as the groundbreaking work of Selma Fraiberg (1977), *Insights from the Blind: Comparative Studies of Blind and Sighted Infants;* yet they provide valuable information that still helps guide families and professionals with regard to the development of children with visual impairments. Sources were chosen that include skills pertaining to listening such as, "Quiets to sound; appears comforted by human voice" from the Oregon Project (2007), or that require listening for development, such as "Engages in discussion about a book/story that is heard" from the *Desired Results Developmental Profile (DRDP)* (2008). A key to the abbreviations for the sources used in the continuum appears at the end of the continuum, along with descriptions of each source.

INFANTS AND TODDLERS

Learning to listen enables infants and toddlers to interpret the world, act and move with intention, and communicate. This act of auditory perception, or, the brain's interpretation of sound, involves much more than merely hearing sound. It requires a form of expectation, of knowing what is about to happen and preparing for it, and thus enables the formation of connections and comprehension. Beginning listening skills are organized in categories of auditory perception (see Chapter 1 of this book for definitions of these categories). The Listening Skills Continuum for infants and toddlers has been divided into the following domains:

- ▶ auditory awareness
- ▶ auditory attention
- ▶ sound localization
- ▶ auditory discrimination
- ▶ auditory memory: concepts and vocabulary

> ▸ receptive and expressive communication skills
> ▸ social listening

Some of the skills relate to more than one domain, such as "Repeats own sound" in both Auditory Awareness and Auditory Discrimination.

AUDITORY AWARENESS

Skill	Age	Sources
Alerts to auditory stimulation	Birth–1 year	Oregon Project
Quiets to sound; appears comforted by a human voice	Birth–1 year	Oregon Project
Smiles to auditory stimulation	Birth–3 months	Carolina Curriculum for Infants
Responds to voice	1 month	Bayley Scales 3
Responds differently to family members and strangers	6–9 months	Carolina Curriculum for Infants
Smiles when examiner speaks	2 months	Bayley Scales 3
Responds pleasurably to the sound of the human voice	Birth–1 year	Oregon Project
Smiles in response to a parent's voice	1 month 3–6 months	Bayley Scales 3 Insights

AUDITORY ATTENTION

Skill	Age	Sources
Habituates to a rattle	1 month	Bayley Scales 3
Quiets when presented with noise	0–3 months	Carolina Curriculum for Infants
Demonstrates a listening attitude; reacts to sound source	Birth–1 year	Oregon Project
Indicates attention to sound by action of hands	7 months	Insights
Bats at toys to hear something (cause and effect)	Birth–1 year	Oregon Project
Repeats own sounds	Birth–1 year	Oregon Project
Responds to name	Birth–1 year	Oregon project
Responds to spoken request	13 months	Bayley Scales 3

AUDITORY ATTENTION (*Continued*)

Skill	Age	Sources
Attends to stories, repeating words or sounds	18–21 months	Carolina Curriculum for Infants
Attends to a story	29–31 months	Bayley Scales 3

SOUND LOCALIZATION

Skill	Age	Sources
Turns head or reaches to sound at ear level while lying on back	Birth–3 months	Carolina Curriculum for Infants
Turns head to sound	4 months	Bailey Scales 3
Turns head to localize sound when in a sitting position	Birth–1 year	Oregon Project
Turns head or reaches to sound at ear level while sitting	3–6 months	Carolina Curriculum for Infants
Turns to the direction from which name is being called	3–6 months	Carolina Curriculum for Infants
Makes slight move toward a familiar sound	6 months	Insights
Orients to a sound source	Birth–1 year	Reynell-Zinkin Scales
Actively listens by localizing to sound source	Birth–1 year	Oregon Project
Opens a container with a lid to find a noisemaker (ticking clock, music box)	Birth–1 year	Oregon Project
Reaches toward a sound source in any direction	Birth–1 year	Reynell-Zinkin Scales
Reaches toward a sound source in correct direction	Birth–1 year	Reynell-Zinkin Scales
Moves to obtain an object using sound cue alone	1–2 years	Oregon Project

AUDITORY DISCRIMINATION

Skill	Age	Sources
Repeats own sounds	Birth–1 year	Oregon Project
Discriminates between bell and rattle	1 month	Bayley Scales 3
Responds differently to a new sound	3–6 months	Carolina Curriculum for Infants

Skill	Age	Sources
Imitates a familiar babbling sound	Birth–1 year	Oregon Project
Demonstrates an adverse reaction to sound of stranger's voice	8 months	Insights
Demonstrates selective response to sound	Birth–1 year	Reynell-Zinkin Scales
Imitates voice intonation patterns of others	Birth–1 year	Oregon Project
Listens selectively to two familiar words	11 months	Bayley Scales 3
Imitates word	14–16 months Birth–1 year	Bayley Scales 3 Oregon Project
Names household objects by their sounds	2–3 years	Oregon Project
Names musical instruments	2–3 years	Oregon Project

AUDITORY MEMORY: CONCEPTS AND VOCABULARY

Skill	Age	Sources
Anticipates familiar daily events based on auditory cues	Birth–1 year	Oregon Project
Anticipates frequently occurring events in familiar games involving sounds after two or three trials	6–9 months	Carolina Curriculum for Infants
Performs a previously learned task on verbal or gestural cue	6–9 months	Carolina Curriculum for Infants
Follows simple verbal direction accompanied by gestures or physical cues ("Give me your hands.")	Birth–1 year	Oregon Project
Has appropriate response for familiar words or phrases	Birth–1 year	Reynell-Zinkin Scales
Responds to "no" (briefly stops activity)	6–9 months	Carolina Curriculum for Infants
Selects a familiar object in response to its name	Birth–1 year	Reynell-Zinkin Scales
Selects named object from a choice of three	Birth–1 year	Reynell-Zinkin Scales
Points to most common objects on request	9–12 months	Carolina Curriculum for Infants
Points to/touches three body parts on request	Birth–1 year 15–18 months	Oregon Project Carolina Curriculum for Infants

AUDITORY MEMORY: CONCEPTS AND VOCABULARY (*Continued*)

Skill	Age	Sources
Has appropriate response to directions such as "Give it to me"	Birth–1 year	Reynell-Zinkin
Responds to "give me"	9–12 months	Carolina Curriculum for Infants
Follows two or more simple commands (one object, one action), spoken	12–15 months	Carolina Curriculum for Infants
Appropriately indicates "yes" or "no" in response to questions	12–15 months	Carolina Curriculum for Infants
Shows recognition of a few familiar sounds	15–18 months	Carolina Curriculum for Infants
Follows directions	20–22 months	Bayley Scales 3
Anticipates parts of rhymes or songs	21–24 months	Carolina Curriculum for Infants
Understands words used to inhibit actions (for example, "wait," "stop," "get down," "my turn")	21–24 months	Carolina Curriculum for Infants
Shows anticipation of events when a verbal cue is provided, such as "Let's go outside"	1–2 years	Oregon Project
Follows commands in familiar context	21–24 months	Carolina Curriculum for Infants
Remembers parts of rhymes or songs	2–3 years	Oregon Project
Says or sings at least parts of rhymes or songs in a group with an adult	24–30 months	Carolina Curriculum for Infants
Independently says or acts out parts of rhymes or songs	30–36 months	Carolina Curriculum for Infants
Notices and reacts to changes in familiar rhymes, songs, or stories	30–36 months	Carolina Curriculum for Infants
When directed, demonstrates concept of just one, in, under, and concept of two	2–3 years	Oregon Project

RECEPTIVE AND EXPRESSIVE COMMUNICATION SKILLS

Skill	Age	Sources
Vocalizes four times	1 month	Bayley Scales 3
Vocalizes when examiner speaks	3 months	Bayley Scales 3
Vocalizes two different vowel sounds	3 months	Bayley Scales 3

Skill	Age	Sources
Vocalizes three different vowel sounds	8 months	Bayley Scales 3
Imitates vocalization	9 months	Bayley Scales 3
Begins to imitate by taking turns in nonvocal noise-making schemes (pats table, shakes rattle)	Birth–1 year	Oregon Project
Jabbers expressively	12 months	Bayley Scales 3
Imitates familiar babbling sound	Birth–1 year	Oregon Project
Imitates voice intonation of others	Birth–1 year	Oregon Project
Repeats vowel-consonant combination	12 months	Bayley Scales 3
Repeats same syllable two to three times ("ma, ma, ma")	Birth–1 year	Oregon Project
Vocalizes five or more syllables in response to speech of another person	Birth–1 year	Oregon Project
Says five different words	1–2 years	Oregon Project
Vocalizes four different vowel-consonant combinations	13 months	Bayley Scales 3
Stops activity at least momentarily when told "no"	Birth–1 year	Oregon Project
Shows anticipation of events when verbal cue is provided ("Let's go outside." Child goes to door.)	Birth–1 year	Oregon Project
Responds to simple phrases with specific nonverbal response	Birth–1 year	Oregon Project
Follows simple verbal direction accompanied by gestures or physical cue	Birth–1 year	Oregon Project
Uses single words appropriately	Birth–1 year	Oregon Project
Responds to spoken request	13 months	Bayley Scales 3
Imitates word	13 months	Bayley Scales 3
Uses one-word sentence as request	1–2 years	Oregon Project
Names one object	20–22 months	Bayley Scales 3
Names familiar objects, people, pets, when asked	1–2 years	Oregon Project
Repeats a series of two digits or words in the same order	2–3 years	Oregon Project
Uses a two-word utterance	23–25 months	Bayley Scales 3
Imitates a two-word sentence	23–25 months	Bayley Scales 3

RECEPTIVE AND EXPRESSIVE COMMUNICATION SKILLS (*Continued*)

Skill	Age	Sources
Uses pronouns	23–25 months	Bayley Scales 3
Says eight different words	23–25 months	Bayley Scales 3
Names three objects	26–28 months	Bayley Scales 3
Uses a three-word sentence	26–28 months	Bayley Scales 3
Speaks in three-word sentence	2–3 years	Oregon Project
Displays verbal comprehension	29–31 months	Bayley Scales 3
Poses questions	32–34 months	Bayley Scales 3
Understands two prepositions	35–37 months	Bayley Scales 3
Produces multiple-word utterances in response to picture book	35–37 months	Bayley Scales 3

SOCIAL LISTENING

Skill	Age	Sources
Shows recognition of family members' voices by vocalizing, smiling, or ceasing to cry	Birth–1 year	Oregon Project
Reaches for familiar person when spoken to	Birth–1 year	Oregon Project
Vocalizes attitude	4 months	Bayley Scales 3
Enjoys social frolic and play	Birth–1 year	Oregon Project
Plays two interactive games (pat-a-cake, peekaboo)	Birth–1 year	Oregon Project
Engages in simple interactive play (pats table, claps hands)	Birth–1 year	Oregon Project
Cooperates in game	10 months	Bayley Scales 3
Repeats activities that get laughter and attention	1–2 years	Oregon Project
Participates in finger plays with adult	1–2 years	Oregon Project
Greets familiar person	1–2 years	Oregon Project
Takes part in simple game with another child and adult (pushing cars, beating drum)	1–2 years	Oregon Project
Shares object or food with one other child when requested	1–2 years	Oregon Project
Spontaneously joins in when familiar song or rhyme is heard	2–3 years	Oregon Project

Skill	Age	Sources
Enjoys hearing familiar stories repeated; tries to participate	2–3 years	Oregon Project
Plays with two or three peers with adult supervision	2–3 years	Oregon Project

PRESCHOOL AND KINDERGARTEN

Children in preschool and kindergarten need to develop listening skills that enable them to successfully understand and relate in the environments of home, school, and some aspects of the community, such as in playgroups, day care, and when out and about with family members. This part of the continuum has been divided into the following domains; they are discussed in Chapter 3:

▶ auditory attention
  • maintaining attention
  • figure-ground discrimination (the ability to focus on foreground sound such as a conversation, while filtering out distracting background noise)
▶ auditory discrimination
▶ auditory memory: concepts and directions
▶ auditory memory: sequence
▶ listening skills for reading readiness
▶ social listening

AUDITORY ATTENTION: MAINTAINING ATTENTION

Skill	Age	Sources
Quiets to listen to adult during caregiving routine	Preschool	DRDP
Responds to people or objects in the environment through actions or sounds	Preschool	DRDP
Attends to familiar adult's voice	Preschool	DRDP
Listens in a quiet environment	3–5 years	Assessment Companion
Listens to materials when presented rapidly	5 years	Assessment Companion

AUDITORY ATTENTION: FIGURE-GROUND DISCRIMINATION

Skill	Age	Sources
Attends to more than one thing at a time	Preschool	DRDP
Listens in a noisy environment	3–5 years	Assessment Companion
Attends in a small group	5 years	Assessment Companion
Attends within a large-group setting, such as a class	5 years	Assessment Companion
Listens to an adult's direction when walking in a noisy environment	5 years	Byrnes

AUDITORY DISCRIMINATION

Skill	Age	Sources
Responds in different ways, depending on the situation	Preschool	DRDP
Matches sound containers	3–4 years	Oregon Project Brigance
Follows one- and two-step directions with action or objects	Preschool	DRDP
Shows awareness and association of sounds to objects, persons, and actions	3–5 years	Listen and Think
Recognizes musical sounds	3–5 years	Listen and Think
Recognizes sounds in context	3–5 years	Listen and Think
Recognizes cause and effect with sounds	3–5 years	Listen and Think
Can identify rhyming words	3–5 years	Listen and Think
Attempts rhythmic movements with instruments	5 years	Brigance
Keeps time to simple tunes	5 years	Brigance

AUDITORY MEMORY: CONCEPTS AND DIRECTIONS

Skill	Age	Sources
When directed, points to 10 body parts	3–4 years	Brigance Oregon Project
When directed, points to 13 body parts	4 years	Brigance
When directed, touches top, bottom, front, and back on object	3–4 years	Oregon Project

Skill	Age	Sources
When directed, demonstrates *over*, *under*, *above*, *below*, *inside*, *through*, and *away from*	3–4 years	Brigance
Demonstrates *high* and *low* (body position) on request	3–4 years	Oregon Project
When directed, places objects in front of or behind other objects	3–4 years	Oregon Project
Responds to a spoken "stop" (for safety)	Preschool	Byrnes
Follows three-step instructions in a sequence involving two to three different objects	4 years	Carolina Curriculum for Preschoolers
When directed, demonstrates *across from*, *next to*, *beside*, *behind*, *in front*, *to the side*, *in back*, *left*, and *right*	5 years	Brigance Oregon Project

AUDITORY MEMORY: SEQUENCE

Skill	Age	Sources
Says or sings at least two nursery rhymes or songs in a group or with an adult	3 years	Carolina Curriculum for Preschoolers
Listens to/sings songs	3 years	Brigance
Repeats sound patterns of voice, clapping, tapping	3 years	Byrnes
Moves different body parts to music	4 years	Brigance
Relates an experience or a creative story in a logical sequence	Preschool	DRDP
Recognizes a sequence	5 years	Listen and Think
Remembers things in the order they are presented	5 years	Assessment Companion

LISTENING SKILLS FOR READING READINESS

Skill	Age	Sources
Repeats new words to self	3 years	Carolina Curriculum for Preschoolers
Gains information from listening to books about real things	3 years	Brigance
Engages in discussion about a book or story that has been heard	Preschool	DRDP

LISTENING SKILLS FOR READING READINESS (*Continued*)

Skill	Age	Sources
Participates in rhymes, songs, and games that play with sounds of language	Preschool	DRDP
Recalls one or two elements from a story just read without prompts	3½–4 years	Carolina Curriculum for Preschoolers
Is interested in different kinds of stories	4 years	Brigance
Likes to follow along in books being read	4 years	Brigance
Recalls most of the essential elements in a story	4½ years	Carolina Curriculum for Preschoolers
Makes rhymes to simple words	4½ years	Carolina Curriculum for Preschoolers
Soon after hearing the meaning of a new word, uses it in his or her own speech	5 years	Carolina Curriculum for Preschoolers
Listens to a story and retells it in own words	5 years	Assessment Companion
Repeats/points to all letters	5 years	Brigance
Answers "What happens if . . ." questions	5 years	Speech and Language Development Chart
Identifies main idea	5–6 years	Listen and Think
Predicts an outcome	5–6 years	Listen and Think
Summarizes a story	5–6 years	Listen and Think
Understands character and setting	5–6 years	Listen and Think
Recognizes speaker's purpose	5–6 years	Listen and Think

SOCIAL LISTENING

Skill	Age	Sources
Shows concern when others are unhappy or upset	Preschool	DRDP
Shows awareness of others	Preschool	DRDP
Reacts to adult's behavior	Preschool	DRDP
Attends to other children's behavior	Preschool	DRDP
Responds to adult guidance in negotiating conflict	Preschool	DRDP
Follows adult request to wait turn	Preschool	DRDP
Sustains conversation for several turns	3 years	Carolina Curriculum for Preschoolers

Skill	Age	Sources
Changes speech depending on listener (for example, talks differently to babies and adults)	3 years	Carolina Curriculum for Preschoolers
Talks on telephone	3 years	Carolina Curriculum for Preschoolers
Follows rules given by adults for new activities or simple games	3½ years	Carolina Curriculum for Preschoolers
Shows interest in conversation	3 years	Brigance
Responds to/verbally greets at appropriate times ("hi," "bye," and the like)	3–4 years	DRDP Brigance
Anticipates/follows multistep daily routines when prompted	3–4 years	DRDP
Follows rules when participating in routine activities	3–4 years	DRDP
Participates in a conversation that develops a thought or idea	3–4 years	DRDP
Responds appropriately to instructions given in a small group	4 years	Carolina Curriculum for Preschoolers
Acknowledges compliments	4 years	Brigance
Localizes and looks at (or faces) speaker when listening	4 years	Byrnes
Answers questions about what was heard in conversation	4–5 years	Assessment Companion
Resists impulsivity and waits for entire message or directions	5 years	Assessment Companion
Listens and waits turn when talking with others	5 years	Assessment Companion
Asks questions to check understanding in a full-class or small-group setting	5 years	Assessment Companion
Participates in a conversation without monopolizing it	5 years	Brigance
Answers telephone and summons person requested	5 years	Brigance Carolina Curriculum for Preschoolers
Answers telephone, takes simple message, and delivers it	5 years	Brigance
Delivers two-part message orally	5 years	Brigance

ELEMENTARY SCHOOL

Students in elementary school need to learn to listen, but also to listen in order to learn. Skilled listening supports the development of literacy skills, in both the development of sound-symbol relationships necessary for reading and the development of listening and reading comprehension. Students with visual impairments need to learn to attend actively and should develop critical listening skills that are essential for curricular instruction. As students learn how to use technology for access to the curriculum and written expression, listening plays an important role. Skilled listening also facilitates the development of social interaction. The listening skills continuum for students in elementary school has been divided into the following domains:

- ▸ listening and literacy skills
  - phonemic and phonological skills
  - listening comprehension of information that is presented or read orally (live reader or recorded)
- ▸ active listening
- ▸ critical listening during oral instruction
- ▸ listening and technology
- ▸ listening and social skills

LISTENING AND LITERACY SKILLS: PHONEMIC AND PHONOLOGICAL SKILLS

Skill	Grade Level	Sources
Discriminates and identifies verbal and nonverbal sounds	Elementary	Harley et al.
Demonstrates understanding of spoken words, syllables, and sounds (phonemes)	1	CCSS
Creates and states a series of rhyming words, including consonant blends	1	CA
Distinguishes initial, medial, and final sounds in single-syllable words	1	CA
Distinguishes long and short vowel sounds in orally stated single-syllable words	1	CA
Adds, deletes, or changes target sounds to change words (for example, changes *cow* to *how*; *pan* to *an*)	1	CA
Blends two to four phonemes into recognizable words (for example, /c/a/t/ = cat; /f/l/a/t/ = flat)	1	CA

Skill	Grade Level	Sources
Segments single-syllable words into their components (for example, /c/a/t/ = cat; /s/p/l/a/t = splat; /r/i/ch/ = rich)	1	CA
Knows and applies grade-level phonics and word analysis in decoding words	1–5	CCSS

LISTENING AND LITERACY SKILLS: LISTENING COMPREHENSION OF INFORMATION THAT IS PRESENTED OR READ ORALLY (LIVE READER OR RECORDED)

Skill	Grade Level	Sources
Recalls fact and details	Elementary	Harley et al.
Identifies sequential order	Elementary	Harley et al.
Selects main idea, summarizes, relates one idea to another, makes inferences	Elementary	Harley et al.
Asks and answers questions about what a speaker says in order to gather additional information or clarify something that is not understood	1	CCSS
Asks and answers questions about key details in a text read aloud or information presented orally or through other media	1	CCSS
Listens to literary texts and performances to appreciate and enjoy literary works; to identify character, setting, and plot; to respond to vivid language; and to identify specific people, places, and events	1	NY
Listens to acquire information from nonfiction text	1	NY
Listens to literary texts and performances to distinguish between a story, a poem, and a play	1–5	NY
Recounts or describes key ideas or details from a text read aloud or information presented orally or through other media	2	CCSS
Identifies elements of character, plot, and setting to understand the author's message with assistance	2	NY
Connects literary texts to previous life experiences to enhance understanding	2	NY
Retells stories, including characters, setting, and plot	2	CA
Connects literary texts to personal experiences and previously encountered texts to enhance understanding and appreciation	3	NY
Determines the main ideas and supporting details of a text read aloud or information presented in diverse media and formats, including visually, quantitatively, and orally	3	CCSS

LISTENING AND LITERACY SKILLS: LISTENING COMPREHENSION OF INFORMATION THAT IS PRESENTED OR READ ORALLY (LIVE READER OR RECORDED) (*Continued*)

Skill	Grade Level	Sources
Identifies elements of character, plot, and setting to understand the author's message or intent	3–4	NY
Paraphrases portions of a text read aloud or information presented in diverse media and formats, including visually, quantitatively, and orally	4	CCSS
Summarizes a text read aloud or information presented in diverse media and formats, including visually, quantitatively, and orally	5	CCSS

ACTIVE LISTENING

Skill	Grade Level	Sources
Identifies and responds to nonverbal sounds, such as school bell, telephone, running water, and the like	Elementary	Harley et al.
Identifies and responds to verbal sounds and voices in the environment	Elementary	Harley et al.
Demonstrates the responsibility of the listener to the speaker: focuses attention on the person who is speaking	Elementary	Harley et al.
Participates in collaborative conversations with diverse partners about class topics and texts with peers and adults in small and large groups	K–2	CCSS
Gives, restates, and follows simple two-step directions	1	CA
Gives and follows three- and four-step oral directions	2	CA
Listens to determine a sequence of steps given	3–4	NY
Participates in collaborative conversations with diverse partners about class topics and texts, building on others' ideas and expressing his or her own clearly	3–5	CCST

CRITICAL LISTENING DURING ORAL INSTRUCTION

Skill	Grade Level	Sources
Listens critically and responds appropriately to oral communication	1	CA
Asks questions for clarification	1	CA

Skill	Grade Level	Sources
Asks and answers questions about what a speaker says in order to clarify comprehension, gather additional information, or deepen understanding of a topic or issue	2	CCSS
Determines the purpose or purposes of listening (for example, to obtain information, to solve problems, for enjoyment)	2	CA
Paraphrases information that has been shared orally by others	2	CA
Recounts experiences in a logical sequence	2	CA
Asks for clarification and explanation of stories and ideas	2	CA
Identifies the musical elements of literary language (for example, rhymes, repeated sounds)	3	CA
Connects and relates prior experiences, insights, and ideas to those of a speaker	3	CA
Retells, paraphrases, and explains what has been said by the speaker	3	CA
Responds to questions with appropriate elaboration	3	CA
Listens to acquire information and understand procedures	4	NY
Asks thoughtful questions and responds to relevant questions with appropriate elaboration	4	CA
Summarizes major ideas and supporting evidence presented in spoken messages and formal presentations	4	CA
Interprets a speaker's verbal and nonverbal messages, purposes, and perspectives	5	CA
Makes inferences or draws conclusions based on an oral report	5	CA
Listens to follow instructions that provide information about a task or assignment	5	NY
Listens to identify essentials for note taking	5	NY

LISTENING AND TECHNOLOGY

Skill	Grade Level	Sources
Listens to audio materials such as books, Internet, radio, and television	Preschool through high school	Postello & Barclay
Listens to curriculum on an interactive audio/tactile learning system	Can begin in pre-kindergarten and be used as long as helpful	Postello & Barclay

LISTENING AND TECHNOLOGY (*Continued*)

Skill	Grade Level	Sources
Listens to an electronic braillewriter	Can begin from preschool to first grade	Postello & Barclay
Listens to to an accessible PDA (electronic notetaker) with braille or speech output or both	Can begin when the student understands the braille code and is an early reader. Student must demonstrate responsibility for care of equipment.	Postello & Barclay
Listens and interacts with auditory games and keyboarding tutor programs on computer	Can begin playing cause-and-effect games as a preschooler; can begin keyboarding in first or second grade	Postello & Barclay
Listens to labels on tactile maps, diagrams, drawings, or courseware	Begins in pre-kindergarten, continuing through elementary school	Postello & Barclay
Listens to screen reader while using the computer	Third grade	Postello & Barclay
Listens to audible literature on digital players or recorders, computers, electronic notetakers, and accessible PDAs	Third grade	Postello & Barclay
Listens while using scanning programs	May begin in fourth or fifth grade or middle school	Postello & Barclay
Listens while using GPS	Depends on student's skill level	Postello & Barclay

LISTENING AND SOCIAL SKILLS

Skill	Grade Level	Sources
Identifies tone of voice, such as humorous, sad, angry, silly	Elementary	Postello & Barclay
Listens for the tone of voice and the content that signal friendly communication	1–5	NY
Follows agreed-upon rules for discussion (for example, listening to others and taking turns speaking about the topics and texts under discussion)	K–5	CCSS
Continues a conversation through multiple exchanges	K	CCSS
Builds on others' talk in conversations by responding to the comments of others through multiple exchanges	1	CCSS

Skill	Age/Grade Level	Sources
Builds on others' talk in conversations by linking their comments to the remarks of others	2	CCSS
Follows agreed-upon rules for discussion (for example, gaining the floor in respectful ways, listening to others with care, speaking one at a time about the topics and texts under discussion)	3–5	CCSS
Maintains appropriate conversation for at least two to five minutes with a beginning, middle, and end	Elementary	Sacks & Barclay
Demonstrates turn-taking ability in conversations and when playing with peers	Elementary	Sacks & Barclay
Listens to locate and identify a specific peer and ask the student to play	4–7 years	TSBVI-IL
Listens to join in a group that is playing or conversing	Elementary	Sacks & Barclay
Recognizes and responds to humor and uses it in social situations	8–11 years	TSBVI-IL
Recognizes sarcasm and responds in an effective manner	8–11 years	TSBVI-IL
Engages in conversation, giving attention and showing interest in others	8–11 years	TSBVI-IL
Recognizes that social communication may include informal language such as jargon	5	NY

MIDDLE AND HIGH SCHOOL

Students in middle school and high school need to refine their ability to listen to classroom instruction actively and critically and engage in collaborative discussions with their teachers and classmates. They must also use fine-tuned listening skills as they utilize assistive technology for many curricular tasks. Middle and high school students will thrive socially if they have learned how to fully interact with their peers because they have learned to listen to what they have to say. This Listening Skills Continuum for middle and high school students has been divided into the following domains:

> ▸ listening in the classroom: active and critical listening
> ▸ listening and organizing information from classroom instruction or read aloud (live reader or recorded)
> ▸ listening and technology
> ▸ listening during social interaction

LISTENING IN THE CLASSROOM: ACTIVE AND CRITICAL LISTENING

Skill	Grade Level	Sources
Listens critically to oral classroom discussion	6–12	Herlich
Engages effectively in a range of collaborative discussions (one-on-one, in groups, and teacher-led) with diverse partners on grade level topics, texts, and issues, building on others' ideas and expressing one's own clearly	6–8	CCSS
Follows rules for collegial discussions, sets specific goals and deadlines, and defines individual roles as needed	6–8	CCSS
Comes to discussions prepared, having read or studied required material; explicitly draws on that preparation by referring to evidence on the topic, text, or issue to probe and reflects on ideas under discussion	6–8	CCSS
Poses and responds to specific questions with elaboration and detail by making comments that contribute to the topic, text, or issue under discussion	6	CCSS
Restates and executes multiple-step oral instructions and directions	6	CA
Identifies the tone, mood, and emotion conveyed in the oral communication	6	CA
Listens attentively, for an extended period of time, to a variety of texts read aloud and oral presentations	6–8	NY
Listens attentively for different purposes, both student determined and teacher determined	6–8	NY
Poses questions that elicit elaboration and responds to others' questions and comments with relevant observations and ideas that bring the discussion back on topic as needed	7	CCSS
Acknowledges new information expressed by others and, when warranted, modifies his or her own views	7	CA
Determines the speaker's attitude toward the subject	7	CA
Responds to persuasive messages with questions, challenges, or affirmations	7	CA
Poses questions that connect the ideas of several speakers and responds to others' questions and comments with relevant evidence, observations, and ideas	8	CCSS
Acknowledges new information expressed by others and, when warranted, qualifies or justifies his or her own views in light of the evidence presented	8	CCSS
Listens to and follows complex directions or instructions	9	NY

Skill	Grade Level	Sources
Recognizes appropriate voice and tone	9	NY
Initiates and participates effectively in a range of collaborative discussions (one-on-one, in groups, and teacher-led) with diverse partners on grade level topics, texts, and issues, building on others' ideas and expressing his or her own clearly and persuasively	9–12	CCSS
Works with peers to set rules for collegial discussions and decision making (for example, informal consensus, taking votes on key issues, presentation of alternate views), clear goals and deadlines, and individual roles as needed	9–10	CCSS
Comes to discussions prepared, having read and researched material under study; explicitly draws on that preparation by referring to the evidence from texts and other research on the topic or issue to stimulate a thoughtful, well-reasoned exchange of ideas	9–12	CCSS
Responds thoughtfully to diverse perspectives, summarizes points of agreement and disagreement, and, when warranted, qualifies or justifies his or her own views and understanding and makes new connections in light of the evidence and reasoning presented	9–10	CCSS
Anticipates the speaker's point and assesses its validity, with assistance	10–12	NY
Recognizes the speaker's use of voice and tone, diction, and syntax in school and public forums, debates, and panel discussions	12	NY

LISTENING AND ORGANIZING INFORMATION FROM CLASSROOM INSTRUCTION OR READ ALOUD (LIVE READER OR RECORDED)

Skill	Grade Level	Sources
Listens to and independently organizes spoken information by summarizing and taking notes about spoken ideas, literature, and curriculum	6–12	Herlich
Reviews the key ideas expressed and demonstrates understanding of multiple perspectives through reflection and paraphrasing	6	CCSS
Determines the speaker's attitude toward the subject	7	CA
Analyzes oral interpretations of literature, including language choice and delivery, and the effect of the information on the listener	8	CA
Paraphrases a speaker's purpose and point of view and asks relevant questions concerning the speaker's delivery and purpose	8	CA

LISTENING AND ORGANIZING INFORMATION FROM CLASSROOM INSTRUCTION OR READ ALOUD (LIVE READER OR RECORDED) (*Continued*)

Skill	Grade Level	Sources
Interprets information from media presentations such as news broadcasts and taped interviews	9	NY
Identifies the speaker's purpose and motive for communicating information	9	NY
Interprets information from media presentations such as documentary films, news broadcasts, and taped interviews	10–12	NY
Determines the need for more information for clarification	10–12	NY
Synthesizes the information from different sources by combining or categorizing data and facts	10–12	NY

LISTENING AND TECHNOLOGY

Skill	Grade Level	Sources
Listens to learn while using appropriate access technology	6–12	Herlich
Selects and uses appropriate technology tools to accomplish a variety of tasks	6–8	NETS
Demonstrates advanced word-processing skills, such as cutting and pasting text, using a spell checker, and using formatting features	6–8	Strategies
Demonstrates advanced use of screen-reading options	6–8	Strategies
Demonstrates effective use of portable notetakers using simple applications, such as word-processing file management, calendar, and calculator functions	6–8	Strategies
Demonstrates effective use of Internet applications as appropriate to student's age level	6–12	Strategies
Selects and applies technology tools for research, information gathering, problem solving, and decision making	9–12	NETS
Demonstrates advanced use of portable notetakers, such as advanced word processing	9–12	Strategies

LISTENING DURING SOCIAL INTERACTION

Skill	Grade Level	Sources
Utilizes effective listening strategies to engage in social interaction	6–12	Herlich
Listens respectfully when others speak	6–8	NY

Skill	Grade Level	Sources
Identifies the tone, mood, and emotion conveyed in oral communication	6	CA
Participates as a listener in social conversation with one or more people	7–8	NY
Maintains a socially appropriate conversation for a minimum of 10 minutes with peers and adults	6–8	Sacks & Barclay
Demonstrates ability to take the role of others and understand others' feelings in various social situations	6–8	Sacks & Barclay
Evaluates social situations to determine appropriate use of specific social behaviors	9–12	Sacks & Barclay
Converses with others on a range of interesting topics without dominating the conversation	9–12	Sacks & Barclay
Compliments others and reciprocates when appropriate	9–12	Sacks & Barclay

KEY TO SOURCES

Source Abbreviation	Full Source	Description
Infants and Toddlers		
Bayley Scales 3	N. Bayley, *Bayley Scales of Infant Development*, 3rd ed. New York: Psychological Corporation, 2005.	A system developed to evaluate the developmental status of young children from ages 1 to 42 months. Consists of three scales: Mental, Motor, and Behavioral Rating. The Mental Scale, which was used as a source of the items in this continuum, assesses skills such as memory, habituation (becoming accustomed to sensory stimulation, such as sound), problem solving, early number concepts, generalization, classification, vocalizations, language, and social skills.
Carolina Curriculum for Infants and Toddlers	N. M. Johnson-Martin, S. M. Attermeier, & B. J. Hacker, *Carolina Curriculum for Infants and Toddlers with Special Needs*, 2nd ed. Baltimore: Paul H.	A curriculum-based assessment developed for use with children from birth to 36 months who have mild to severe disabilities; includes items that cover developmental skills in that age range. In addition to the assessment checklist, there is a

Source Abbreviation	Full Source	Description
	Brookes Publishing Co., 2004.	complete curriculum for each area assessed that includes recommended teaching adaptations for children with special learning requirements as a result of specific disabilities, including visual impairment.
Insights	S. Fraiberg, *Insights from the Blind*. New York: Basic Books, 1977.	The findings from one of the first studies to discover how the human personality develops without vision. The study of 27 infants who were blind covered early development in the areas of self-concept, language acquisition, mobility, object relationship, and the formation of human attachments.
Oregon Project	S. Anderson, S. Boignon, K. Davis, & C. deWaard, *Oregon Project for Visually Impaired and Blind Preschool Children*, 6th ed. Medford: Southern Oregon Education Service District, 2007.	An assessment and curriculum guide developed for students with visual impairments. The Skills Inventory, one segment of the guide, consists of 800 behavioral statements organized in eight developmental areas: cognitive, language, socialization, vision, compensatory, self-help, fine motor, and gross motor. Each of these eight areas contains skills that have been developmentally sequenced and arranged in the following age categories: birth–1, 1–2, 2–3, 3–4, 4–5, and 5–6 years. The Skills Inventory enables educators to find the performance level of a child who is visually impaired or blind, select long- and short-term objectives, and record the acquisition of skills.
Reynell-Zinkin Scales	J. Reynell, *Manual for the Reynell-Zinkin Developmental Scales for Young Visually Handicapped Children*. Windsor, UK: NFER-Nelson, 1983.	System designed to provide guidelines and developmental guidance to parents and educators of students with visual impairment. Covers the developmental range from 2 months to 5 years and includes scales on social adaptation, sensorimotor understanding, exploration of the environment, response to sound and verbal comprehension, and expressive language. A special subscale for communication is available for assessing people who

Source Abbreviation	Full Source	Description
		have cerebral palsy, deafness, or specific language difficulties or who are deaf-blind. The scales were standardized on children who are visually impaired, including those with multiple handicaps.

Preschool and Kindergarten

Source Abbreviation	Full Source	Description
Assessment Companion	R. Huisingh, M. Barrett, L. Zachman, J. Orman, & C. Blagden, *The Assessment Companion: Communication Checklists for Speech and Language Pathologists, Teachers, and Parents*. East Moline, IL: LinguiSystems, 1993.	Includes checklists, questionnaires for teachers and parents, information handouts, and data-collection forms for the following communication areas: early language, vocabulary and semantics, syntax and morphology (the structure and content of word forms), pragmatics (language as it is used in a social context), thinking and problem solving, listening and processing, articulation and phonology, voice, fluency, and metalinguistics (the ability to use and talk about language).
Brigance	A. H. Brigance, *Brigance Diagnostic Inventory of Early Development*. North Billerica, MA: Curriculum Associates, 2004.	A criterion-referenced developmental inventory (states what students can do and what they know, not how they compare to others at specific ages) that evaluates the development of normally sighted children up to the age of 7. Evaluates gross-motor, fine-motor, pre-speech, speech and language, general knowledge, readiness, basic reading, manuscript writing, and basic math skills. Test results are expressed as developmental ages.
Byrnes	K. A. Byrnes, "Preschool and Kindergarten: Early Skill Development" in L. A. Barclay, Ed., *Learning to Listen/Listening to Learn: Teaching Listening Skills to Students with Visual Impairments*. New York: AFB Press, 2011.	See Chapter 3 of this book.
Carolina Curriculum for Preschoolers	N. M. Johnson-Martin, S. M. Attermeier, & B. J. Hacker, *Carolina Curriculum for Preschoolers*	A curriculum-based assessment developed for use with children who have mild to severe disabilities from 24 months to 5 years of age for determining the child's

Source Abbreviation	Full Source	Description
	with Special Needs. Baltimore: Paul H. Brookes Publishing, 2004.	mastery of important social, cognitive, language, motor, and adaptive skills; includes items that cover developmental skills. In addition to the assessment checklist, there is a complete curriculum for each area assessed that includes recommended teaching adaptations for children with special learning requirements as a result of specific disabilities, including visual impairment.
DRDP	*Desired Results Developmental Profile-Revised (DRDP)*. Sacramento: California Department of Education, Child Development Division, in collaboration with the Center for Child and Family Studies, 2008. www.wested.org/desiredresults/training/form_drdp.htm.	An assessment tool for 3-, 4-, and 5-year-old children who have Individualized Education Programs (IEPs) for preschool services in California. Helps the California Department of Education evaluate its programs for young children to document children's progress in areas such as learning, getting along with others, and being safe and healthy.
Listen and Think	E. Pester, *Listen and Think Auditory Readiness (AR) Level*. Louisville, KY: American Printing House for the Blind, 1972. (Original work produced by Educational Developmental Laboratories and adapted in 1972.)	Although originally written in 1969, one of the few curricular resources specific to listening available. *Listen and Think* was adapted for visually impaired students to learn basic listening skills. It includes concepts such as understanding placement (for example, up and down), using the senses, comparing, and classifying.
Speech and Language Development Chart	American Speech-Language-Hearing Association. www.asha.org/public/speech/development/chart.htm.	This series of charts from the American Speech-Language-Hearing Association (ASHA) provide a listing of hearing, understanding, and talking skills that infants and toddlers will develop from birth through 5 years of age.

Elementary, Middle, and High School

Source Abbreviation	Full Source	Description
CA	California Department of Education. *English–Language Arts Content Standards for California Public Schools, Kindergarten through Grade Twelve*. Sacramento, CA: CDE Press, 1997.	Standards and skills were chosen from this state because they represent specific examples of elementary-level listening skills and the variety of listening skills required for learners in middle and high school, and therefore provide additional guidance for choosing skills to target for development.

Source Abbreviation	Full Source	Description
CCSS	Common Core State Standards Initiative. *Common Core State Standards for English Language Arts and Literacy in History/Social Studies, Science, and Technical Subjects.* 2010.' Retrieved from http://www.corestandards.org/the-standards.	Common Core State Standards have been developed by the Common Core State Standards Initiative, a state-led effort coordinated by the National Governors Association Center for Best Practices and the Council of Chief State School Officers in collaboration with teachers, school administrators, and experts "to provide a clear and consistent framework to prepare children for college and the workforce" and have been adopted by most states across the country. Skills were chosen from the Common Core State Standards to illustrate the variety of listening skills that are required for all learners throughout elementary school.
Harley et al.	R. K. Harley, M. B. Truan, & L. D. Sanford, "Developing Listening Skills," *Communication Skills for Visually Impaired Learners*, 2nd ed., Chapter 9. Springfield, IL: Charles C Thomas, 1997.	Outlines many aspects of the development of listening skills for students who are visually impaired.
Herlich	S. Herlich, "Middle School and High School: Advanced Skill Development" in L. A. Barclay, Ed., *Learning to Listen/Listening to Learn: Teaching Listening Skills to Students with Visual Impairments*. New York: AFB Press, 2011.	See Chapter 5 of this book.
NETS	International Society for Technology in Education National Education Technology Standards, *NETS for Students: National Curriculum/Content Area Standards*. Eugene, OR: International Society for Technology in Education, 2007.	The primary goal of the (NETS) project is to help develop national standards for educational use of technology.

Source Abbreviation	Full Source	Description
NY	*English Language Arts Core Curriculum*. Albany: University of the State of New York, State Education Department, 2005.	Standards and skills were chosen from this state because they represent specific examples of elementary-level listening skills and the variety of listening skills required for learners in middle and high school, and therefore provide additional guidance for choosing skills to target for development.
Postello & Barclay	T. Postello & L. A. Barclay, "Elementary School: Developing and Refining Listening Skills," in L. A. Barclay, Ed., *Learning to Listen/Listening to Learn: Teaching Listening Skills to Students with Visual Impairments*, Table 4.1. New York: AFB Press, 2011.	See Chapter 4 of this book.
Sacks & Barclay	S. Z. Sacks & L. A. Barclay, Benchmarks for Social Skills of Students with Visual Impairments, in "Social Skills Assessment," in S. Z. Sacks & K. E. Wolffe, Eds., *Teaching Social Skills to Students with Visual Impairments: From Theory to Practice* (pp. 282–285). New York: AFB Press, 2006.	This checklist includes basic social skills that children of various ages who are visually impaired need to learn.
Strategies	F. M. D'Andrea & K. Barnicle, "Access to Information: Technology and Braille," in D. P. Wormsley & F. M. D'Andrea, Eds., *Instructional Strategies for Braille Literacy* (pp. 269–307). New York: American Foundation for the Blind, 1997.	This chapter contains a breakdown of what technology to introduce at different grade levels.
TSBVI-IL	R. Loumiet & N. Levack, *Independent Living*, Vol. 1, *Social Competence*. Austin: Texas School for the Blind and Visually Impaired, 1993.	A living skills curriculum, written by educators from Texas School for the Blind and Visually Impaired, that focuses on skills presented in developmental sequence for learners with visual impairments.

Appendix B

Informal Checklist for Listening Skills Development

This informal checklist can be used in tandem with the Listening Skills Continuum (Appendix A) to document a student's growth in listening skill development. It will also provide ongoing guidance for selecting skills to target for development. It can be used by parents and caregivers, teachers, and other professionals to ensure that listening skills are addressed as an important aspect of each student's expanded core curriculum from infancy through high school.

Decisions regarding which skills to prioritize for emphasis and instruction need to be part of students' Individualized Family Service Plan (IFSP) or Individualized Education Program (IEP) process. For listening skills that can be considered as goals for students with visual and multiple disabilities, see Appendix 7A in this book, which lists alternate functional listening skills that align with standards-based core curricula.

INFANTS AND TODDLERS

Child's Name: _____　**Evaluator's Name:** _____

Directions: Insert the date of the IFSP or IEP year in which the skill is targeted at the top of the chart. Record the child's level of development in the targeted skills using the following key:

    – Not yet mastered
    +/– Emerging
    + Mastered and generalized

AUDITORY AWARENESS

Skill	Date			
Alerts to auditory stimulation				
Quiets to sound; appears comforted by a human voice				
Smiles to auditory stimulation				
Responds to voice				
Responds differently to family members and strangers				
Smiles when examiner speaks				
Responds pleasurably to the sound of the human voice				
Smiles in response to a parent's voice				

AUDITORY ATTENTION

Skill	Date			
Habituates to a rattle				
Quiets when presented with noise				
Demonstrates a listening attitude; reacts to sound source				
Indicates attention to sound by action of hands				
Bats at toys to hear something (cause and effect)				
Repeats own sounds				
Responds to name				
Responds to spoken request				
Attends to stories, repeating words or sounds				
Attends to a story				

SOUND LOCALIZATION

Skill	Date			
Turns head or reaches to sound at ear level while lying on back				
Turns head to sound				
Turns head to localize sound when in a sitting position				
Turns head or reaches to sound at ear level while sitting				
Turns to the direction from which name is being called				
Makes slight move toward a familiar sound				
Orients to a sound source				
Actively listens by localizing to sound source				
Opens container with lid to find a noisemaker (ticking clock, music box)				
Reaches toward a sound source in any direction				
Reaches toward a sound source in correct direction				
Moves to obtain object using sound cue alone				

AUDITORY DISCRIMINATION

Skill	Date			
Repeats own sounds				
Discriminates between bell and rattle				
Responds differently to a new sound				
Imitates a familiar babbling sound				
Demonstrates adverse reaction to sound of stranger's voice				
Demonstrates selective response to sound				
Imitates voice intonation patterns of others				
Listens selectively to two familiar words				
Imitates word				
Names household objects by their sounds				
Names musical instruments				

AUDITORY MEMORY: CONCEPTS AND VOCABULARY

Skill	Date			
Anticipates familiar daily events based on auditory cues				
Anticipates frequently occurring events in familiar games involving sounds after two or three trials				
Performs a previously learned task on verbal or gestural cue				
Follows simple verbal direction accompanied by gestures or physical cues ("Give me your hands.")				
Has appropriate response for familiar words or phrases				
Responds to "no" (briefly stops activity)				
Selects a familiar object in response to its name				
Selects named object from a choice of three				
Points to most common objects on request				
Points to/touches three body parts on request				
Has appropriate response to directions such as "Give it to me"				
Responds to "give me"				
Follows two or more simple commands (one object, one action), spoken				
Appropriately indicates "yes" or "no" in response to questions				
Shows recognition of a few familiar sounds				
Follows directions				
Anticipates parts of rhymes or songs				
Understands words used to inhibit actions (for example, "wait," "stop," "get down," "my turn")				
Shows anticipation of events when a verbal cue is provided, such as "Let's go outside"				
Follows commands in familiar context				
Remembers parts of rhymes or songs				
Says or sings at least parts of rhymes or songs in a group with an adult				
Independently says or acts out parts of rhymes or songs				
Notices and reacts to changes in familiar rhymes, songs, or stories				
When directed, demonstrates concept of just one, in, under, and concept of two				

RECEPTIVE AND EXPRESSIVE COMMUNICATION SKILLS

Skill	Date			
Vocalizes four times				
Vocalizes when examiner speaks				
Vocalizes two different vowel sounds				
Vocalizes three different vowel sounds				
Imitates vocalization				
Begins to imitate by taking turns in nonvocal noise-making schemes (pats table, shakes rattle)				
Jabbers expressively				
Imitates familiar babbling sound				
Imitates voice intonation of others				
Repeats vowel-consonant combination				
Repeats same syllable two to three times ("ma, ma, ma")				
Vocalizes five or more syllables in response to speech of another person				
Says five different words				
Vocalizes four different vowel-consonant combinations				
Stops activity at least momentarily when told "no"				
Shows anticipation of events when verbal cue is provided ("Let's go outside." Child goes to door.)				
Responds to simple phrases with specific nonverbal response				
Follows simple verbal direction accompanied by gestures or physical cue				
Uses single words appropriately				
Responds to spoken request				
Imitates word				
Uses one-word sentence as request				
Names one object				
Names familiar objects, people, pets, when asked				
Repeats a series of two digits or words in the same order				
Uses a two-word utterance				
Imitates a two-word sentence				
Uses pronouns				

RECEPTIVE AND EXPRESSIVE COMMUNICATION SKILLS (*Continued*)

Skill	Date			
Says eight different words				
Names three objects				
Uses a three-word sentence				
Speaks in three-word sentence				
Displays verbal comprehension				
Poses questions				
Understands two prepositions				
Produces multiple-word utterances in response to picture book				

SOCIAL LISTENING

Skill	Date			
Shows recognition of family members' voices by vocalizing, smiling, or ceasing to cry				
Reaches for familiar person when spoken to				
Vocalizes attitude				
Enjoys social frolic and play				
Plays two interactive games (pat-a-cake, peekaboo)				
Engages in simple interactive play (pats table, claps hands)				
Cooperates in game				
Repeats activities that get laughter and attention				
Participates in finger plays with adult				
Greets familiar person				
Takes part in simple game with another child and adult (pushing cars, beating drum)				
Shares object or food with one other child when requested				
Spontaneously joins in when familiar song or rhyme is heard				
Enjoys hearing familiar stories repeated; tries to participate				
Plays with two or three peers with adult supervision				

PRESCHOOL AND KINDERGARTEN

Student's Name: **Evaluator's Name:**

Directions: Insert the date of the IEP year in which the skill is targeted at the top of the chart. Record the child's level of development in the targeted skills using the following key:

    – Not yet mastered
    +/– Emerging
    + Mastered and generalized

AUDITORY ATTENTION: MAINTAINING ATTENTION

Skill	Date			
Quiets to listen to adult during caregiving routine				
Responds to people or objects in the environment through actions or sounds				
Attends to familiar adult's voice				
Listens in a quiet environment				
Listens to materials when presented rapidly				

AUDITORY ATTENTION: FIGURE-GROUND DISCRIMINATION

Skill	Date			
Attends to more than one thing at a time				
Listens in a noisy environment				
Attends in a small group				
Attends within a large-group setting, such as a class				
Listens to an adult's direction when walking in a noisy environment				

AUDITORY DISCRIMINATION

Skill	Date			
Responds in different ways, depending on the situation				
Matches sound containers				
Follows one- and two-step directions with action or objects				
Shows awareness and association of sounds to objects, persons, and actions				

AUDITORY DISCRIMINATION (*Continued*)

Skill	Date			
Recognizes musical sounds				
Recognizes sounds in context				
Recognizes cause and effect with sounds				
Can identify rhyming words				
Attempts rhythmic movements with instruments				
Keeps time to simple tunes				

AUDITORY MEMORY: CONCEPTS AND DIRECTIONS

Skill	Date			
When directed, points to 10 body parts				
When directed, points to 13 body parts				
When directed, touches top, bottom, front, and back on object				
When directed, demonstrates *over*, *under*, *above*, *below*, *inside*, *through*, and *away from*				
Demonstrates *high* and *low* (body position) on request				
When directed, places objects in front of or behind other objects				
Responds to a spoken "stop" (for safety)				
Follows three-step instructions in sequence involving two to three different objects				
When directed, demonstrates *across from*, *next to*, *beside*, *behind*, *in front*, *to the side*, *in back*, *left*, and *right*				

AUDITORY MEMORY: SEQUENCE

Skill	Date			
Says or sings at least two nursery rhymes or songs in a group or with an adult				
Listens to/sings songs				
Repeats sound patterns of voice, clapping, tapping				
Moves different body parts to music				
Relates an experience or a creative story in a logical sequence				

Skill	Date			
Recognizes a sequence				
Remembers things in the order they are presented				

LISTENING SKILLS FOR READING READINESS

Skill	Date			
Repeats new words to self				
Gains information from listening to books about real things				
Engages in discussion about a book or story that has been heard				
Participates in rhymes, songs, and games that play with sounds of language				
Recalls one or two elements from a story just read without prompts				
Is interested in different kinds of stories				
Likes to follow along in books being read				
Recalls most of the essential elements in a story				
Makes rhymes to simple words				
Soon after hearing the meaning of a new word, uses it in his or her own speech				
Listens to a story and retells it in own words				
Repeats/points to all letters				
Answers "What happens if . . ." questions				
Identifies main idea				
Predicts an outcome				
Summarizes a story				
Understands character and setting				
Recognizes speaker's purpose				

SOCIAL LISTENING

Skill	Date			
Shows concern when others are unhappy or upset				
Shows awareness of others				
Reacts to adult's behavior				

SOCIAL LISTENING (*Continued*)

Skill	Date			
Attends to other children's behavior				
Responds to adult guidance in negotiating conflict				
Follows adult request to wait turn				
Sustains conversation for several turns				
Changes speech depending on listener (for example, talks differently to babies and adults)				
Talks on telephone				
Follows rules given by adults for new activities or simple games				
Shows interest in conversation				
Responds to/verbally greets at appropriate times ("hi," "bye," and the like)				
Anticipates/ follows multistep daily routines when prompted				
Follows rules when participating in routine activities				
Participates in a conversation that develops a thought or idea				
Responds appropriately to instructions given in a small group				
Acknowledges compliments				
Localizes and looks at (or faces) speaker when listening				
Answers questions about what was heard in conversation				
Resists impulsivity and waits for entire message or directions				
Listens and waits turn when talking with others				
Asks questions to check understanding in a full-class or small-group setting				
Participates in a conversation without monopolizing it				
Answers telephone and summons person requested				
Answers telephone, takes simple message, and delivers it				
Delivers two-part message orally				

ELEMENTARY SCHOOL

Student's Name: **Evaluator's Name:**

Directions: Insert the date of the IEP year in which the skill is targeted at the top of the chart. Record the child's level of development in the targeted skills using the following key:
  – Not yet mastered
  +/– Emerging
  + Mastered and generalized

LISTENING AND LITERACY SKILLS: PHONEMIC AND PHONOLOGICAL SKILLS

Skill	Date			
Discriminates and identifies verbal and nonverbal sounds				
Demonstrates understanding of spoken words, syllables, and sounds (phonemes)				
Creates and states a series of rhyming words, including consonant blends				
Distinguishes initial, medial, and final sounds in single-syllable words				
Distinguishes long and short vowel sounds in orally stated single-syllable words				
Adds, deletes, or changes target sounds to change words (for example, changes *cow* to *how*; *pan* to *an*)				
Blends two to four phonemes into recognizable words (for example, /c/a/t/ = cat; /f/l/a/t/ =flat)				
Segments single-syllable words into their components (for example, /c/a/t/ = cat; /s/p/l/a/t = splat; /r/i/ch/ = rich)				
Knows and applies grade-level phonics and word analysis in decoding words				

LISTENING AND LITERACY SKILLS: LISTENING COMPREHENSION OF INFORMATION THAT IS ORALLY PRESENTED OR READ (LIVE READER OR RECORDED)

Skill	Date			
Recalls fact and details				
Identifies sequential order				
Selects main idea, summarizes, relates one idea to another, makes inferences				
Asks and answers questions about what a speaker says in order to gather additional information or clarify something that is not understood				

LISTENING AND LITERACY SKILLS: LISTENING COMPREHENSION OF INFORMATION THAT IS ORALLY PRESENTED OR READ (LIVE READER OR RECORDED) (*Continued*)

Skill	Date			
Asks and answers questions about key details in a text read aloud or information presented orally or through other media				
Listens to literary texts and performances to appreciate and enjoy literary works; to identify character, setting, and plot; to respond to vivid language; and to identify specific people, places, and events				
Listens to acquire information from nonfiction text				
Listens to literary texts and performances to distinguish between a story, a poem, and a play				
Recounts or describes key ideas or details from a text read aloud or information presented orally or through other media				
Identifies elements of character, plot, and setting to understand the author's message with assistance				
Connects literary texts to previous life experiences to enhance understanding				
Retells stories, including characters, setting, and plot				
Connects literary texts to personal experiences and previously encountered texts to enhance understanding and appreciation				
Determines the main ideas and supporting details of a text read aloud or information presented in diverse media and formats, including visually, quantitatively, and orally				
Identifies elements of character, plot, and setting to understand the author's message or intent				
Paraphrases portions of a text read aloud or information presented in diverse media and formats, including visually, quantitatively, and orally				
Summarizes a text read aloud or information presented in diverse media and formats, including visually, quantitatively, and orally				

ACTIVE LISTENING

Skill	Date			
Identifies and responds to nonverbal sounds, such as school bell, telephone, running water, and the like				
Identifies and responds to verbal sounds and voices in the environment				
Demonstrates the responsibility of the listener to the speaker: focuses attention on the person who is speaking				
Participates in collaborative conversations with diverse partners about class topics and texts with peers and adults in small and large groups				
Gives, restates, and follows simple two-step directions				
Gives and follows three- and four-step oral directions				
Listens to determine a sequence of steps given				
Participates in collaborative conversations with diverse partners about class topics and texts, building on others' ideas and expressing his or her own clearly				

CRITICAL LISTENING DURING ORAL INSTRUCTION

Skill	Date			
Listens critically and responds appropriately to oral communication				
Asks questions for clarification				
Asks and answers questions about what a speaker says in order to clarify comprehension, gather additional information, or deepen understanding of a topic or issue				
Determines the purpose or purposes of listening (for example, to obtain information, to solve problems, for enjoyment)				
Paraphrases information that has been shared orally by others				
Recounts experiences in a logical sequence				
Asks for clarification and explanation of stories and ideas				
Identifies the musical elements of literary language (for example, rhymes, repeated sounds)				
Connects and relates prior experiences, insights, and ideas to those of a speaker				

CRITICAL LISTENING DURING ORAL INSTRUCTION (*Continued*)

Skill	Date			
Retells, paraphrases, and explains what has been said by the speaker				
Responds to questions with appropriate elaboration				
Listens to acquire information and understand procedures				
Asks thoughtful questions and responds to relevant questions with appropriate elaboration				
Summarizes major ideas and supporting evidence presented in spoken messages and formal presentations				
Interprets a speaker's verbal and nonverbal messages, purposes, and perspectives				
Makes inferences or draws conclusions based on an oral report				
Listens to follow instructions that provide information about a task or assignment				
Listens to identify essentials for note taking				

LISTENING AND TECHNOLOGY

Skill	Date			
Listens to audio materials such as books, Internet, radio, and television				
Listens to curriculum on an interactive audio/tactile learning system				
Listens to an electronic braillewriter				
Listens to an accessible PDA (electronic notetaker) with braille or speech output or both				
Listens and interacts with auditory games and keyboarding tutor programs on computer				
Listens to labels on tactile maps, diagrams, drawings, or courseware				
Listens to screen reader while using the computer				
Listens to audible literature on digital players or recorders, computers, electronic notetakers, and accessible PDAs				
Listens while using scanning programs				
Listens while using GPS				

LISTENING AND SOCIAL SKILLS

Skill	Date			
Identifies tone of voice, such as humorous, sad, angry, silly				
Listens for the tone of voice and the content that signal friendly communication				
Follows agreed-upon rules for discussion (for example, listening to others and taking turns speaking about the topics and texts under discussion)				
Continues a conversation through multiple exchanges				
Builds on others' talk in conversations by responding to the comments of others through multiple exchanges				
Builds on others' talk in conversations by linking their comments to the remarks of others				
Follows agreed-upon rules for discussion (for example, gaining the floor in respectful ways, listening to others with care, speaking one at a time about the topics and texts under discussion)				
Maintains appropriate conversation for at least two to five minutes with a beginning, middle, and end				
Demonstrates turn-taking ability in conversations and when playing with peers				
Listens to locate and identify a specific peer and ask the student to play				
Listens to join in a group that is playing or conversing				
Recognizes and responds to humor and uses it in social situations				
Recognizes sarcasm and responds in an effective manner				
Engages in conversation, giving attention and showing interest in others				
Recognizes that social communication may include informal language such as jargon				

MIDDLE AND HIGH SCHOOL

Student's Name: **Evaluator's Name:**

Directions: Insert the date of the IEP year in which the skill is targeted at the top of the chart. Record the child's level of development in the targeted skills using the following key:

    – Not yet mastered
    +/– Emerging
    + Mastered and generalized

LISTENING IN THE CLASSROOM: ACTIVE AND CRITICAL LISTENING

Skill	Date			
Listens critically to oral classroom discussion				
Engages effectively in a range of collaborative discussions (one-on-one, in groups, and teacher-led) with diverse partners on grade level topics, texts, and issues, building on others' ideas and expressing one's own clearly				
Follows rules for collegial discussions, sets specific goals and deadlines, and defines individual roles as needed				
Comes to discussions prepared, having read or studied required material; explicitly draws on that preparation by referring to evidence on the topic, text, or issue to probe and reflects on ideas under discussion				
Poses and responds to specific questions with elaboration and detail by making comments that contribute to the topic, text, or issue under discussion				
Restates and executes multiple-step oral instructions and directions				
Identifies the tone, mood, and emotion conveyed in the oral communication				
Listens attentively, for an extended period of time, to a variety of texts read aloud and oral presentations				
Listens attentively for different purposes, both student determined and teacher determined				
Poses questions that elicit elaboration and responds to others' questions and comments with relevant observations and ideas that bring the discussion back on topic as needed				
Acknowledges new information expressed by others and, when warranted, modifies his or her own views				
Determines the speaker's attitude toward the subject				

Skill	Date			
Responds to persuasive messages with questions, challenges, or affirmations				
Poses questions that connect the ideas of several speakers and responds to others' questions and comments with relevant evidence, observations, and ideas				
Acknowledges new information expressed by others and, when warranted, qualifies or justifies his or her own views in light of the evidence presented				
Listens to and follows complex directions or instructions				
Recognizes appropriate voice and tone				
Initiates and participates effectively in a range of collaborative discussions (one-on-one, in groups, and teacher-led) with diverse partners on grade level topics, texts, and issues, building on others' ideas and expressing his or her own clearly and persuasively				
Works with peers to set rules for collegial discussions and decision making (for example, informal consensus, taking votes on key issues, presentation of alternate views), clear goals and deadlines, and individual roles as needed				
Comes to discussions prepared, having read and researched material under study; explicitly draws on that preparation by referring to the evidence from texts and other research on the topic or issue to stimulate a thoughtful, well-reasoned exchange of ideas				
Responds thoughtfully to diverse perspectives, summarizes points of agreement and disagreement, and, when warranted, qualifies or justifies his or her own views and understanding and makes new connections in light of the evidence and reasoning presented				
Anticipates the speaker's point and assesses its validity, with assistance				
Recognizes the speaker's use of voice and tone, diction, and syntax in school and public forums, debates, and panel discussions				

LISTENING AND ORGANIZING INFORMATION (CLASSROOM INSTRUCTION OR READ [LIVE READER OR RECORDED])

Skill	Date			
Listens to and independently organizes spoken information by summarizing and taking notes about spoken ideas, literature, and curriculum				
Reviews the key ideas expressed and demonstrates understanding of multiple perspectives through reflection and paraphrasing				
Determines the speaker's attitude toward the subject				
Analyzes oral interpretations of literature, including language choice and delivery, and the effect of the information on the listener				
Paraphrases a speaker's purpose and point of view and asks relevant questions concerning the speaker's delivery and purpose				
Interprets information from media presentations such as news broadcasts and taped interviews				
Identifies the speaker's purpose and motive for communicating information				
Interprets information from media presentations such as documentary films, news broadcasts, and taped interviews				
Determines the need for more information for clarification				
Synthesizes the information from different sources by combining or categorizing data and facts				

LISTENING AND TECHNOLOGY

Skill	Date			
Listens to learn while using appropriate access technology				
Selects and uses appropriate technology tools to accomplish a variety of tasks				
Demonstrates advanced word-processing skills, such as cutting and pasting text, using a spell checker, and using formatting features				
Demonstrates advanced use of screen-reading options				
Demonstrates effective use of portable notetakers using simple applications, such as word-processing file management, calendar, and calculator functions				

Skill	Date			
Demonstrates effective use of Internet applications as appropriate to student's age level				
Selects and applies technology tools for research, information gathering, problem solving, and decision making				
Demonstrates advanced use of portable notetakers, such as advanced word processing				

LISTENING DURING SOCIAL INTERACTION

Skill	Date			
Utilizes effective listening strategies to engage in social interaction				
Listens respectfully when others speak				
Identifies the tone, mood, and emotion conveyed in oral communication				
Participates as a listener in social conversation with one or more people				
Maintains a socially appropriate conversation for a minimum of 10 minutes with peers and adults				
Demonstrates ability to take the role of others and understand others' feelings in various social situations				
Evaluates social situations to determine appropriate use of specific social behaviors				
Converses with others on a range of interesting topics without dominating the conversation				
Compliments others and reciprocates when appropriate				

Resources

The listings in this section include a sampling of the many sources of information about developing the listening skills of children with visual impairments. They include additional information and resources on the topics discussed in this volume; websites that provide resources for teachers and parents; sources of electronic books and digital media, assessments, and curricula; and recommended readings and references.

For additional information and more detailed listings of organizations, products, and services, see the *AFB Directory of Services for Blind and Visually Impaired Persons in the United States and Canada*, published by the American Foundation for the Blind and available on its website, www.afb.org.

NATIONAL ORGANIZATIONS AND AGENCIES

American Foundation for the Blind (AFB)
2 Penn Plaza, Suite 1102
New York, NY 10121
(212) 502-7600; (800) 232-5463
TDD: (212) 502-7662
Fax: (212) 502-7777
www.afb.org
info@afb.org

A national organization serving as an information clearinghouse for people who are visually impaired and their families, professionals, schools, organizations, corporations, and the public. Operates a toll-free information hotline; conducts research and mounts program initiatives to promote the inclusion of visually impaired persons, especially in the areas of literacy, technology, aging, and employment; and advocates for services and legislation. Through AFB Press, its publishing arm, publishes books, pamphlets, DVDs, and electronic and online products including the *Directory of Services for Blind and Visually Impaired Persons in the United States and Canada,* the *Journal of Visual Impairment & Blindness,* and *AccessWorld: Technology and People with Visual Impairments.* Maintains a number of web-based initiatives, including FamilyConnect (www .FamilyConnect.org), an online, multimedia community for parents and families of visually impaired children created with the National Association for Parents of Children with Visual Impairments, and CareerConnect (www.CareerConnect.org), a free resource for people who want to learn about the range and diversity of jobs performed by adults who are blind or visually impaired throughout the United States and Canada.

American Printing House for the Blind (APH)
1839 Frankfort Avenue
P.O. Box 6085
Louisville, KY 40206
(502) 895-2405; (800) 223-1839
www.aph.org
info@aph.org

A national organization that publishes books in braille, large-print, and audiotape formats; manufactures educational aids for persons who are blind or visually impaired; modifies and develops computer-access equipment and software; maintains an educational research and development program concerned with educational methods and aids; and provides a reference catalog service for volunteer-produced textbooks in all media for students who are visually impaired and for information about other sources of related materials. Maintains the M.C. Migel Library, a centralized source of materials related to blindness and visual impairment.

Council for Exceptional Children (CEC)

2900 Crystal Drive, Suite 1000
Arlington, VA 22202
(703) 620-3660; (800) 224-6830
www.cec.sped.org
Division of Early Childhood
www.decsped.org
Division on Visual Impairments
www.cecdvi.org

A professional organization for practitioners serving infants, children, and youths who have disabilities. Holds an annual national conference and publishes *Exceptional Children* and *Teaching Exceptional Children*, which contain articles on strategies and practices. The Division on Visual Impairments (DVI) publishes *DVI Quarterly*. The Division of Early Childhood (DEC) has a separate annual conference and state chapters and publishes *Journal of Early Intervention* and *Young Exceptional Children*.

National Clearinghouse for English Language Acquisition (NCELA)

2011 Eye Street NW, Suite 300
Washington, DC 20006
(800) 321-6223; (202) 467-0867
Fax: (800) 531-9347
www.ncela.gwu.edu/
askncela@gwu.edu

Collects, analyzes, synthesizes, and disseminates information about language instruction educational programs for English language learners and related programs.

National Consortium on Deafblindness (NCDB)

Western Oregon University
Teaching Research Institute
345 North Monmouth Avenue
Monmouth, OR 97361
(800) 438-9376
TTY/TDD: (800) 854-7013
Fax: (503) 838-8150
www.nationaldb.org

A national technical assistance and dissemination center for children and youth who are deaf-blind. Formerly known as NTAC, NCDB is home to DB-LINK, the largest collection of information related to deaf-blindness worldwide.

National Dissemination Center for Children and Youth with Disabilities (NICHCY)

1825 Connecticut Avenue NW, Suite 700
Washington, DC 20009
Voice/TTY/TDD: (800) 695-0285
Fax: (202) 884-8441
www.nichcy.org
nichcy@aed.org

A national information clearinghouse on subjects related to children and youths with disabilities. Provides information and referrals to national, state, and local resources and disseminates numerous free publications.

National Early Childhood Technical Assistance Center (NECTAC)

Campus Box 8040
UNC Chapel Hill
Chapel Hill, NC 27599-8040
(919) 962-2001
Fax: (919) 966-7463
www.nectac.org
nectac@unc.edu

A national early childhood technical assistance center supported by the U.S. Department of Education's Office of Special Education Programs. Provides an array of services and supports to improve service systems and outcomes for infants, toddlers, and preschool-age children (birth through 5 years) with special needs and their families. Provides access to a wide range of information on evidence-based practices and provision of services under federal laws.

TASH

1001 Connecticut Avenue NW, Suite 235
Washington, DC 20036
(202) 540-9020
Fax: (202) 540-9019
www.tash.org
info@TASH.org

An advocacy organization for professionals who work with infants, children, and youths who have severe disabilities and their families. TASH holds an annual national conference, publishes *Research and Practice for Persons with Severe Disabilities* and *TASH Connections*, and has a committee on early childhood that meets at the annual conference. There are state and regional TASH chapters.

Zero to Three: National Center for Infants, Toddlers, and Families

2000 M Street NW, Suite 200
Washington, DC 20036
(202) 638-1144
Fax: (202) 638-0851

A national nonprofit, multidisciplinary organization that informs, educates, and supports professionals, policy makers, and parents to promote the healthy development and well-being of infants, toddlers, and their families. Offers on-site training across the country; publishes educational and instructional books, curricula, assessment tools, videos, and practical guidebooks for professionals.

WEBSITES

The following websites provide resources for parents and teachers; some provide activities and recreational opportunities for listening for students and young children.

Center for Early Literacy Learning (CELL)

www.earlyliteracylearning.org

Promotes the adoption and sustained use of evidence-based early literacy learning practices. Provides resources for early childhood intervention practitioners, parents, and other caregivers of children, birth to 5 years of age, with identified disabilities or developmental delays or who are at risk for poor outcomes. Offers many listening activities and games.

Early Intervention Training Center for Infants and Toddlers with Visual Impairments

www.fpg.unc.edu/~edin/index.htm

Houses the interactive multimedia training modules and information and resources developed at the FPG Child Development Institute, University of North Carolina, Chapel Hill, including *Family Centered Practices for Infants and Toddlers with Visual Impairments*, *Visual Conditions and Functional Vision: Early Intervention Issues*, *Developmentally Appropriate Orientation and Mobility*, *Communication and Emergent Literacy: Early Intervention Issues*, and *Assessment of Infants and Toddlers with Visual Impairments*.

Hark the Sound

http://harkthesound.org/

An online collection of free audio games for students with visual impairments (from University of North Carolina at Chapel Hill).

Interesting Things for ESL Students

www.ManyThings.org

Offers quizzes, word games, word puzzles, proverbs, slang expressions, anagrams, a random-sentence generator, and other computer-assisted language learning activities that teachers can use with their ESL students.

The Internet TESL Journal
http://iteslj.org

A website about teaching English as a second language, including articles, research papers, lesson plans, classroom handouts, and teaching ideas as well as activities for students, including listening quizzes and activities with sounds and corresponding questions and answers.

Intervention Central
www.interventioncentral.org

Provides teachers, schools, and school districts with free articles and tools to successfully implement Response to Intervention, a method of academic intervention designed to provide early, effective assistance to children who are having difficulty learning.

Learning through Listening
www.learningthroughlistening.org/

A website for teachers from Learning Ally (see entry under "Sources of Digital and Electronic Books") offering a variety of free, downloadable lesson plans, strategies (including graphic organizers), and activities devoted to teaching listening. Also features the 2008 Listening Skills Inventory based on the 1996 New York Learning Standards for English and Language Arts.

Music Together
www.musictogether.com

An internationally recognized early childhood music and movement program for babies, toddlers, preschoolers, and kinder-

garteners. The website offers information, classes, recordings, and musical instruments for children.

National Reading Panel
www.nichd.nih.gov/health/topics/national_reading_panel.cfm

Information dissemination site for the National Reading Panel, created by Congress in 1977 to review research on how children learn to read and determine the most effective evidence-based methods for teaching children to read. Offers information about the importance of the development of phonemic and phonological skills as well as comprehension, which are dependent upon the development of listening skills.

Talk to Your Baby
www.talktoyourbaby.org.uk

Offers ideas, games, and resources for both parents and professionals devoted to the importance of talking to their baby.

What Works Clearinghouse
http://ies.ed.gov/ncee/wwc/

The U.S. Department of Education Institute of Education Sciences website that includes articles and resources about many educational topics and a searchable database of interventions in areas including language development.

SOURCES OF DIGITAL AND ELECTRONIC MEDIA

Accessible Book Collection
www.accessiblebookcollection.org/

Provides children's books in accessible formats for schools or other nonprofit organizations that provide specialized services relating to training, education, or adaptive reading or information access needs of persons who are blind or other persons with disabilities.

Bookshare
www.bookshare.org

Offers a searchable online library of approximately 90,000 digital books, including best sellers and new releases, textbooks, teacher-recommended reading, and periodicals for free to students in the United States with qualifying disabilities.

Canadian National Institute for the Blind Library
www.cnib.ca/en/services/library/

Canada's largest producer of materials in alternate formats. Offers downloadable e-text, audio formats, and braille books for members.

Described and Captioned Media Program (DCMP)
www.dcmp.org/

Provides a library of free-loan described and captioned educational videos for grades K–12. These videos are available on DVD, and many can be streamed instantly from the DCMP website.

International Braille Research Center
www.braille.org/papers/index.htm

Maintains the Electronic Braille Book Library and provides numerous books, including many classic literature titles, in electronic format. Also houses several research articles and publications on braille literacy.

Learning Ally
www.learningally.org/

Provides digitally recorded textbooks and literature titles to students who cannot read standard print due to blindness, visual impairment, dyslexia, or other learning disabilities. Formerly Recording for the Blind & Dyslexic (RFB&D).

National Center for Accessible Media at WGBH (NCAM)
http://ncam.wgbh.org/

Research and development organization specializing in accessible media. Offers a list of resources for accessible media on its website.

National Library Service (NLS) for the Blind and Physically Disabled
Library of Congress
www.loc.gov/nls

Through a national network of cooperating libraries, NLS administers a free library program of braille and digital audio materials circulated to eligible borrowers in the United States by postage-free mail. Also maintains an electronic library for e-text for registered users.

Project Gutenberg Literary Archive Foundation
www.gutenberg.org/wiki/Gutenberg: The_Audio_Books_Project

Makes audio e-books of numerous literary works available in plain text. Listings are divided into two categories: human-read and computer-generated audiobooks.

University of Virginia Scholars' Lab
http://etext.lib.virginia.edu/

Provides electronic text of many classic literary works, college-level reading materials, and foreign-language materials.

RECOMMENDED READINGS AND RESOURCES

Infants, Toddlers, and Preschool

Anthony, T. L., Armenta-Schmitt, F., Chen, D., Fazzi, D. L., Hughes, M. A., McCann, M. E., et al. (1993). *First steps: A handbook for teaching young children who are visually impaired.* Los Angeles: Blind Childrens Center.

Blakely, K., Lang, M. A., & Kushner-Sosna, B. (1995). *Toys and play: A guide to fun and development for children with impaired vision.* New York: Lighthouse International.

Casey-Harvey, D. G. (1995*). Early communication games: Routine-based play for the first two years.* Tucson, AZ: Communication Skill Builders.

Early Beginnings: Early Literacy Knowledge and Instruction: A guide for early childhood administrators and professional development providers. Washington, DC: National Institute for Literacy. Available from http://lincs.ed.gov/publications/pdf/NELPEarlyBeginnings09.pdf.

Ferrell, K. A. (2011). *Reach out and teach: Helping your child who is visually impaired learn and grow.* New York: AFB Press.

Lueck, A. H., Chen, D., Kekelis, L. S., & Hartmann, E. S. (2008). *Developmental guidelines for infants with visual impairments: A guidebook for early intervention* (2nd ed.). Louisville, KY: American Printing House for the Blind.

Margetik, C., Calvello, G., Bernas-Pierce, J., & Murphy, D. (1999). *Off to a good start: Access to the world for infants and toddlers with visual impairments.* San Francisco: Blind Babies Foundation.

Petersen, B., & Nielsen, J. (2005). *Vision program: Vision skills in the natural environment: An intervention guide for use with children birth to three with blindness or vision impairment.* Logan: SKI*HI Institute, Department of Communication Disorders, Utah State University.

Pogrund, R. L., & Fazzi, D. L. (Eds.). (2002). *Early focus: Working with young, blind, and visually impaired children and their families* (2nd ed.). New York: AFB Press.

Teaching Strategies. *Observing young children: Learning to look, looking to learn* [Video]. Van Nuys, CA: Child Development Media.

Trief, E. (1992). *Working with visually impaired young students: A curriculum guide for birth–3 year olds.* Springfield, IL: Charles C Thomas.

Wright S., & Stratton, J. M. (2007). *On the way to literacy* (2nd ed.). Louisville, KY: American Printing House for the Blind.

Elementary and High School

Beck, I. L., McKeown, M. G., & Kucan, L. (2002*). Bringing words to life: Robust vocabulary instruction.* New York: Guilford Press.

Carreon, J., Kuns, J., Amandi, A., & Anderson, J. (2009). *CSB technology curriculum guides.* Fremont: California School for the Blind.

Harley, R. K., Truan, M. B., & Sanford, L. D. (1997). *Communication skills for visually impaired learners: Braille, print, and listening skills for students who are visually impaired* (2nd ed.). Springfield, IL: Charles C Thomas.

Holbrook, C., & Koenig, A. (2000). *Foundations of Education* (2nd ed.). New York: AFB Press.

Lybolt, J. (2007). *Building language throughout the year.* Baltimore, MD: Paul H. Brookes.

McLaughlin, M. (2010). *Guided comprehension in the primary grades* (2nd ed.). Newark, DE: International Reading Association.

McLaughlin, M., & Allen, M. B. (2009). *Guided comprehension in grades 3–8* (combined 2nd ed.). Newark, DE: International Reading Association.

Presley, I., & D'Andrea, F. M. (2009). *Assistive technology for students who are blind or visually impaired: A guide to assessment.* New York: AFB Press.

Wiig, E. H., & Wilson, C. C. (2002). *The learning ladder: Assessing and teaching text comprehension.* Eau Claire, WI: Thinking Publications.

Students with Multiple Disabilities

Anthony, T. L. (2004). Individual sensory learning profile interview. In I. Topor, L. P. Rosenblum, & D. D. Hatton, *Visual conditions and functional vision: Early intervention issues,* Session 4: Functional Vision Assessment and Developmentally Appropriate Learning Media Assessment, Handout K. Chapel Hill: Early Intervention Training Center for Infants and Toddlers with Visual Impairments, FPG Child Development Institute, University of North Carolina, Chapel Hill.

Blaha, R. (2001). *Calendars: For students with multiple impairments including deafblindness.* Austin: Texas School for the Blind and Visually Impaired.

Chen, D. (Ed.). (1999). *Essential elements in early intervention: Visual impairment and multiple disabilities.* New York: AFB Press.

Chen, D., & Dote-Kwan, J. (1995). *Starting points: Instructional practices for young children whose multiple disabilities include visual impairment.* Los Angeles: Blind Childrens Center.

Hagood, L. (1997). *Communication: A guide for teaching students with visual and multiple impairments.* Austin: Texas School for the Blind and Visually Impaired.

O'Sail, B., Levack, N., Donovan, L., & Sewell, D. (2001). *Elementary concepts.* Austin: Texas School for the Blind and Visually Impaired.

Rowland, C., & Schweigert, P. (2000). *Tangible symbols systems manual.* Portland, OR: Design to Learn.

Sensory Learning Kit. Louisville, KY: American Printing House for the Blind. Kit for use in the development of skills for learners with the most significant challenges. Contains tools to help create daily schedules, lesson plans, and alternative assessments for play or functional routines.

SKI*HI Institute. (1993). *A resource manual for understanding and interacting with infants, toddlers, and preschool age children with deaf-blindness.* Logan, UT: Hope.

Smith, M. (2005). How to use the sensory learning kit. In *SLK guidebook and assessment forms: Using the sensory learning kit* [Video]. Louisville, KY: American Printing House for the Blind.

Listening Curricula and Activities

The following curricular materials and games utilize and support the development of listening skills.

McDonald, M., & Shaw-King, A. (2007). *Learning to listen, listening to learn.* Austin, TX: Pro-Ed. An activity book to develop effective listening skills, especially phonological awareness and critical listening, for students in pre-kindergarten through sixth grade.

101 games for social skills. Castro Valley, CA: Exceptional Teaching Aids. Games that teach looking, listening, speaking, thinking, and concentration skills and help develop positive relationships.

Perkins Panda early literacy kit. (2002). Watertown, MA: Perkins School for the Blind. Kit for teaching fundamental early literacy skills to children from birth through 8 years old. Includes storybooks in uncontracted braille and large print, activity guides, cassettes, and other materials.

Pester, E. (1972). *Listen and think.* Louisville, KY: American Printing House for the Blind. A curriculum for developing and improving listening comprehension and thinking skills for students from birth to 8 years of age. Covers basic listening skills such as understanding on CD-ROM with braille and print answer sheets, progress charts, and a teacher's handbook.

Phonemic awareness listening lotto. Carson, CA: Lakeshore Learning Materials. Activities for phonemic awareness concepts from rhyming patterns to phoneme blending for children from pre-kindergarten through first grade, with CD and 16 lotto cards.

Language and Listening Assessments

The following assessments are typically administered by a speech and language pathologist to students who exhibit weakness in listening, attention, auditory comprehension, or phonological awareness. Teachers of students with visual impairments need to be involved in the administration of such assessments to ensure the application of appropriate modifications and accommodations to test materials and to help interpret results.

Barrett, M., Huisingh, R., Zachman, L., Blagden, C., & Orman, J. (2006). *The listening test–2.* East Moline, IL: LinguiSystems. Norm-referenced assessment for students ages 6 to 11 years testing auditory comprehension.

Gardner, M. (2005). *Test of auditory-perceptual skills–3.* Novato, CA: Academic Therapy Publications. Norm-referenced assessment for students ages 4 to 18 years focusing on phonological awareness, auditory comprehension, and auditory memory.

Keith, R. W. (2009). *SCAN–3: Test for auditory processing disorders in children.* San Antonio, TX: PsychCorp, Pearson Educational. Norm-referenced assessment for students ages 5 to 12.11 years focusing on auditory processing.

Robertson, C., & Salter, W. (2007). *The phonological awareness test–2.* East Moline, IL: LinguiSystems. Norm-referenced assessment for students 5 to 9 years focusing on phonological awareness.

Semel, E., Wiig, E. H., & Secord, W. A. (2003). *Clinical evaluation of language fundamentals* (4th ed.) *(CELF–4).* San Antonio, TX: PsychCorp, Pearson Educational. Norm-referenced assessment for students ages 5 to 21 testing auditory comprehension and auditory memory.

Sheslow, D., & Adams, W. (2003). *Wide range assessment of memory and learning 2 (WRAML 2).* Austin, TX: Pro-Ed. Norm-referenced assessment for students ages 5 to 90 years focusing on auditory memory and auditory comprehension.

Phonemic/Phonological Screening

Crumrine, L., & Lonegan, H. (2000). *Phonemic-awareness skills screening (PASS).* Austin, TX: Pro-Ed. Un-normed skills survey focusing on pre-reading skills of phonological/ phonemic awareness: rhyme, segmentation, blending, deletion, isolation, substitution.

Robertson, C., & Salter, W. (1995). *The phonological awareness profile.* East Moline, IL: LinguiSystems. Un-normed skills survey focusing on pre-reading and early reading skills of phonological awareness and development of sound-symbol connections.

Orientation and Mobility

Anthony, T. L., Shier Lowry, S., Brown, C. J., & Hatton, D. D. (2004). *Developmentally appropriate orientation and mobility.* Chapel Hill: Early Intervention Center for Infants and Toddlers with Visual Impairments, FPG Child Development Institute, University of North Carolina, Chapel Hill. Available from www.fpg.unc.edu/~edin/Resources/ modules/OM1.cfm.

Brothers, R.J., & Huff, R.A. (2008). *The sound localization guidebook* (4th ed.). Louisville, KY: American Printing House for the Blind.

Guérette, H., & Zabihaylo, C. (2011). *Mastering the environment through audition, kinesthesia, and cognition: An O&M approach to training for guide dog travel* [DVD]. New York: AFB Press.

Kish, D. (2009). Flash sonar program: Helping blind people learn to see. Encino, CA: World Access for the Blind. Retrieved from www.worldaccessfortheblind.org/node/131. Provides strategies for teaching auditory space perception.

O'Mara, B. (1989). *Pathways to independence: Orientation and mobility skills for your infant and toddler.* New York: Lighthouse International.

Pogrund, R., Healy, G., Jones, K., Levack, N., Martin-Curry, S., Martinez, C., Marz, J., Roberson-Smith, B. & Vrba, A. (1995). *TAPS—Teaching age-appropriate purposeful skills: An orientation and mobility curriculum for students with visual impairments* (2nd ed.). Austin: Texas School for the Blind and Visually Impaired.

Index

Printed by BoD™in Norderstedt, Germany

9 780891 284918